Herbal Supplements—
Drug Interactions

Herbal Supplements— Drug Interactions

Scientific and Regulatory Perspectives

edited by

Y. W. Francis Lam
University of Texas Health Science Center
San Antonio, Texas, U.S.A.

Shiew-Mei Huang
FDA Center for Drug Evaluation and Research
Silver Spring, Maryland, U.S.A.

Stephen D. Hall
Indiana University School of Medicine
Wishard Memorial Hospital
Indianapolis, Indiana, U.S.A.

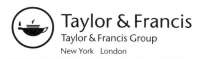

Taylor & Francis
Taylor & Francis Group
New York   London

Taylor & Francis is an imprint of the
Taylor & Francis Group, an informa business

Published in 2006 by
Taylor & Francis Group
270 Madison Avenue
New York, NY 10016

© 2006 by Taylor & Francis Group, LLC

No claim to original U.S. Government works
Printed in the United States of America on acid-free paper
10 9 8 7 6 5 4 3 2 1

International Standard Book Number-10: 0-8247-2538-7 (Hardcover)
International Standard Book Number-13: 978-0-8247-2538-9 (Hardcover)

Library of Congress Cataloging-in-Publication Data

Catalog record is available from the Library of Congress

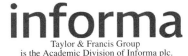
Taylor & Francis Group
is the Academic Division of Informa plc.

**Visit the Taylor & Francis Web site at
http://www.taylorandfrancis.com**

Preface

Although the potential of an interaction between concurrently administered botanical and pharmaceutical products is not unexpected, this topic has received increased attention and scrutiny over the past several years. The widespread use of botanical products in Western societies and the potency of modern pharmaceuticals have led to numerous reports of interaction, sometimes with significant adverse effects.

While no one would argue for the need of another book related to drug interaction, this book differs from available books in several aspects. This book is not a standard book listing numerous reported botanical product-drug interactions organized by examples. Rather, the focus is to provide a timely discussion and perspective on the complex scientific and regulatory issues associated with investigating, reporting, and assessing these interactions in humans.

From the beginning, our goal has been to provide information that is not readily available in other books covering the same topic. In addition to regulatory and industry perspectives, we have included a chapter describing interactions involving the more commonly used traditional Chinese medicine, and discussion regarding specific issues unique to this group of medicinal products that needs to be taken into consideration when assessing the potential and significance of interaction. In contrast to single active components in modern pharmaceuticals, the presence of multiple active ingredients commonly present in botanical products underscores the importance of quality assurance and standardization in this emerging industry. The relevance and challenges of standardization for documentation and evaluation of botanical product-drug interactions are presented in depth in one chapter and, where applicable, discussed throughout the book.

We realize that the terms *herbs*, *herbal products*, *botanical products*, and *dietary supplements* are often used interchangeably in the literature or sometimes even within the same context by consumer. While dietary supplements may be more easily recognized by consumers, the term includes vitamins, minerals, and other nutritional products that are not the focus of this book. On the other hand, it is generally accepted that herbs and botanical products also encompass different concentrated forms including extracts, powders, and formulated products containing a combination of different herbs. We used the term *botanical products* where applicable throughout the book because it denotes a more extensive scope than the more commonly used term *herbs* or *herbal products*, and it enables the inclusion of interaction involving citrus products as well.

The book chapters are organized into five major sections. Section 1 (Chapters 1 to 3) provides background information regarding botanical usage and discusses several of the mechanisms in which botanical products can interfere with drug disposition and effect. The complex nature of botanical product-drug interaction and the different variables associated with interpretation of the reported interaction are highlighted in this section as well. The second section (Chapters 4 to 7) focuses on botanical products that have been documented to interact with pharmaceutical products and, where applicable, their purported mechanism of interaction. Where possible, the contributors use specific examples in this section to illustrate the complexity of the issues in assessing the potential and significance of the interaction. The next section (Chapters 8 and 9) provides an overview of the pharmacokinetics of different botanical products, and discusses the importance of quality assurance and standardization. The fourth section on regulatory viewpoints (Chapters 10 to 13) outlines the Food and Drug Administration's approach to utilize the MedWatch program for documenting and evaluating reported botanical product-drug interactions. The last section (Chapters 14 and 15) provides industry and regulatory perspectives on developing botanical products as pharmaceutical agents.

This book is intended not only for scientists involved in the study of botanical product-drug interactions, but also for practitioners who advise patients on the safety concerns involved with using these products concurrently. It is our sincere hope that the use of this book will serve to improve understanding of the complex issues associated with evaluating botanical product-drug interactions, which is an essential component in further developing botanical products and obtaining regulatory approval as pharmaceutical agents.

Y. W. Francis Lam
Shiew-Mei Huang
Stephen D. Hall

Contents

Contributors

John T. Arnason   Centre for Research in Biopharmaceuticals and Biotechnology, University of Ottawa, Ottawa, Ontario, Canada

Colin J. Briggs   Faculty of Pharmacy, University of Manitoba, Winnipeg, Manitoba, Canada

Veronika Butterweck   Department of Pharmaceutics, Center for Food Drug Interaction Research and Education, University of Florida, Gainesville, Florida, U.S.A.

Lucas R. Chadwick   Program for Collaborative Research in the Pharmaceutical Sciences, WHO Collaborating Center for Traditional Medicine and UIC/NIH Center for Botanical Dietary Supplements Research, College of Pharmacy, University of Illinois, Chicago, Illinois, U.S.A.

Min-Chu Chen   Office of Drug Safety, Center for Drug Evaluation and Research (CDER), Food and Drug Administration, Silver Spring, Maryland, U.S.A.

Shaw T. Chen   Center for Drug Evaluation and Research (CDER), Food and Drug Administration, Silver Spring, Maryland, U.S.A.

W. V. De Castro   Department of Pharmaceutics, Center for Food Drug Interaction Research and Education, University of Florida, Gainesville, Florida, U.S.A.

Hartmut Derendorf   Department of Pharmaceutics, Center for Food Drug Interaction Research and Education, University of Florida, Gainesville, Florida, U.S.A.

E. Ernst   Complementary Medicine, Peninsula Medical School, University of Exeter, Exeter, and University of Plymouth, Plymouth, U.K.

Harry H. S. Fong   Program for Collaborative Research in the Pharmaceutical Sciences, WHO Collaborating Center for Traditional Medicine and UIC/NIH Center for Botanical Dietary Supplements Research, College of Pharmacy, University of Illinois, Chicago, Illinois, U.S.A.

Brian C. Foster   Therapeutic Products Directorate, Health Canada and Centre for Research in Biopharmaceuticals and Biotechnology, University of Ottawa, Ottawa, Ontario, Canada

J. Christopher Gorski   Division of Clinical Pharmacology, Department of Medicine, Indiana University School of Medicine, Indianapolis, Indiana, U.S.A.

Stephen D. Hall   Division of Clinical Pharmacology, Department of Medicine, Indiana University School of Medicine, Indianapolis, Indiana, U.S.A.

Freddie Ann Hoffman   HeteroGeneity, LLC, Washington, D.C., U.S.A.

Shiew-Mei Huang   Office of Clinical Pharmacology and Biopharmaceutics, Center for Drug Evaluation and Research (CDER), Food and Drug Administration, Silver Spring, Maryland, U.S.A.

Y. W. Francis Lam   Departments of Pharmacology and Medicine, University of Texas Health Science Center at San Antonio, San Antonio, and College of Pharmacy, University of Texas at Austin, Austin, Texas, U.S.A.

Lawrence J. Lesko   Office of Clinical Pharmacology and Biopharmaceutics, Center for Drug Evaluation and Research (CDER), Food and Drug Administration, Silver Spring, Maryland, U.S.A.

Lori A. Love   Office of Regulatory Affairs, Food and Drug Administration, Rockville, Maryland, U.S.A.

S. U. Mertens-Talcott   Department of Pharmaceutics, Center for Food Drug Interaction Research and Education, University of Florida, Gainesville, Florida, U.S.A.

Andrew Morris   Department of Pharmacy Practice, Purdue University, West Lafayette and Regenstrief Institute, Inc., Indianapolis, Indiana, U.S.A.

Michael D. Murray   Department of Pharmacy Practice, Purdue University, West Lafayette and Regenstrief Institute, Inc., Indianapolis, Indiana, U.S.A.

Ming Ou   Guangzhou University of Traditional Chinese Medicine, Guangzhou, P.R. China

Toni Piazza-Hepp   Division of Surveillance, Research and Communication Support Office of Drug Safety, Center for Drug Evaluation and Research (CDER), Food and Drug Administration, Silver Spring, Maryland, U.S.A.

Robert Temple   Office of Medical Policy, Center for Drug Evaluation and Research (CDER), Food and Drug Administration, Silver Spring, Maryland, U.S.A.

I. Zadezensky   Department of Pharmaceutics, Center for Food Drug Interaction Research and Education, University of Florida, Gainesville, Florida, U.S.A.

1

The Landscape of Botanical Medicine Utilization and Safety

Andrew Morris and Michael D. Murray

Department of Pharmacy Practice, Purdue University, West Lafayette and Regenstrief Institute, Inc., Indianapolis, Indiana, U.S.A.

INTRODUCTION

Comprehending the use and safety of botanical dietary supplements is challenging largely owing to the lack of regulation and the paucity of data on their utilization, effectiveness, and safety. The literature describing the utilization of botanical products tends to be poorly documented and incomplete and evidence in the form of clinical trials is sparse; safety data are largely derived from anecdotal case reports. Medications from botanical sources have been described as far back as 60 millennia and most of the medications used throughout the world were derived from plants until the early 1900s (1). It is estimated that 35,000 to 70,000 plants have been used for medical purposes (2). For example, opium and willow bark have long been used for the treatment of pain (3). It was not uncommon for over-the-counter medications to contain opium without warnings or legal restrictions (4). Willow bark may still be purchased over the counter as an extract to relieve pain and many other prescriptions medications are currently derived from botanical sources.

Prescriptions Derived from Botanical Sources

Today, it is estimated that 25% of the Western pharmacopoeia contains chemical entities that were first isolated from plants and another 25% are derived from chemical entities modified from plant sources (1,2). In 1999, 121 prescription medicines worldwide came directly from plant extracts and it is now a $10 billion-a-year industry (1). These medicines are not dietary supplements but rather are botanical products that have passed the more rigorous process of approval to be used as a prescription drug. The World Health Organization estimates that 75% to 80% of the developing world continues to rely heavily on botanicals for medication (1,5). However, most products available are considered dietary supplements in the United States.

Botanical Dietary Supplements

The use of botanicals in the industrialized world is growing. In the United States, it has been estimated that about 20,000 products are in use (6), with the top ten botanical products comprising 50% of the commercial botanical market (7). In China, approximately 80% of medications are obtained from between 5000 and 30,000 types of plants (2). In the era of increased globalization, many botanical products are available to people all over the world through the Internet, imported for sale by botanical shops catering to high-use ethnic populations, or imported (often illegally) by individuals returning from global travel (8). Utilization of these products has dramatically increased in the past decade (2,9–18). In 1991, the U.S. Congress passed legislation to establish the National Institutes of Health Office of Alternative Medicine, which later became the National Center for Complementary and Alternative Medicine, to better understand how Americans are embracing the use of unconventional therapies.

UTILIZATION OF BOTANICAL DIETARY SUPPLEMENTS IN THE UNITED STATES

Although physicians in the United States infrequently prescribe botanicals, they receive little formal training on the benefits and risks of these and other complementary and alternative medications (CAM) (19). This is disturbing because a significant proportion of patients take botanical dietary supplements. More than 37 million Americans utilize botanical remedies and some estimates put forth a much higher (20–23). Since the Dietary Supplement Health and Education Act (DSHEA) of 1994, growth of the botanical market has been dramatic. However, the industry is fragmented, with a few large corporations manufacturing the bulk of botanical products and many smaller companies targeting specific herbs. Market research organizations have traditionally avoided analyzing botanical products because the market was too small (24), but this has changed recently because botanicals are now profitable to analyze. As a result of DSHEA, the public now has many botanical dietary supplements from which to choose. With the increasing number of products competing against one another, corporations have taken action to distinguish their products from one another. As such, dietary supplement manufacturers have taken a page from the pharmaceutical industry and have begun branding botanical products to develop a market following for their product (25–34). Many products also consist of combinations of dietary supplements and at least one of them also uses a nonprescription medication in combination with the botanical dietary supplement. At least one pharmaceutical manufacturer has also entered the branded botanical market (32).

Direct-to-consumer advertising of branded botanical dietary supplements appears to be quite effective, judging from the number of advertisements appearing in the print and electronic media. Many of these products claim to improve conditions that are refractory to conventional medical treatment or they are touted to be natural and, as such, purported to be safer than conventional pharmaceuticals and free of side effects. The public is well aware of dietary supplements, because many of these have appeared on late-night infomercials. Some examples of branded products touted for weight loss include Metabolife® (33), Leptoprin® (29), and Cortislim™ (30). Most weight loss products in the United States contained ephedra before the Food and Drug Administration (FDA) banned ephedra-containing dietary supplements. It appears that weight loss products are now being reformulated with other stimulants that have not received the intense scrutiny of the FDA, such as bitter orange (synephrine), green tea extract (caffeine), and guarana (methylxanthines: caffeine, theobromine, and theophylline). Other branded combination botanical products such as Enzyte® (25) and Avlimil® (26) are touted for treatment of sexual dysfunction and are advertised in a manner similar to sexual dysfunction pharmaceuticals. Still other formulations are advertised for breast enhancement—Bloussant™ (28), hair loss—Avacor™ (34), depression—Amoryn™ (27), nourishing the brain—Focus Factor™ (31), and sleep—Alluna™ Sleep (32). All of these contain one or more botanical constituents and are sold under the auspices of DSHEA, and therefore are not regulated by the FDA and the Federal Trade Commission as rigorously as prescription pharmaceuticals or food additives.

Sizing up the economics of the botanical dietary supplements market in the United States is challenging because the market is prodigiously dynamic. The market has been estimated to represent a demand between $0.6 and $5.1 billion (9,13,23,24,35–41). Estimated retail sales in the United States by year can be seen in Figure 1. It is important to note that each study sampled a different population. Growth in the market occurred rapidly between 1991 and 1998, but recent sales appear to have reached a plateau. Americans usually pay for botanical dietary supplements as well as other CAM therapies out of their own pockets because most health insurance programs do not cover CAM therapies (9,42). In 1997, total CAM out-of-pocket expenses exceeded $27 billion (43), with the expenditure on botanical products estimated at greater than $5 billion (9). Insurance coverage that covered CAM therapies would also likely result in

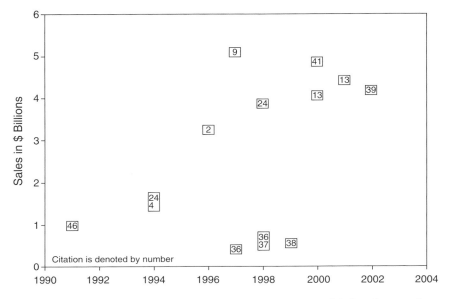

Figure 1   Estimates for U.S. retail botanical sales in billions of dollars by year from multiple citations.

growth in the botanical industry. One study found that full insurance coverage for botanical dietary supplements predicted an increase in usage of fivefold and partial insurance coverage predicted a threefold increase in botanical utilization (44).

Rapid growth in the botanical dietary supplement industry occurred within the first four years of DSHEA and there was also a concurrent growth spurt in the U.S. economy in the mid-1990s. DSHEA relaxed regulatory restrictions on dietary supplements, thus lowering the barrier to enter the market. As a result, growth in CAM likely is a result of deregulation by DSHEA and may reflect the disposable income available. This would explain the rapid growth in the mid-1990s and leveling of spending on botanical products at the turn of the century. Also, Eisenberg et al. found that the increase in botanical product utilization between 1990 and 1997 was likely due to an increase in the proportion of the population using botanicals rather than an increase in per patient utilization (9). In contrast to the growth of botanical products in the mid-1990s reported by Eisenberg et al., growth of the botanical market in early 2000 was reported to be from patients already using sundry botanical products according to the Natural Marketing Institute (NMI) (18). This indicates that botanical dietary supplement market expansion among new patients has moderated, which would explain the apparent stabilization of sale around the year 2000, as shown in Figure 1.

Market Analyses

Several major surveys of dietary supplement utilization have been conducted recently. The Saskatchewan Nutriceutical Network (SNN) (13), National Nutritional Food Association (NNFA) (14), Consumer Healthcare Products Association (CHPA) (11), Landmark Healthcare, Inc. (16), The NMI (18), individual investigators (9,12), Centers for Disease Control and Prevention (CDC) (15), and FDA (10) have all recently either conducted or contracted market analyses of CAM utilization in the United States, which included botanicals. Each survey is presented individually because the data are so heterogeneous among studies.

Saskatchewan Nutriceutical Network (13)

The SSN estimated U.S. botanical sales in 1999 to be $4 billion. The network further quantified where consumers buy their botanical products. Forty-seven percent are sold in retail stores, 30% are sold in multilevel distribution systems, 8% are sold by mail order or practitioners, 6% was sold by Asian herbal shops, and only 1% was purchased on the Internet (13). Notwithstanding these findings, it is important to note that the Internet was the fastest growing sales market for botanical products, at 150% per year (45).

National Nutritional Food Association (14)

The NNFA commissioned a telephone survey of 736 adults in October of 2001. The key finding was that women (25%) were more likely to take botanical products than men (15%). The survey emphasizes the importance of accurate labeling. Seventy percent agreed with the statement "Labels on supplements' bottles or packages are carefully read by most: they help the majority of older adults choose the right supplement and to determine the correct dosage." Only 22% disagreed with that statement. Fifty-five percent of respondents agreed with this statement: "Labels on dietary supplements help me understand if this is the right supplement for me," while 64% agreed with the following statement: "Labels on dietary supplements help me determine the dosage I need to take." The more educated patients were less likely to agree with this statement (14).

Consumer Healthcare Products Association (11)

The CHPA commissioned a study entitled "Self-Care in the New Millenium: American Attitudes Toward Maintaining Personal Health and Treatment." They conducted 1505 telephone interviews in January of 2001, using random telephone numbers. African-Americans and Hispanics were oversampled to conduct in-depth subgroup analysis. Of particular interest is the finding that 96% of respondents felt confident that they could take care of their own health. This might explain why so many people want access to pharmacologically active botanicals. These products do not require a prescription and thus allow patients to treat themselves.

Many of these products are being used for specific medical conditions. The top five conditions, in many cases are refractory to conventional medicine, namely menopausal symptoms, colds, allergies/sinus, muscle/joint/back pain, and premenstrual/menstrual symptoms.

The demographics of utilization in the past six months were reported. Thirty percent of women reported using a dietary supplement and 23% of men used a dietary supplement in the six-month period. Results for the effect of age on utilization have been mixed across studies. Patients who were between 50 and 64 years old had the highest reported use of dietary supplements, and 59% and those who were 18 to 34 years old had the lowest use at 48%. Income may be reflected in the utilization-by-age category. Utilization of dietary supplements by ethnicity was characteristic of other studies. Forty-four percent of African-Americans and 42% of Hispanics reportedly used dietary supplements, as compared to 53% of the general population. Although the study did not report Caucasian dietary supplement utilization rates, we can infer that Caucasians increased the overall utilization rate for the population. Health insurance status was associated with greater dietary supplement use, 56% versus 45%. This likely reflected the fact that patients who had health insurance also had more income. Those with some college education reported the highest utilization rate of 60%. People with college degrees used dietary supplements slightly less, 57%, but those with high school education or lesser educational qualification reported 48% utilization of dietary supplements in the past six months (11).

Landmark Healthcare Inc. (16)

In 1997, Landmark Healthcare Inc. commissioned a report entitled "The Landmark Report on Public Perceptions of Alternative Care." They conducted 1500 telephone interviews in November 1997, using random digit selection. The survey included a representative sample of minority patients—85% Caucasian, 8% African-Americans, and 3% Hispanic. The survey found that 17% of the U.S. population used botanical dietary supplements in the past year and even more striking, 75% of the U.S. population was most likely to use botanical products. Eighty-five percent of those reported to have taken a botanical supplement self-prescribed and self-administered the products. Three-fourths of patients who used alternative forms of care did so in conjunction with conventional medicine, yet 15% of patients replaced their conventional treatment with alternative care (16).

Natural Marketing Institute (18)

The NMI surveyed by mail 2002 households, July through August 2001. Only 53% of botanical supplement users were satisfied with botanical supplements. Despite the low satisfaction for botanical products, supplement users accounted for most of the increase in the previous year: 46% of botanical users increased utilization while only 10% of the general population increased utilization of botanical dietary supplements. Consumers took botanical supplements primarily for general health benefits, 59% versus 40% for a specific condition. Only 6% took botanicals products for short-term benefits, whereas 80% took them for daily or long-term benefit. Many have recently started, with only 50% having used an herb for more than three years (18).

Independent Investigators (9,12)

Eisenberg et al. surveyed 1539 adults in 1990 and 2055 adults in 1997. Botanical use in the prior 12 months increased from 2.5% in 1990 to 12.1% in 1997—a 4.8-fold increase. They estimated, in 1997, that 15 million adults took a botanical product or high-dose vitamins with other medications, which represented approximately 18.4% of those taking medications in the United States. Growth in botanicals was found to be from an increase in the percentage of the population taking botanicals and not due to an increase in utilization per patient. More than 60% of patients did not discuss CAM use with their doctor. Patients spent an estimated $5.1 billion on botanical medications (9). Kaufman surveyed 2590 patients, February 1998 through December 1999. Fourteen percent of the U.S. population reported using botanical supplements. Concurrent use with medication was highest with patients on fluoxetine, 22%; overall, 16% of those taking medication reported using botanical medications (12).

Centers for Disease Control and Prevention (15)

The Division of Health Interview Statistics, National Center for Health Statistics, CDC conducted a survey entitled "Utilization of Complementary and Alternative Medicine by United States Adults" in 1999. The survey attempted to obtain a representative sample of minorities and also patients without telephones. This is important because these demographic groups tend to report lower utilization of botanicals products than Caucasians and those of higher socioeconomic status. The CDC found that 9.6% of the population took botanical medicines. Hispanics reported the lowest use of CAM followed by African-Americans, and then Caucasians: 19.9%, 24.1%, and 30.8%, respectively. The western part of the United States reported the highest use of CAM (15).

Food and Drug Administration (10)

FDA commissioned a study of dietary supplement sales in the United States in 1999. Samples of products were purchased from a representative sample of retail establishments, catalogs, and the Internet. The authors looked at the consistency of botanical products purchased. Forty percent to 46% of botanicals and botanical products were consistent with the ingredients listed on the label. Botanical extracts were even less consistent with the label, only 12% to 24% (depending on where purchased) were found to be consistent with the label. They also gave the mean, minimum, and maximum price paid for dietary supplements by source of purchase. Interestingly, the mean purchased price on the Internet was the most expensive at $23.34, followed by the mean catalog price, $16.40. The mean retail price was less than half the cost of the mean Internet price, at $11.62 (10).

Utilization Summary

Patients who use botanicals tend to have attained higher education, be female, be older persons, have higher incomes, and have a recalcitrant chronic disease unresponsive to conventional medicine. There is also evidence that cultural differences have a strong impact on the use of botanicals. Certain subpopulations may defy these generalizations to the U.S. population. Asian-Americans have a long history of using botanicals as medication and often consider botanicals a conventional form of treatment (2). Southern rural poor are also reported to have a higher utilization profile of plant-derived products (46). Rural poor may treat illness with botanical products while the U.S. population as a whole tends to use botanical products for general health benefits rather than to treat a specific illness (18,46). Table 1 summarizes frequently used botanical products and what the patients are using them for.

SAFETY OF BOTANICAL PRODUCTS

As a result of DSHEA, the majority of botanical drug products are used in the United States without medical supervision. Only 8% of those who use botanicals do so under medical supervision (13) and 85% of those who treat themselves with herbs do not seek professional guidance or advice (16). Even if patients utilizing botanical dietary supplements were medically supervised, adulteration and misbranding are prevalent and so little is known about the supplements that many untoward events could not be prevented or recognized in a timely fashion (47,48). Despite the widespread acceptance of CAM by the lay public, clinicians possess little scientific information about the practices of CAM relative to conventional western medicine. This is particularly unsettling because it is estimated that 16% to 18% of prescription medication users took botanical and supplements coincidentally (9,12). Medication–botanical interactions are largely unknown (42). Even more alarming is a report that 14.5% of women used botanical products during pregnancy and 23.5% of children under 16 may be taking botanical products. Neonatal heart failure has been attributed to the use of Blue cohosh during pregnancy (47).

Up to 60% of patients using alternative therapies are reported to have never informed their physician of their botanical or CAM use (9,22,49,50). Furthermore, only 40% of physicians ask their patients about alternative therapy (22). The 60% of physicians who do not ask about the use of

Table 1 Estimates for Botanical Utilization, Sales Data in the United States, and Reasons for Patient Use of Botanical Products

Herbal product	United States herbal rank (7)	United States herbal rank (13)	United States sales in $ 1998 (36), 1998–1999 (13), 1999 (7,39), 1999–2000 (67), 2000 (38), 2000–2001 (68)	Possibly effective uses (66)	Ineffective uses (66)
Aloe Vera	10		49.37 million (7)	Burns, frostbite tissue survival, psoriasis	
Bilberry	8		97.21 (7)	Retinopathy	Night vision
Capsicum (cayenne)	16		36.29 million (7)	Pain, fibromyalgia, prurigo nodularis	HIV-associated peripheral neuropathy
Chinese herbs	18		33.57 million (7)		
Chondroitin		8		Eye surgery, osteoarthritis, dry eyes	
Cranberry	17		34.27 million (7)	Urinary odor, urinary tract infections	Diabetes
Creatine		9		Athletic performance, congestive heart failure, gyrate atrophy of the choroid and retina, McArdle's disease, muscular dystrophy	Amyotrophic lateral sclerosis, rheumatoid arthritis, athletic conditioning
Garlic	2	3	61.21 million (38), 84 million (36),	Atherosclerosis, colon cancer prevention, gastric	Breast cancer prevention, diabetes prevention and

(Continued)

Table 1 Estimates for Botanical Utilization, Sales Data in the United States, and Reasons for Patient Use of Botanical Products (*Continued*)

Herbal product	United States herbal rank (7)	United States herbal rank (13)	United States sales in $ 1998 (36), 1998–1999 (13), 1999 (7,39), 1999–2000 (67), 2000 (38), 2000–2001 (68)	Possibly effective uses (66)	Ineffective uses (66)
			280.85 million (7), 100 million (68)	cancer prevention, hyperlipidemia treatment, hypertension treatment, prostate cancer prevention, tick bite prevention, tinea corporis treatment, tinea cruris prevention, tinea pedis treatment	treatment, *Helicobacter pylori* treatment, familial hypercholesterolemia treatment, lung cancer prevention, peripheral artery disease treatment
Ginger	20		27.48 million (7)	Chemotherapy-induced nausea, morning sickness, postoperative nausea and vomiting, vertigo	Motion sickness
Ginkgo	1	2	151 million (36), 395.68 million (7)	Age-related macular degeneration treatment, age-related memory impairment, altitude sickness, cognitive performance, dementia, diabetic retinopathy,	Antidepressant-induced sexual dysfunction, seasonal affective disorder, tinnitus

Botanical			Annual retail sales	Conditions	Conditions
Ginseng	6	1	96 million (36), 159.32 million (7), 56.27 million (66), 62.5 million (38)	glaucoma, premenstrual syndrome, Raynaud's disease, vetigo, Cognitive performance, diabetes, erectile dysfunction, premature ejaculation	Athletic performance, menopausal symptoms, quality of life
Glucosamine	4		871.8 million (39)	Osteoarthritis, temporomandibular joint arthritis	
Goldenseal	14		39.01 million (7)		Urine drug testing
Grape seed	7		122.41 million (7)	Chronic venous insufficiency, ocular stress	Allergic rhinitis
Green tea (extract)	15		37.68 million (7), 3.15 million (38)	Bladder cancer, esophageal cancer, pancreatic cancer, breast cancer, cervical dysplasia, cognitive performance, gastric cancer, hyperlipidemia, leukoplakia, ovarian cancer, Parkinson's disease	Colon cancer
Echinacea	5		70 million (36), 193.03 million (7), 58.42 million (38)	Common cold, vaginal candidiasis	Herpes simplex, influenza, leukopenia
Horse chestnut	11		49.24 million (7)	Chronic venous insufficiency	

(Continued)

Table 1 Estimates for Botanical Utilization, Sales Data in the United States, and Reasons for Patient Use of Botanical Products (*Continued*)

Herbal product	United States herbal rank (7)	United States herbal rank (13)	United States sales in $ 1998 (36), 1998–1999 (13), 1999 (7,39), 1999–2000 (67), 2000 (38), 2000–2001 (68)	Possibly effective uses (66)	Ineffective uses (66)
Kava	12		17 million (36), 45.25 million (7), 14.68 million (38)	Anxiety, benzodiazepine withdrawal, menopausal anxiety	
Lecithin		7		Hepatic steatosis, dermatitis, dry skin	Gallbladder disease, hypercholesterolemia, Alzheimer's disease and dementia, extrapyramidal disorders
Milk thistle	9		56.70 million (7), 8.91 million (38)		
Pygeum	19		28.21 million (38)	Benign prostatic hyperplasia, prostatic adenoma	
Saw palmetto	4	10	32 million (36), 193.17 million (7), 43.85 million (38)	Benign prostatic hyperplasia	Prostatitis and chronic pelvic pain syndrome
St. John's	3	5	140 million (36), 209.34 million (7),	Depression, anxiety	Hepatitis C virus

(*Continued*)

Wort		55.98 million (38)	HIV/AIDS, polyneuropathy
Valerian	13	44.21 million (7), 16.82 million (38)	Anxiety, insomnia

Note: In column 2 (7), sales rankings, by dollars, for the top 20 sold in the United States for the year 1999 are given. Column 3 (12) gives the top 10 products in 2002 in an ambulatory adult population (13). Reported sales in dollars are present in column 4. Columns 5 and 6 (66) give the conditions the botanicals have been used for. The Natural Medicines Comprehensive Database at http://www.naturaldatabasc.com (66) distinguishes gradations of evidence for effectiveness, which we have not done here. There is much variability in the data from report to report; even data within the same trade journal data are inconsistent with that from previous reports. This in no way endorses the utilization of dietary supplements for treatment of these conditions. Patients should always seek the advice of their health care provider.

botanical supplements and other CAM are unlikely be informed of alternative therapies their patients are using. Clearly, there is a lack of communication between patients and providers. Some patients may fear disapproval by physicians and wish to give socially desirable answers. However, the majority of patients express a lack of concern about their physician's approval, rather they were more concerned with their physician's inability to understand and incorporate CAM into their medical management (51). Patients are not using alternative therapy because they are dissatisfied with conventional medicine but instead because they value both types of therapy (51).

Many botanical dietary supplements are potentially unsafe because of adulteration and misbranding. Thirty-two percent of botanical medications collected in California contained an undeclared pharmaceutical or heavy metal (8,48). Pharmaceuticals adulterating botanical products are one of the most frequent reasons botanical dietary supplements are placed on the FDA MedWatch site, and this is undoubtedly a small fraction of what actually occurs. Table 2 gives the botanical products placed on MedWatch in the past five years (52). Many of these adulterants are not detected until patient illnesses are first detected. Consumers often do not recognize that many imported products, purported to be traditional medications, are actually recognized pharmaceuticals. For example, a "Mexican asthma cure" had a claim on the label that said it contained no corticosteroids and was free of adverse effects, but the product was found to contain triamcinolone, a moderately potent corticosteroid with well-documented systemic adverse effects common to all glucocorticoids. In another example, a patient used an illegally imported Chinese medicine; it was reported to last much longer than the medication the physician had prescribed. The label on the Chinese medicine said it contained astemizole, a long-acting antihistamine withdrawn from the United States as a result of its effect of prolonging the cardiac QTc interval (8). In many cases, patients may not recognize pharmaceuticals that are sold as traditional medicines. In the past, consumers have had difficulty distinguishing between vitamins and botanical products (9,23). It is likely no different for botanicals and pharmaceuticals. This may be problematic because corporations are creating proprietary botanical blends and branding them for use in specific medical conditions. Patients could inadvertently assume they are treating themselves with a medication that has undergone the same rigorous clinical testing as other FDA-approved medications. Patients readily read and trust the directions on labels of dietary supplements (14). In fact 59% of the public incorrectly thought a government body reviewed and approved botanical supplements before they are sold (6,53,54).

There are other risks of contamination to botanical and botanical supplements. Due to stress on the supply of cultivars for botanical supplements, products may vary greatly in their active content. In the era of limited resources, with increasing utilization and decreasing wild production, there is pressure to produce a product. Raw material costs may override the

Table 2 Dietary Supplement Information from MedWatch for Herbal Products from 1999–2003

Product	Company	Date	Reason for action
Ancom antihypertensive compound tablets	Herbbsland, Inc., Tai Chien Inc.	01/17/2003	Contains unapproved reserpine, diazepam, promethazine, and hydrochlorothiazide
Viga tablets	Best of Life International	05/29/2003	Contains unlabeled drug sildenafil
Viga or Viga for women	Health Nutrition (RMA Labs)	06/27/2003	Contains unlabeled drug sildenafil
Vinarol tablets	Ultra Health Laboratories, Inc.	04/09/2003	Contains unlabeled drug sildenafil
Kava (*Piper methysticum*)	All products containing kava	03/26/2002	Kava is associated with liver-related injury including hepatitis, cirrhosis, and liver failure
Nettle capsules	Nature's Way Products, Inc.	07/03/2002	Contains high concentrations of lead
PC SPES and SPES	BotanicaLab	02/08/2002	Contains undeclared amounts of warfarin and alprazolam
Aristolochic acid	All products containing aristolochic acid	04/16/2001	Aristolochic acid is associated with renal interstitial fibrosis with atrophy and loss of tubules, and the development of end-stage renal failure
Kava (*Piper methysticum*)	All products containing kava	12/19/2001	Kava-containing products have been implicated in serious liver toxicity
Lipokinetix	Syntrax innovations, Inc.	11/20/2001	Lipokinetix has been implicated in several cases of serious liver injury
Neo Concept Aller Relief	BMK International	01/22/2001	Contains trace amounts of aristolochic acid, a carcinogen and nephrotoxin

(Continued)

Table 2 Dietary Supplement Information from MedWatch for Herbal Products from 1999–2003 (*Continued*)

Product	Company	Date	Reason for action
Aristolochic acid	All products containing aristolochic acid	06/01/2000	Aristolochic acid has been associated with nephropathy
St. John's Wort	All products containing St. John's Wort	02/10/2000	Hypericum perforatum can decrease indinavir plasma concentrations due to the induction of the P-450 metabolic pathway
Tiratricol	All products containing tiratricol	11/22/2000	Tiratricol also known as triiodothyroacetic acid or TRIAC, is a potent thyroid hormone that may result in serious health consequences
Asian remedy for menstrual cramps—KooSar	Tien Sau Tong	01/25/1999	One case report of lead poisoning from a woman who was taking 6 pills per day. There were no other reports of lead poisoning and the product was not recalled
GBL	All products containing GBL	01/22/1999 05/11/1999 08/25/1999	GBL is converted to GHB in vivo. At that time GHB was banned outside of clinical trials approved by the FDA. GHB has been implicated as a potential "date rape" drug

Abbreviations: FDA, Food and Drug Administration; GBL, gamma-butyrolactone; GHB, gamma-hydroxybutyrate.
Source: From Ref. 52.

quality and purity of the product. There are few barriers to bringing new products to the market and many newer entrants may lack expertise to prevent quality issues and contamination in their product (24). This creates the potential for inadvertent poisoning as a result of overdosing or contamination as well as treatment failure through underdosing. Indeed, a study of botanical consistency found that only 43% of the products tested were consistent for ingredients and dose with the benchmark or recommended daily dose. Twenty percent had the correct ingredient but not the stated dose and 37% were not consistent with either ingredients; dose or the labeling was too vague to draw conclusions (37,55). The FDA also found that many botanical products were inconsistent with the ingredients listed on the label and estimated that only 12% to 24% of botanical extracts and 40% to 46% of botanical products contained what was on the label (10).

Adulteration was found to be a problem in another dietary supplement containing androstenedione; although not strictly a botanical, it is regulated in a similar fashion under the auspices of DSHEA. Ingestion of androstenedione contaminated with trace amounts of 19-norandrosterone resulted in a positive test for 19-norandrosterone, a metabolite used to detect nandrolone. Other samples were also found to be contaminated with testosterone (56). The FDA has been cautious in its enforcement of DSHEA after its experience with the passage of The Nutritional Labeling and Education Act of 1990. This act severely restricted unproven claims on foods and dietary supplements. Fearful of the loss of the ability to conduct business as usual, the dietary supplement industry responded with forceful lobbying to the Congress, which responded with DSHEA, exempting dietary supplements from the earlier law.

DSHEA severely limited when the FDA could take action to protect the public and what actions could be taken. The burden of proof to show harm is now placed on the FDA. Moreover, dietary supplement manufacturers are not required to report adverse dietary supplement events. In fact, between 1994 and 1999 fewer than 10 of the 2500 adverse events associated with dietary supplements and reported to the FDA were reported by the manufacturer (53). The Office of Inspector General concluded the spontaneous adverse event reporting "system has difficulty generating signals of possible public health concern" due to "limited medical information, product information, manufacturer information, consumer information, and ability to analyze trends" (57). One weight loss supplement manufacturer is reported to have withheld from the FDA 14,684 complaints of adverse events regarding ephedra, which included heart attacks, strokes, seizures, and deaths (53).

Recently, the FDA has begun to enforce DSHEA more assertively. Ephedra was banned as a dietary supplement in April of 2004 because ephedra presented an "unreasonable risk." However, this ban does not include foods containing ephedra, approved drugs, or Asian medicines, which are allowed to contain ephedra under the final rule (58). It appears that FDA may address androstenedione in the near future (59,60). In March of 2004, FDA sent warning letters to 23 manufactures or distributors of androstenedione threatening enforcement if they do not immediately cease distribution of androstenedione and within 15 days advise the FDA, in writing, of actions taken (61). The FDA did this on the grounds that androstene dione was not marketed on October 15, 1994 and as such is not presumed safe under DSHEA. Furthermore, the FDA has stated that androstenedione consumption would be considered an unreasonable risk, given what is now known (61–63).

Other botanical products are receiving FDA attention. The acting commissioner of the FDA, Lester Crawford, told members at the American Society for Pharmacology and Experimental Therapeutics in April 2004 that the FDA was compiling data on other botanical products that have been associated with safety issues (64). Kava, used as an anxiolytic, and usnic acid, used for weight loss, have both been associated with liver disease; bitter orange is used as a sympathomimetic in weight loss products to replace ephedra; all the pyrrolizidine alkaloids have the eye of the FDA (64). There are other products that could receive scrutiny of the FDA in the future. Examples profiled in Consumer Reports include a list of what they call "the dirty dozen herbs listed by risk." The botanicals are broken down as follows: "definitively hazardous": aristolochic acid; "very likely hazardous": comfrey, androstenedione, chaparral, germander, and kava; and "likely hazardous": bitter orange, organ/glandular extracts, lobelia, pennyroyal oil, skullcap, and yohimbe (53). These are products with potent pharmacological actions and poorly documented toxicities, and as long as they are available safety will clearly be an issue.

As a result of DSHEA, botanical supplements are presumed safe by virtue of being "grandfathered" by the FDA if the product was marketed before October 15, 1994. Products brought to market after that date only require 75-day premarket notification to the FDA with information that substantiates that the ingredients will reasonably be expected to be safe (65). FDA cannot take action until patients are injured but it is increasingly clear relatively rare adverse events may not be detected until a significant number of patients are killed or injured.

Safety Summary

With little knowledge of dietary supplements, many physicians do not ask patients about botanical products and patients are also not disclosing the consumption of these products. Some of these products also have substantial pharmacologic activity that interacts with prescription medications and disease states while other are devoid of any biological activity. Many patients may actually think they are taking something that is rigorously tested and regulated by the FDA when in fact some have been reported have serious issues with contaminants. Safety has been presumed as a result of DSHEA despite common misbranding, and adulteration. Several dietary supplements have been linked to cancer, renal and liver failure, and even death. The vast majority of products are probably safe but many likely have low level undocumented adverse effects. This leaves the possibility most adverse events likely go unrecognized and untreated. Under current practices, the situation is unlikely to change.

CONCLUSIONS

The profile of the patient who uses a botanical product will likely be someone with higher education, be female, have higher socioeconomic status, have more disposable income, and be older. The market is estimated to be in excess of $5 billion in the United States with an estimated 10% to 20% of the population using botanicals. Utilization of botanical dietary supplements will continue to grow under the deregulation of DSHEA and as they gain acceptance by the public and medical establishment. With increasing stress on the harvesting of wild foliage, corporations must resort to harvesting domestically grown botanical dietary supplements to meet the demand. This should result in a more consistent product base. By increasing direct-to-consumer marketing and branding of specific products, there will likely be an acceleration of market growth. New ads for branded botanicals have already appeared as this chapter was being published. Products will continue to be imported and Internet sales will continue to grow. As more patients use these products and regulatory issues remain, safety will continue to be a concern and the market will likely be difficult to define. Drug–botanical interactions and disease–botanical interactions are only now beginning to be recognized by health care professionals as a potential source of harm, as the prevalence of botanical dietary supplement utilization increases.

REFERENCES

1. Barrett B, Kiefer D, Rabago D. Assessing the risks and benefits of herbal medicine: an overview of scientific evidence. Altern Ther Health Med 1999; 5(4):40–49.
2. Iqbal M. International trade in non-wood forest products: an overview. XI Medicinal Plants, 1993. Rome: Food and Agriculture Organization of the United Nations, 1993. http://www.fao.org/docrep/X5326E/x5326e0e.htm#xi.%20medicinal%20plants (accessed 2–16–04).
3. Angell M, Kassirer JP. Alternative medicine—the risks of untested and unregulated remedies. N Engl J Med 1998; 339(12):839–841.
4. Opium. DEA, 2004. http://www.dea. gov/concern/opium.htm (accessed 2–16–2004).
5. Gedif T, Hahn HJ. Epidemiology of herbal drugs use in Addis Ababa, Ethiopia. Pharmacoepidemiol Drug Saf 2002; 11(7):587–591.

6. Bent S, Ko R. Commonly used herbal medicines in the United States: a review. Am J Med 2004; 116(7):478–485.

7. Popovich B. What is the cure for leveling botanicals sales? Chemical Market Reporter 2000. http://www.findarticles.com/cf_0/m0FVP/13_258/65951203/p1/article, jhtml (accessed 2–2004).

8. Dreskin SC. A prescription drug packaged in China and sold as an ethnic remedy. JAMA 2000; 283(18):2393.

9. Eisenberg DM, Davis RB, Ettner SL, et al. Trends in alternative medicine use in the United States, 1990–1997: results of a follow-up national survey. JAMA 1998; 280(18):1569–1575.

10. Muth MK, Domanico JL, Anderson DW, Siegel PH, Bloch LJ. Dietary Supplement Sales Information Final Report. RTI Project Number 6673.004. 1999. Research Triangle Park, North Carolina, Research Triangle Institute, Center for Economics Research. http://vm.cfsan.fda.gov/~acrobat/ds-sales.pdf (accessed 5–18–2004).

11. Self-care in the new millennium, 2001. Roper Starch Worldwide Inc. http://www.chpa-info.org/web/press_room/statistics/consumer_survey.aspx (accessed 2–13–2004).

12. Kaufman DW, Kelly JP, Rosenberg L, Anderson TE, Mitchell AA. Recent patterns of medication use in the ambulatory adult population of the United States: the Slone survey. JAMA 2002; 287(3):337–344.

13. Nutraceutical market and industry information. Saskatchewan Nutraceutical Network, 2002. Saskatchewan Nutraceutical Network. http://www.nutranet.org/subpages/markets.htm (accessed 3–2004).

14. Strategy One/NNFA Dietary Supplements Usage Survey. 1–10. 10–22–2001. http://www.nutranet.org/subpages/markets.htm (accessed 3–2004).

15. Ni H, Simile C, Hardy AM. Utilization of complementary and alternative medicine by United States adults: results from the 1999 national health interview survey. Med Care 2002; 40(4):353–358.

16. The Landmark report on public perceptions of alternative care, 1998. Sacramento, California, Landmark Healthcare, Inc. 1998. www.landmarkhealthcare.com (accessed 3–2004).

17. Wetzel MS, Kaptchuk TJ, Haramati A, Eisenberg DM. Complementary and alternative medical therapies: implications for medical education. Ann Intern Med 2003; 138(3):191–196.

18. Blumenthal M. Natural marketing institute measures consumer use of herbal products. Herbalgram 2004; (50). http: www.herbalgram.com/herbalgram/articleview.asp?a=2295 (accessed 2–18–2004).

19. Adams KE, Cohen MH, Eisenberg D, Jonsen AR. Ethical considerations of complementary and alternative medical therapies in conventional medical settings. Ann Intern Med 2002; 137(8):660–664.

20. Dietary supplement facts and figures. Consumer Healthcare Products Association. 4–12–2002. http://www.chpa-info.org/web/press_room/statistics/supplement_facts_figures.aspx (accessed 2–13–2004).

21. Johnston BA. Prevention magazine assesses use of dietary supplements. Herbalgram 2004; (48):65. http://www.herbalgram.com/herbalgram/articleview.asp?a=378 (accessed 2–18–2004).

22. Halsted CH. Dietary supplements and functional foods: 2 sides of a coin? Am J Clin Nutr 2003; 77(suppl 4):1001S–1007S.
23. Blumenthal M. Harvard study estimates consumers spend $5.1 billion on herbal products? Herbalgram 2004; 45:68. http://www.herbalgram.com/herbalgram/articleview.asp?a=760 (accessed 2–19–2004).
24. Brevoort P. The booming U.S. botanical market a new overview. Herbalgram 1998; (44):33–46.
25. Enzyte: the once-a-day tablet for natural male enhancement. World Wide Web, 4–10–2004. http://www.enzyte.com (accessed 4–10–2004).
26. Reclaim your sensuality, Avlimil. World Wide Web, 2004. http://www.avlimil.com (accessed 4–10–2004).
27. Introducing Amoryn. World Wide Web, 2004. http://www.amoryn.com (accessed 4–10–2004).
28. Bloussant product.com. World Wide Web, 2004. http://www.bloussantproduct.com/?campaign=google&kw=bloussant (accessed 4–19–2004).
29. Leptoprin-SF: the first stimulant-free weight control compound available! World Wide Web, 2004. http://www.leptoprin.com/contactus.asp?sid=654693403 (accessed 4–10–2004).
30. Dr. Talbott links daily stress to hormone that stores FAT! (Cortislim). World Wide Web, 2004. http://www.cortisol.com (accessed 4–10–2004).
31. Welcome to the official focus factor web site! World Wide Web, 2004. http://www.focusfactor.com/?id=2 (accessed 4–10–2004).
32. Alluna A to ZZZ. World Wide Web, 2004. http://www.allunasleep.com/atoz.asp (accessed 4–10–2004).
33. Metabolife get back into your wardrobe. World Wide Web. http://www.metabolife.com (accessed 4–19–2004).
34. Wellness guide to dietary supplements. UC Berkley wellness letter. http://www.berkeleywellness.com/html/ds/dsAvacor.php (accessed 5–14–2004).
35. Miller LG. Herbal medicinals: selected clinical considerations focusing on known or potential drug-herb interactions. Arch Intern Med 1998; 158(20):2200–2211.
36. Blumenthal M. Herb market levels after five years of boom: 1999 sales in mainstream market up only 11% in first half of 1999 after 55% increase in 1998. Herbalgram 1999; 47:64–65. http://www.herbalgram.org/herbalgram/articleview.asp?a=254 (accessed 4–17–2004).
37. Garrard J, Harms S, Eberly LE, Matiak A. Variations in product choices of frequently purchased herbs: caveat emptor. Arch Intern Med 2003; 163(19):2290–2295.
38. Kane JR. Nutritional supplements are under the weather. (Sales decline) (Statistical data included). Chemical Market Reporter Pub 6/2001. http://www.findarticles.com/cf_dls/m0FVP/26_260/76495868/p1/article.jhtml (accessed 2–01–2004).
39. Challener C. Specialty dietary supplement ingredients are the hot spot. Chemical Market Reporter 2000. http://www.findarticles.com/cf_dls/m0FVP/13_258/65951204/p1/article.jhtml (accessed 2–14–2004).
40. Grünwald J. The European phytomedicines market figures, trends, analysis. Herbalgram 1995; (35):60–65.

41. Health Strategy Consulting LLC (HSC). The $16.7 billion U.S. dietary supplement market is led in size by vitamins, but in growth by specialty supplements. http://www.health-strategy.com/contentmgr/showdetails.php/id/21 (accessed 2–02–2004).

42. Huang SM, Hall SD, Watkins P, et al. Drug interactions with herbal products and grapefruit juice: a conference report. Clin Pharmacol Ther 2004; 75(1): 1–12.

43. Woolf AD. Herbal remedies and children: do they work? Are they harmful? Pediatrics 2003; 112(1 Pt 2):240–246.

44. Wolsko PM, Eisenberg DM, Davis RB, Ettner SL, Phillips RS. Insurance coverage, medical conditions, and visits to alternative medicine providers: results of a national survey. Arch Intern Med 2002; 162(3):281–287.

45. Blumenthal M. Herb sales up 1% for all channels of trade in 2000. Herbalgram 2001; (53):63. http://www.herbalgram.com/herbalgram/articleview.asp?a= 2216 (accessed 4–18–2004).

46. Frate DA. Self-treatment with herbal and other plant-derived remedies—rural Mississippi, 1993. MMRW Morb Mortal Wkly Rep 2004; 44:204–207 (accessed 3–2004).

47. Boullata JI, Nace AM. Safety issues with herbal medicine. Pharmacotherapy 2000; 20(3):257–269.

48. Ko RJ. Adulterants in Asian patent medicines. N Engl J Med 1998; 339(12):847.

49. Foster DF, Phillips RS, Hamel MB, Eisenberg DM. Alternative medicine use in older Americans. J Am Geriatr Soc 2000; 48(12):1560–1565.

50. Navo MA, Phan J, Vaughan C, et al. An assessment of the utilization of complementary and alternative medication in women with gynecologic or breast malignancies. J Clin Oncol 2004; 22(4):671–677.

51. Eisenberg DM, Kessler RC, Van Rompay MI, et al. Perceptions about complementary therapies relative to conventional therapies among adults who use both: results from a national survey. Ann Intern Med 2001; 135(5):344–351.

52. MedWatch FDA. http://www.fda.gov/medwatch/safety.htm (accessed 3–1–2004).

53. Dangerous supplements. Consumer Reports, 12, 2004. http://www.consumer-reports.org/main/content/display_report.jsp?FOLDER%3C%3_Efolder_id= 419341&ASSORTMENT%3C%3East_id=333141 (accessed 5–3–2004).

54. Wong N. Widespread ignorance of regulation and labeling of vitamins, minerals and food supplements, according to a National Harris Interactive Survey. Harris Interact 2002; 2(23). http://www.harrisinteractive.com/news/allnews bydate. asp?NewsID=560 (accessed 4–20–2004).

55. Erickson AK. Not all herbal products are created equal. Pharm today 2004; 10(2):4.

56. Catlin DH, Leder BZ, Ahrens B, et al. Trace contamination of over-the-counter androstenedione and positive urine test results for a nandrolone metabolite. JAMA 2000; 284(20):2618–2621.

57. Adverse event reporting for dietary supplements, an inadequate safety valve, 2001. http://oig.hhs.gov/oei/reports/oei-01-00-00180.pdf (accessed 4–20–2004).

58. Final rule declaring dietary supplements containing ephedrine alkaloids adulterated because they present an unreasonable risk; final rule. 21 CFR 119. 2004.

http://www.fda.gov/oc/initiatives/ephedra/february2004/finalsummary.html (accessed 2–11–2004).

59. Matiak AW. FDA plans move against sports supplement. Wall Street Journal 2004; B1.

60. Questions and answers androstenedione. 3–11–2004. FDA/Center for Food Safety and Applied Nutrition. http://vm.cfsan.fda.gov/~dms/androqa.html (accessed 4–02–2004).

61. HHS launches crackdown on products containing andro. FDA warns manufacturers to stop distributing such products. 3–11–2004. United States Department of Health and Human Services. http://www.fda.gov/bbs/topics/news/2004/hhs_031104.html (accessed 5–18–2004).

62. FDA white paper health effects of androstenedione. 3–11–2004. http://www.fda.gov/oc/whitepapers/andro.html (accessed 4–11–2004).

63. FDA/Center for Food Safety and Applied Nutrition. Sample warning letter on androstenedione. http://vm.cfsan.fda.gov/~dms/andltr.html (accessed 4–11–2004).

64. Heavey S. Corrected-update 1-US FDA may act on ephedra substitutes, others. Reuters. http://www.alertnet.org/thenews/newsdesk/N22590286.htm (accessed 4–22–2004).

65. FDA. Dietary Supplement Health and Education Act of 1994. 12–1–1995. http://vm.cfsan.fda.gov/~dms/dietsupp.html (accessed 5–18–2004).

66. Jellin JM, Batz F, Hitchens K. Pharmacist's letter/prescriber's letter natural medicines comprehensive database. Stockton, California: Therapeutic Research Faculty, 1999. http://www.naturaldatabase.com.

67. Blumenthal M. Ginseng sales down 27% in mainstream markets; sales follow decreasing trend for total herb category. Herbalgram 2004; (52):58–59. http://www.herbalgram.org/herbalgram/articleview.asp?a=2241.

68. Garlic industry statistics. The Horticultural Web. http://www.horticulture.com.au/australian+horticulture/industries+and+statistics/garlic/garlic+industry+statistics.htm (accessed 2–16–2004).

2

Drug Interactions with Botanical Products

Y. W. Francis Lam

*Departments of Pharmacology and Medicine,
University of Texas Health Science Center at San Antonio, San Antonio, and
College of Pharmacy, University of Texas at Austin, Austin,
Texas, U.S.A.*

Shiew-Mei Huang

*Office of Clinical Pharmacology and Biopharmaceutics,
Center for Drug Evaluation and Research (CDER), Food and Drug Administration,
Silver Spring, Maryland, U.S.A.*

Stephen D. Hall

*Division of Clinical Pharmacology, Department of Medicine,
Indiana University School of Medicine, Indianapolis,
Indiana, U.S.A.*

OVERVIEW OF BOTANICAL–DRUG INTERACTIONS

The use of botanicals by consumers in North American and European countries has significantly increased over the last decade, with one survey showing an almost 10% increase in usage from 1990 to 1997 (1). Although the efficacy of some botanicals has been documented (2), there is concern regarding the perceived safety of these products, particularly with respect to the lack of research and knowledge on botanical–drug interaction potential and significance (3). As more consumers use botanicals for various purposes, the likelihood of concurrent use of botanicals with prescription

and/or over-the-counter medications, as well as the potential of pharmacokinetic and/or pharmacodynamic botanical–drug interactions will increase.
The survey conducted by Eisenberg et al. (1) reported that as many as
15 million adults in 1997 took botanical supplements concurrently with prescription drugs. Over the subsequent years, there has been no change in this
usage pattern, with as many as 16% of consumers surveyed indicating concurrent use of botanical dietary supplements and prescription drugs (4).

This continued trend of concurrent use of drug and botanical supplements (5), together with an underreporting of such use (6,7) and a general
lack of knowledge of the interaction potential (8), poses a challenge for the
health care professionals and a safety concern for patients and/or consumers. Indeed, several clinically important botanical–drug interactions have
been reported and some have resulted in altered efficacy and/or toxicity of
the drug (3). The purpose of this chapter is to present an overview of common mechanisms of botanical–drug interactions, and using specific
literature examples, discuss challenges associated with the interpretation
of available study data or reports, and the of prediction of botanical–drug
interactions. Detailed information for specific botanicals, and their interactions with drugs, appears in Chapters 4 to 7.

MECHANISMS OF BOTANICAL–DRUG INTERACTIONS

In essence, interactions between pharmacologically active botanicals and
drugs involve the same pharmacokinetic and pharmacodynamic mechanisms as drug–drug interactions. Pharmacokinetic interactions may involve
alteration in absorption, distribution, metabolism, or excretion of the
affected drug or botanical. Pharmacodynamic interactions, on the other
hand, alter the relationship between the drug concentration and the pharmacological response for a drug or botanical. Although most pharmacodynamic interactions reported in the literature and reviewed in this
chapter focus on adverse effects as an outcome, not all pharmacodynamic
botanical–drug interactions result in an undesirable effect. Animal studies
have shown that the combination of an extract of the Chinese medicinal
plant, *Tripterygium wilfordi*, and cyclosporine significantly increased the
heart and kidney allograft survival compared to cyclosporine administered
alone. The effective cyclosporine dose required for 100% kidney allograft
survival was reduced by 50% to 75% in the presence of the botanical
extract (9). The immunosuppressive activity associated with the use of
the botanical extract needs to be studied further in humans in order to
explore the clinical potential of their combined use, perhaps by a mechanism similar to that for the ketoconazole and cyclosporine interaction.

Most pharmacokinetic and pharmacodynamic botanical–drug interaction studies and clinical cases in the literature evaluated the quantitative

effect or reported the consequence of adding a specific botanical to a drug regimen, and not the other way around. This likely represents the challenge of not knowing the identify and constitution of the botanical or botanical product, the difficulty of measuring concentration of a specific botanical or its active ingredient(s), and the more common scenario of patients using botanical preparations on a sporadic basis, while being stabilized on a drug regimen. Nevertheless, the pharmacokinetic profiles of different botanical products are currently being investigated (Chapter 9). A better understanding of botanical pharmacokinetics in humans is needed if the prediction of botanical–drug interactions is to be successful.

ALTERED PHARMACOKINETICS

Drug Absorption

While reduction in the extent of drug absorption can potentially occur as a result of increased intestinal transit time, secondary to the use of botanicals containing anthranoid laxatives (e.g., aloe; *Aloe* spp.) or as a result of complex formation between botanical constituents (e.g., polyphenols in green tea), clinical cases of these types of interaction have not been reported. Nevertheless, based on the well-documented chelation of fluoroquinolones by different divalent and trivalent cations (e.g., sucralfate and didanosine) with the resultant significant decrease in fluoroquinolone concentrations and potential treatment failure, there remains the possibility that natural product supplements containing cations might also exert the same undesirable effect. Indeed, concurrent administration of an aqueous extract of fennel, the fruit of *Foeniculum vulgare*, in rats was shown to reduce maximum blood concentration, area under the concentration time curve (AUC), and urinary recovery of ciprofloxacin by 83%, 48%, and 43%, respectively. None of the phenolic or terpene constituents were reported to have an interacting effect, and the most likely mechanism is chelation of ciprofloxacin by metal cations present in the extract. The dose of the extract employed (2 g/kg) is unlikely to be consumed by humans, but the potential of impaired absorption of ciprofloxacin and other fluoroquinolones needs to be considered when patients take concurrent botanical products containing large amount of inorganic materials; staggering administration times of the two products should be considered when such physical interactions are possible (10).

Interestingly, there was a report of an interaction between aspirin and tamarind, an Asian fruit used not only as an Ayurvedic medicine, but also as a flavoring ingredient for cooking. In six healthy volunteers, tamarind significantly increased the extent of absorption of a single 600 mg dose of aspirin, which might result in toxicity if a large amount of acetylsalicylate was ingested concurrently with tamarind (11).

The more significant botanical–drug interaction resulting in altered extent of drug absorption involves modulation of P-glycoprotein within the gastrointestinal tract. Originally discovered by Juliano and Ling (12), P-glycoprotein has been primarily known for its association with drug resistance to chemotherapeutic agents. However, P-glycoprotein also possesses a physiological protective role by transporting toxic xenobiotics or metabolites out of normal cells. In humans, P-glycoprotein is also expressed in several tissues including the gastrointestinal tract, liver, and blood–brain barrier. The presence of this efflux transporter on the luminal surface of the intestinal mucosa suggests a possible role in limiting drug bioavailability after oral administration (13).

In early 2000, several reports publicized the now well-recognized interaction between St. John's wort (*Hypericum perforatum*) and commonly used drugs such as cyclosporine, some with significant clinical consequences, e.g., organ transplant rejection (14). Because cyclosporine is primarily metabolized by cytochrome P-450 3A4 (CYP3A4) (15), induction of CYP3A4 was originally thought to be the primary mechanism of the interaction. However, there is substantial overlapping drug selectivity between CYP3A4 and P-glycoprotein (16), and it has been demonstrated that St. John's wort is an inducer of P-glycoprotein (17). P-glycoprotein induction results in reduced oral absorption and at least partially accounts for the reduced systemic concentration of cyclosporine when St. John's wort is coadministered. Indeed, demonstration of correlation between pharmacokinetic parameters of cyclosporine and intestinal P-glycoprotein level in kidney transplant recipients suggests a significant role of P-glycoprotein in reducing cyclosporine absorption after oral administration (18). St. John's wort has also been reported to reduce concentration of other P-glycoprotein substrates such as digoxin (19,20). Current evidence strongly indicates that long-term administration of St. John's wort (longer than 14 days) induces both intestinal CYP3A4 and P-glycoprotein (21,22), secondary to activation of the nuclear factor pregnane X receptor (PXR) by the hyperforin component of St. John's wort (23). Further examples of St. John's wort–mediated reduction in drug absorption can be found in Chapter 4.

Based on the same principle of modulation of drug absorption, other less known botanicals could produce similar or different effects compared to St. John's wort. Rosemary (*Rosemarinus officinalis* Labiatae) is a commonly used dietary botanical that has been found to have a chemopreventive effect (24). Furthermore, in drug-resistant MCF-7 human breast cancer cells expressing P-glycoprotein, methanol extracts of Rosemary at two concentrations (16.5 and 85 µg/mL) inhibited the efflux and increased intracellular accumulation of doxorubicin and vinblastine, two chemotherapeutic drugs that are known substrates of P-glycoprotein. Treatment of drug-resistant cells with the extracts also increased the cytotoxic effects of doxorubicin. On the other hand, in wild-type MCF-7 cells that do not express

P-glycoprotein, the extracts did not affect accumulation or efflux of doxorubicin. Binding of azidopine, an analog of vinblastine, to P-glycoprotein was also reduced by the extract. The investigators concluded that Rosemary extracts appear to exert an inhibitory effect on P-glycoprotein activity via inhibition of drug binding to P-glycoprotein, with the responsible constituent(s) yet to be identified (25). Therefore, despite no reported interaction with cyclosporine, this botanical has the potential to increase plasma concentration of cyclosporine via an increase in its oral bioavailability.

Similarly, green tea (*Camellia sinensis*), a commonly consumed dietary supplement in many Asian countries, contains catechins, which have been shown to inhibit the activity of P-glycoprotein (26) and the efflux of doxorubicin by a carcinoma cell line (27). Although currently there is no literature report of an interaction between green tea and prescription or over-the-counter drug based on modulation of P-glycoprotein, a potential interaction between green tea and warfarin was reported and is described in Chapter 6.

Drug Distribution

Changes in distribution of drugs resulting from altered protein binding of highly protein-bound drugs have been studied intensively. However, the clinical significance of interactions based on this mechanism is usually minor and transient, unless accompanied by impaired metabolism and/or excretion that almost always result in persistently elevated blood concentrations of the affected drug. Examples of botanical–drug interactions involving changes in drug distribution and/or protein binding have not been reported in the literature.

Drug Metabolism

Inhibition

More than half of the drugs in current use or in development are eliminated primarily by metabolism, and the most common cause of clinically significant drug–drug interaction is a result of drug-metabolizing enzyme inhibition or induction. Botanicals can have similar effects on drug-metabolizing enzymes, and therefore it is not surprising that most of the reports of botanical–drug pharmacokinetic interactions involve altered drug metabolism. The most common pathway of drug metabolism is oxidation by the cytochrome P-450 (CYP) super family of enzymes located in the endoplasmic reticulum of the hepatocytes. Although there are many subfamilies in the human CYP superfamily, only three are responsible for the majority of drug oxidations in humans, namely CYP1, CYP2, and CYP3. Nine individual CYPs make contributions to drug oxidation in humans: CYP1A2, CYP2B6, CYP2C8, CYP2C9, CYP2C19, CYP2D6, CYP2E1, CYP3A4, and CYP3A5.

However, a simpler outlook is often useful because the majority of drug interactions are seen with substrates of just four enzymes. CYP2C9, CYP2D6, and CYP3A4/5 metabolize 15%, 20%, and 60%, respectively, of the drugs that are principally eliminated by metabolism.

Considerable effort has been focused on understanding and predicting the inhibition of CYPs in vivo. Over the past decade, an impressive arsenal of gene- and protein-based tools has been brought to bear on this issue and significant advances have been made in the use of in vitro data to identify the specific CYPs involved in a given biotransformation and to predict clinically important drug interactions. These techniques have recently been extended to characterize botanical–drug interactions. All new drugs are required by the Food and Drug Administration to have the extent of metabolism defined, the CYPs responsible for major metabolite formation to be identified, and the potency of CYP inhibition to be quantified. These regulatory requirements are in part a response to the need to withdraw several drugs from the marketplace due to an unacceptable level of adverse events that stemmed from drug interactions. Whenever two substrates are cometabolized, there is the potential for a metabolic drug interaction, but in most cases a clinically important event does not occur because sufficient systemic blood concentrations of inhibitor are not achieved.

In some cases, drug interactions occur in the wall of the small intestine as well as in the liver. To date, this has only been described for drugs metabolized by CYP3A4/5, because these are the only enzymes expressed at a high level in the gut wall. The balance between the rates of absorption through the intestinal epithelium and the rates of metabolism will determine the net availability at the gut wall. Thus a CYP3A substrate that is either rapidly absorbed or not efficiently metabolized will not experience significant gut wall metabolism, e.g., alprazolam. For a drug such as midazolam, the complete inhibition of intestinal CYP3A4/5 alone could increase the oral AUC of midazolam by 2.5-fold. However, it has been speculated that the remarkable sensitivity of some CYP3A substrates, such as lovastatin, simvastatin, and buspirone, to drug interactions reflects a very low gut wall availability. The clinically important inhibitors of CYP3A4/5 share the capability to completely inhibit the enzymes in the intestinal wall, as illustrated by the high intestinal wall availability of oral midazolam in the presence of clarithromycin and ketoconazole. This is not unexpected because there are high concentrations of inhibitor at the gut wall during absorption. A similar pattern should be anticipated for botanical products that contain strong inhibitors of CYP3A enzymes.

We often rationalize drug interactions as reflecting the reversible competition of two substrates for an active site. However, it is becoming increasingly clear that other mechanisms of inhibition are operational in vivo. For example, some mechanism-based inhibitors are activated during metabolism and form a complex with the heme of CYP3A, known as a metabolite intermediate complex, or make a covalent modification of enzymes and result in irreversible loss of enzyme activity. These irreversible mechanisms appear to contribute to the inhibition of CYPs that occurs following exposure to bergamottins (in grapefruit juice), capsaicin (in chili peppers), glabridin (in licorice root), isothiocyanates (from cruciferous vegetables), oleuropein (from olive oil), diallyl sulfone (from garlic), and resveratrol, a red wine constituent [for review see Ref. (28)]. An important consequence of this irreversible inhibition is that interactions take one to two weeks to resolve on termination of the drug because this is how long the CYP3A takes to resume its predrug steady state (29). This is one reason why a good medical history should include questions about drugs and botanical products that have been discontinued in the past two weeks, when addressing possible botanical–drug interactions.

Induction

The term "induction" has evolved to include any mechanism that results in increased tissue concentration of catalytically active protein involved in drug metabolism. This increased enzyme activity results in greater systemic clearance and lower bioavailability of extensively metabolized drugs. The resulting lower drug concentrations often result in therapeutic failure. For example, it is well known that oral contraceptive pills become ineffective when rifampin is coprescribed.

In general, induction may result from enhanced gene transcription rates, increased mRNA stability or translational efficiency, and protein stabilization induced by substrate binding or posttranslational modifications. However, the most common mechanism of induction is binding to and activation of discrete nuclear factors that act in the form of protein heteromers to enhance rates of gene transcription. It is clear that a single nuclear factor may modulate the expression of numerous genes and this mechanism of induction most likely applies to all drug-metabolizing enzymes but the extent of induction, tissue selectivity, and ligand selectivity vary widely between genes. Some degree of predictability has arisen from the discovery of the nuclear factors primarily responsible for the effects of the clinically important inducers. It is worth noting that some inducers, such as ritonavir for CYP3A4, are also potent inhibitors of at least some of the enzymes induced. Therefore, despite greater concentrations of enzyme, the net interaction maybe inhibition prior to full induction, followed by induction or even no effect. The transcriptional regulation of drug-metabolizing enzymes is commonly cell-type and tissue selective. Thus, tissues that express low concentrations of nuclear factors do not experience significant induction. In contrast, both liver and intestines express significant concentrations of nuclear factors such as the PXR and experience profound induction in the presence of its ligands. The best example of a botanical product altering drug metabolism efficiency is that of St. John's wort, which is a potent inducer of CYP3A4 (30) and causes accelerated metabolism of cyclosporine (14) and indinavir (31). Details of these and other examples of CYP3A4 induction by St. John's wort are presented in Chapter 4.

Of equal importance but less studied is the effect of botanicals on oral contraceptive disposition, which can potentially affect a large number of subjects. Recently, Hall et al. reported that St. John's wort induced the metabolism of both ethynyl estradiol and norethindrone in 12 healthy women via enhanced CYP3A4 activity. The incidence of breakthrough bleeding was higher with concurrent use of St. John's wort (seven subjects) than without (two subjects), and subjects with breakthrough bleeding had a higher CYP3A4 activity, as measured by midazolam clearance (32). Therefore, this study provides supportive evidence and explanation for case reports of unexpected menstrual bleedings in women taking concurrent oral contraceptive and St. John's wort (33,34). Although Hall et al. (32) did not find evidence of loss of oral contraceptive efficacy or ovulation, breakthrough bleeding is well known as a contributory factor for discontinuance of oral contraceptive use that may lead to a higher incidence of pregnancy (35). Schwartz et al. reported the loss of contraceptive efficacy associated with the use of St. John's wort with resultant unwanted pregnancies (36). This issue of oral contraceptive–botanical interaction requires further studies.

The effect of garlic (*Allium sativum*)–containing botanicals on drug metabolism has also been studied in vitro, and in vivo in both animal and human studies. Using human liver microsome as an in vitro drug-metabolism model, Foster et al. showed that raw garlic constituents inhibit CYP3A4-mediated drug metabolism (37). In rats, acute administration of a single dose of garlic oil produced significant reduction in the activity of several enzymes, including CYPs. However, chronic administration for five days produced the opposite effect—a significant increase in CYP activity (38). Gurley et al. (39) reported that chronic administration of garlic oil for 28 days in humans reduced CYP2E1 activity by 39%, possibly a result of inhibition of the CYP by diallyl sulfone (40), a metabolic product of alliin, the major component of garlic. A pharmacokinetic study in healthy volunteers showed that a three-week course of garlic tablets taken twice daily resulted in a 51% reduction in AUC of the protease inhibitor saquinavir, a CYP3A4 substrate (41). Details of these human studies are summarized in Chapter 5.

In view of the multiplicity of CYPs and the many possible botanical–drug interactions, highly efficient clinical study designs using CYP probe cocktails have been explored. Following successful application to St. John's wort, other botanicals that have been evaluated in this fashion include *echinacea* (42), saw palmetto (43), garlic (39), peppermint oil, and ascorbyl palmitate (44). The results are summarized in Table 1. Curbicin, a botanical

Table 1 Effect of Selected Botanical Products on CYP Probe Markers

Botanical products	Effect on CYP activity
Echinacea purpurea, 400 mg q.i.d. × 8 days, 6 male and 6 female healthy volunteers	• 29% ↑ in AUC of caffeine (CYP1A2)[a] • 14% ↑ in AUC of tolbutamide (CYP2C9)[a] • 2% ↑ in AUC of dextromethorphan (CYP2D6)[a] in EM • 42% ↑ in AUC of dextromethorphan (CYP2D6) in PM ($n = 1$) • 25% ↓ in AUC of intravenous midazolam (CYP3A4)[a]
Saw palmetto, 320 mg q.i.d. × 14 days, 6 male and 6 female healthy volunteers	• 8% ↑ in AUC of alprazolam (CYP3A4)[b] • 26% ↑ in urinary metabolic ratio of dextromethorphan (CYP2D6)[c]
Peppermint oil, 600 mg single dose, 9 male and 3 female healthy volunteers	• 40% ↑ in AUC of felodipine (CYP3A4)

[a]Based on geometric mean ratio of *echinacea* to control.
[b]Based on geometric mean ratio of baseline condition to saw palmetto.
[c]Based on mean ratio of baseline condition to saw palmetto.
Abbreviations: CYP, cytochrome P-450; CYP3A4, cytochrome P-450 3A4; AUC, area under the concentration time curve; EM, extensive metabolizer; PM, poor metabolizer.
Source: From Refs. 42–44.

remedy taken by patients for the management of prostate enlargement, contains saw palmetto as one of the ingredients. Elevated international normalized ratio (INR) values were reported in two patients taking curbicin, and one of the patients also took warfarin (45). Cheema et al. (46) also reported a patient who suffered from severe intraoperative hemorrhage with doubling of the bleeding time value after taking saw palmetto. The prolonged bleeding times were normalized after the botanical use was discontinued. Although the effect of saw palmetto on CYP2C9, the enzyme responsible for metabolism of the active *S*-isomer of warfarin, has not been studied, it is of note that the prothrombin time (PT) and activated partial thromblastin time were both within normal limits before, during, and after the surgical procedure. It is also not known whether the bleeding abnormality observed in the patient might be related to the reported inhibitory effect of the botanical on cyclooxygenase in animal studies (47). The differential effect of *echinacea* on CYP3A4 will be discussed later in this chapter. With the exception of garlic (41), at present there are no reported drug interactions with the other three botanicals, but based on available data, potential interaction, especially with drugs metabolized by CYP3A4, could be expected.

Drug Excretion

While theoretically it is possible that botanicals with diuretic effects can increase drug excretion, most botanical diuretics are not as potent as furosemide and are unlikely to result in significant interactions. Most botanicals also do not affect urinary pH significantly, and hence are unlikely to affect renal tubular reabsorption of drugs. Nevertheless, lithium toxicity was thought to be related to the use of a botanical diuretic mixture in a patient. If the toxicity indeed is related to the use of the botanical diuretic, the mechanism of action or the responsible constituent(s) is not known (48).

ALTERED PHARMACODYNAMICS

In addition to pharmacokinetic botanical–drug interaction, pharmacodynamic interactions can also occur, resulting in either an augmented or attenuated response. These effects can occur without any significant changes in either the systemic or tissue concentrations of the affected drug or botanical, and generally are more difficult to predict. In addition, unlike pharmacokinetic botanical–drug interactions, most pharmacodynamic interactions reported in the literature are mostly based on patient cases or clinicians' experience and seldom involve clinical or experimental study. For example, combining St. John's wort and selective serotonin reuptake inhibitors have been reported to result in an additive pharmacological effect and possibly serotonin syndrome (49), but there were no clinical studies or literature reports of changes in the pharmacokinetics of the selective serotonin reuptake inhibitors when combined with St. John's wort. The most commonly reported pharmacodynamic botanical–drug interactions primarily involve anticoagulants and antiplatelet agents.

Augmented Pharmacological Effect

Warfarin

Most literature reports of pharmacodynamic botanical–drug interaction involve the anticoagulant warfarin, likely because it has therapeutic end points such as the INR and PT, which are routinely closely monitored. In addition, most botanicals possess anticoagulant and/or antiplatelet activities, and their combined use with warfarin provides a good example of pharmacodynamic interaction with additive pharmacological effect.

Botanicals such as garlic can inhibit platelet aggregation (50), likely accounting for episodes of spontaneous spinal epidural hematoma (51) and postoperative bleeding reported in the literature (52,53). Currently, there are no reports of an interaction between garlic and warfarin, but based on the inhibitory effect of garlic on platelet aggregation, one would expect that there is at least a risk of additive pharmacological response to warfarin when the two compounds are taken concurrently. In fact, such interactions have been reported with other botanicals that also inhibit platelet aggregation, including ginkgo and the traditional Chinese medicines, dong quai (*Angelica sinensis*) and dan shen (*Salvia miltiorrhiza*).

In a patient who had been stabilized on warfarin for five years, recent use of ginkgo was reported to result in intracerebral hemorrhage (54). In an in vitro model using human liver microsomes, the activity of CYP2C9, which metabolizes the active *S*-isomer of warfarin, was inhibited by commercial ginkgo extracts (55). Therefore, the interaction between ginkgo and warfarin potentially involves both pharmacokinetic and pharmacodynamic mechanisms. Dong quai also inhibits platelet aggregation, and there have been several reports of increased INR in patients taking concurrent warfarin and dong quai (56). Despite the elevated INR, the patient did not experience any bleeding episodes. It is not known whether the lack of clinical consequence in this report is a result of intersubject variability in the magnitude of interaction or the absence of a pharmacokinetic component, as an animal study demonstrated that warfarin pharmacokinetics was unchanged by dong quai. Further details of the interaction between warfarin and dong quai can be found in Chapter 6.

Antiplatelet Drugs

Although no pharmacokinetic antiplatelet drug–botanical interactions have been reported in the literature, there is the potential of an additive pharmacodynamic effect with concurrent use of antiplatelet drugs or botanicals that possess antiplatelet activity or contain salicylates, such as willow bark (*Salix* spp.) and meadowsweet (*Filipendula ulmaria*). The ginkgolide constituents, found in ginkgo, are known to exhibit platelet-activating factor antagonistic activity. In an elderly patient who was prescribed aspirin therapy after a coronary bypass surgery, self-initiation of ginkgo use resulted in spontaneous bleeding within the eye and blurred vision. On cessation of ginkgo use, the bleeding stopped and the visual changes resolved (57).

Drugs Acting on the Central Nervous System

Selective Serotonin Reuptake Inhibitors

The similar pharmacological profile of selective serotonin reuptake inhibitors and St. John's wort would suggest the potential of a pharmacodynamic interaction due to an additive effect. A case of concurrent use of sertraline and St. John's wort, resulting in mania, was reported for a patient with a history of depression who was prescribed sertraline and who also took St. John's wort against medical advice (58). A similar potentiation of serotonergic effect was reported by Gordon (49).

Benzodiazepines

Kava (*Piper methysticum*) is a popular botanical product used for management of anxiety and insomnia. Almeida and Grimsley (59) reported a case of potentiation of the central nervous system (CNS)-depressant effect of alprazolam by kava extract and/or kavalactones in a 54-year-old, male patient who became lethargic and disoriented after taking kava for three days. Kava ingestion was concurrent with his usual medications, including alprazolam, cimetidine, and terazosin, but the patient denied overdose of any of his medications. The physicians attributed the patient's mental state to a kava–alprazolam interaction. Both kava extract and kavalactones have been shown in vitro to inhibit several CYPs, including CYP3A4 (60,61). However, it is possible that in this case, the enhanced effect involves not just a pharmacokinetic component but also a pharmacodynamic basis secondary to synergistic activity at the gamma-aminobutyric acid (GABA) receptor.

Miscellaneous Central Nervous System Acting Drugs

Ephedra (ma huang) is a popular botanical incorporated into a variety of formulations for weight loss, "energy" or "performance" enhancement, and symptomatic control of asthma. A pharmacodynamic interaction leading to a fatality has been reported with concurrent use of caffeine and ephedra (62), possibly as a result of additive adrenergic agonist effect of the ephedrine alkaloids and caffeine on the cardiovascular system and the CNS (63). Ephedra was recently withdrawn from the market (64).

A botanical–drug interaction postulated to have both pharmacokinetic and pharmacodynamic mechanisms was reported in an elderly Alzheimer's patient, who developed coma likely as a result of concurrent use of ginkgo leaf extract 80 mg twice daily and the antidepressant trazodone 20 mg twice a day (65). The pharmacodynamic mechanism was suggested because the coma was reversed by flumazenil, indicating increased activity at GABA-activated receptors; ginkgo flavonoids possess GABA agonist activity on the benzodiazepine receptor (66). A pharmacokinetic basis of the interaction was also proposed to be a result of CYP3A4 induction, and subsequent increased conversion of trazodone, to *m*-chlorophenylpiperazine, an active metabolite with GABA agonist activity (67).

Digoxin

The use of botanicals containing laxatives has not been reported to result in altered drug absorption to date. However, excessive use of laxative-containing botanicals such as cascara (*Rhamnus purshiana*), senna leaves, and/or pods from *Cassia senna* can potentially decrease serum potassium and other electrolyte concentrations, and therefore enhance toxicity of digoxin. To date, no clinical interactions have been reported between digoxin and these botanicals, but given the narrow therapeutic range of digoxin, it would be prudent to monitor for signs and symptoms of digitalis toxicity with long-term, excessive use of these botanical laxatives. The concurrent administration of these botanicals with prescription diuretics should be approached with caution.

The narrow therapeutic index of digoxin necessitates the monitoring of serum digoxin concentration as an aid for optimizing drug therapy in patients, and an in vitro laboratory interaction between digoxin and several botanicals such as danshen and ginseng products have been reported in the literature. These "cardioactive" botanicals possess active constituents with structures similar to digoxin, and therefore can demonstrate digoxin-like immunoreactivity. Chow et al. (68) reported that small amounts (2–5 μL) of aqueous extracts of these "cardioactive" botanicals interfered with immunoassays used to determine digoxin concentration, both in vitro and ex vivo. Patients taking digoxin might also take these "cardioactive" botanicals and this laboratory interference could result in falsely elevated digoxin concentrations in patients. McRae (69) reported a 74-year-old man who had been stabilized on digoxin for about 10 years with therapeutic concentrations between 0.9 and 2.2 ng/mL. Ingestion of Siberian ginseng resulted in a serum concentration of 5.2 ng/mL, even though the patient was asymptomatic with no electrocardiographic changes. The digoxin concentration returned to normal after the patient stopped taking the ginseng product.

Oral Hypoglycemic Agents

In a brief report, a potential interaction between curry and chlorpropamide, leading to reduction in chlorpropamide dose in a 40-year-old woman was attributed to the garlic and karela components of this complex mixture (70). Garlic reportedly can lower blood glucose. However, there was no information provided regarding the estimated amount of garlic intake in this patient. To date, there are no formal studies that confirm the initial clinical observation or evaluate the likely mechanism.

ANTAGONISTIC PHARMACODYNAMIC EFFECT

While dong quai and possibly garlic have an additive effect on the pharmacological action of warfarin, an antagonistic interaction between warfarin and coenzyme Q_{10} had been reported. Spigset (71) reported three elderly patients who were all stabilized on different warfarin dosage regimens. All experienced a decrease in INR to values below 2 after taking ubidecarenone (coenzyme Q_{10}). The dose of coenzyme Q_{10} was documented as 30 mg/day in two of the patients. In both patients, the warfarin dose was temporarily increased and coenzyme Q_{10} discontinued. The INR returned to the patients' previous stabilized values prior to taking the coenzyme Q_{10}. Because coenzyme Q_{10} is structurally similar to vitamin K_2, the authors suggested that one potential mechanism might be related to the enhanced coagulation effect of coenzyme Q_{10}. Animal data showed that antagonism of coenzyme Q_{10} resulted in increased PT, suggesting that coenzyme Q_{10} might have an opposite pharmacological effect to that of warfarin (72).

Two patients stabilized on a phenytoin regimen suffered a loss of seizure control after taking shankhapushpi, an Ayurvedic antiepileptic medicine, three times a day. There was also a significant decrease in serum phenytoin concentration from 9.6 to 5.1 mg/L. To investigate the possible mechanisms, multiple doses of shankhapushpi were administered to rats and resulted in decreased plasma phenytoin concentrations, whereas single-dose administration was reported to interfere with the antiplatelet effect of phenytoin, thereby implying both a pharmacokinetic and pharmacodynamic basis for the interaction (73).

There are several botanicals that have purported immunostimulating effects. These include *Panax ginseng* and *Echinacea purpurea* (74), which have both been used as an immune stimulant. Any potential adverse effect on the pharmacological activity of immunosuppressants has not been reported in patients or evaluated in clinical studies. Given the lack of data, it would be prudent to advise against concurrent intake of these botanicals, and closely monitor changes in efficacy in patients who self-administer these botanicals.

EVALUATING BOTANICAL–DRUG INTERACTION

Overall, an accurate assessment of the reliability of reported botanical–drug interactions with a pharmacodynamic basis or mechanism is usually more difficult than the assessment of those with a pharmacokinetic basis. This likely reflects the fact that the former reports are usually case reports, whereas the later reports are often accompanied with objectively measured end points. Also, despite a common belief that botanical–drug interactions are underreported, the overall incidence of this phenomenon is difficult to define. This partly reflects the lack of a mechanism for reporting the interactions, and difficulty in obtaining reliable information to assess clinical relevance or to establish a definitive causality relationship. For example, even with the evidence of St. John's wort increasing the metabolism of oral contraceptive hormone (32) and possibly contributing to reports of breakthrough bleeding and pregnancy (36), it is well established that pregnancy can occur with oral contraceptive used alone or with other drugs, and a definitive causality relationship has not been established. Nevertheless, there is sufficient clinical evidence that interaction involving commonly used drugs such as cyclosporine and protease inhibitors with St. John's wort can be serious and sometimes life threatening. In addition, the lack of fatalities resulting from the various reports of botanical–anticoagulant interaction likely reflects close clinical and laboratory monitoring with appropriate dosage adjustment, if necessary, in the patients.

Challenges of Predicting Botanical–Drug Interaction

While defining the overall pharmacokinetic or pharmacodynamic basis of botanical–drug interactions may be relatively straightforward, attempts to explain the underlying mechanism of altered drug concentrations or to predict the magnitude and significance of the interaction is certainly not easy. There are several factors that contribute to this difficulty, and they are briefly discussed below.

Lack of Definition of Active Constituents

First and foremost, it must be emphasized that botanicals or botanical preparations are not pure synthetic molecules but are composed of many constituents, sometimes from multiple botanicals, and some or many of them can be biologically active. Although altered drug concentration can be caused by induction or inhibition of intestinal and hepatic drug-metabolizing enzymes as well as P-glycoprotein, the identity of the biologically active constituent(s) that is responsible for these effects is usually not known. Without this knowledge, most investigations are restricted to studying the commercially available products containing multiple constituents with potentially different modulating effects on these proteins. Commercial preparations of St. John's wort used in most clinical and interaction studies are usually standardized to contain specific amounts of hypericin, but it is another constituent, hyperforin, which was shown to be responsible for induction of CYP3A4 (23). Similarly, although administration of milk thistle 175 mg (containing 153 mg of silymarin) three times a day for three weeks resulted in 9% and 25% reduction in AUC and trough concentration, respectively, of indinavir (75,76), its differential effect on CYP3A4 and P-glycoprotein needs to be further studied. In addition, while the overall study result suggested a minimal clinical consequence for AIDS patients receiving indinavir, whether botanical constituents other than silymarin would have a greater modulating effect remains unknown.

   In addition, very few studies provide information on the content of important constituents of the botanical or botanical preparation. This obviously poses a problem of general applicability in terms of predicting interaction across different preparations with variable content of constituents, or extrapolating the result of one study to the overall interaction potential. For example, one of the active constituents in garlic is allicin, which gives garlic its specific, well-known odor. Although allicin has been suggested to enhance production of CYP (77), there is no data to confirm or refute the possibility, let alone the identity of the specific enzyme that is induced. It is clear, however, that commercial garlic preparations have highly variable contents ranging from no allicin (Kyolic Aged Garlic Extract, Wakunaga) (77) to maximum standardized allicin content (GarliPure, Maximum Allicin

Formula, Natrol) used in the garlic-saquinavir study described above (41). In the study by Gurley et al. (39) garlic oil 500 mg did not result in appreciable differences in the 1-hydroxymidazolam/midazolam phenotypic ratio for CYP3A4, the enzyme that mediates the metabolism of saquinavir. Both studies administered the garlic preparations for at least three weeks, and therefore it is unlikely that the duration of therapy would account for the difference between studies. On the other hand, if allicin content is a critical issue, it may be that one of the reasons for the conflicting results between the two studies is potential variability in this active constituent in the two garlic preparations used.

Lack of Standardization of Known Active Constituents

Even though the active constituent responsible for the interaction has been identified, conflict in study results can still occur due to variable content of the known active constituent(s). In the study by Piscitelli et al. (41), the investigators took extra effort in analyzing the allicin and allin content of the commercial garlic caplets administered to the subjects. They reported that the allicin and allin contents were 4.64 and 11.2 mg per caplet, which were different from the labeled content. This study highlights the challenge associated with evaluating any aspect of pharmacology or therapeutic use of dietary supplement, including botanicals. While consumers increasingly are aware of the fact that dietary supplements and botanical products do not have to be proven to be efficacious or to be safe, they are less aware of the lack of standardization among products.

Although dietary supplements and botanical products are required to state exactly the content of active ingredients and their amounts on the label, the manufacturers do not necessarily comply. More importantly, the labels are not routinely checked for compliance by any government agency. In addition, unlike prescription drugs, dietary supplement and botanical products are not required to be manufactured under standardized conditions. This has led to substantial variability in the amount of active constituent(s) between batches. Prime examples of this include *echinacea* (78) and ginseng products (79). Gilroy analyzed different single botanical *echinacea* preparations purchased from retail stores and reported that only 10 of 19 preparations (53%), labeled as standardized, had an assayed content consistent with the labeled content. There were only weak correlations between labeled milligram content of *echinacea* versus measured milligram for the standardized preparations ($r = 0.49$, $p = 0.02$) and the correlation was even lower for nonstandardized preparations ($r = 0.21$, $p = 0.28$) (78). Similar discrepancies in content were reported in a study conducted by the Consumer Unions, in which they tested the content of 10 marketed ginseng preparations, and found significant differences in the amount of the active constituent ginsenosides (range: 0.4–23.2 mg) (79).

Of particular concern is that this inconsistency in product and active constituent occurs even within the same batch. As part of a clinical study with St. John's wort, Hall et al. analyzed 10 capsules of St. John's wort from the same lot (lot # 13207) and found the mean total weight to be 444 mg (4.6% CV) versus 300 mg as stated on the label. In addition, the dosage form was supposed to be standardized to contain 900 µg of hypericin, but the mean content was found to be 840 µg (6.6% CV). There was also variability of the hyperforin content (mean 11 mg and 5.7% CV), which was not stated on the label (21). Our experience (Lam YWF, unpublished data) with two random capsules from one batch of kava-kava also showed the same extent of undesirable variance: the total content of the pharmacologically active kavalactone was 47.3 mg in one capsule and 39.4 mg in the second one.

CONFOUNDING ISSUES RELATED TO STUDY DESIGN

Extrapolation of Result from In Vitro Study

Similar to evaluation of potential inhibitory effect of different drugs on the CYPs, in vitro preparations such as human liver microsomes have also been used to evaluate the potential of a botanical to cause interaction. Nevertheless, there are numerous reasons why in vitro results based on human liver microsomes do not necessarily agree with in vivo study results. One reason is the inability of human liver microsomes to evaluate and predict enzyme induction. St. John's wort serves as an excellent example to illustrate this limitation. In vitro, St. John's wort has been shown to inhibit CYP2C9, CYP2D6, and CYP3A4 (80,81). However, as discussed above and also in Chapter 4, St. John's wort has been shown in numerous human studies to induce CYP3A4. This may be due to the finding of hyperforin, a constituent of St. John's wort, binding to the PXR and upregulating CYP3A4 gene expression. Importantly, microsomal preparations lack the capability to synthesize new protein and cannot be expected to provide any insight into the potential for induction to occur in vivo.

Differential Effect on Intestinal and Hepatic CYP3A4

Another confounding issue specific to CYP3A4 would be the potential differential effect of a specific botanical or botanical constituent on intestinal and hepatic CYP3A4. The clinical study by Gorski et al. (42) elegantly showed that, consistent with in vitro inhibition of CYP3A4 by *echinacea* tinctures (81), administration of *echinacea* 400 mg four times a day for eight days in healthy volunteers inhibited intestinal CYP3A4 and resulted in an 85% increase in systemic bioavailability. However, hepatic CYP3A4 activity, as measured by systemic clearance of midazolam after intravenous administration, was increased by 34%. Therefore predicting potential interaction between *echinacea* and CYP3A4 substrate would depend on whether the substrate has high oral bioavailability, in which case the likely pharmacokinetic and clinical outcome would be increased clearance secondary to hepatic CYP3A4 induction and lower serum drug concentration versus substrate with a low bioavailability secondary to extensive intestinal first-pass effect, in which case the likely pharmacokinetic and clinical outcome would be decreased oral clearance secondary to intestinal CYP3A4 inhibition and increased serum drug concentration. One can only imagine the difficulty of predicting the potential and extent of interaction between *echinacea* and CYP3A4 substrates if a patient who is receiving CYP3A4 substrate for medical conditions also treats a cold at the same time by taking *echinacea* and drinking grapefruit juice, which potently inhibit intestinal CYP3A4.

Single-Dose Administration vs. Multiple Dosing

Results from single-dose studies could be different from chronic dose administration. Although St. John's wort administered as a single 900 mg dose to healthy volunteers was found to increase the maximum plasma concentration and decrease the oral clearance by 45% and 20%, respectively, of the P-glycoprotein substrate fexofenadine (22), the opposite effects (35% decrease in maximum plasma concentration and 47% increase in oral clearance) were observed after daily administration of the same dose of St. John's wort for two weeks (82). Similar differential effects between single versus chronic dose administration have been shown before with CYP3A4: single-dose ritonavir caused inhibition of CYP3A4 and chronic administration resulted in CYP3A4 induction (83).

FUTURE

In our effort to understand the potential therapeutic role of botanicals and promote their safe use for the consumers, one must not only focus on evaluating mechanism of action and identifying the active ingredients. As indicated by the few clinical reports outlined in this chapter, the issue of botanical–drug interaction has not been well appreciated and is definitely under-studied. Likewise, as discussed in the Chapter 9, the pharmacokinetic profiles of most botanicals are not known, and knowledge in this area would provide better understanding in botanical–drug interactions. To this end, funding initiatives such as the National Center for Complementary and Alternative Medicine are critical.

REFERENCES

1. Eisenberg DM, Davis RB, Ettner SL, et al. Trends in alternative medicine use in the United States, 1990–1997: results of a follow-up national survey. JAMA 1998; 280:1569–1575.
2. Ernst E. Herbal medicine: where is the evidence? BMJ 2000; 321:395–396.
3. Fugh-Berman A. Herb-drug interactions. Lancet 2000; 355:134–138.
4. Kaufman DW, Kelly JP, Rosenberg L, Anderson TE, Mitchell AA. Recent patterns of medication use in the ambulatory adult population of the United States. JAMA 2002; 287:337–344.
5. Tsen LC, Segal S, Pothier M, Bader AM. Alternative medicine use in presurgical patients. Anesthesiology 2000; 93:148–151.
6. Hensrud DD, Engle DD, Scheitel SM. Underreporting the use of dietary supplements and nonprescription medications among patients undergoing a periodic health examinations. Mayo Clin Proc 1999; 74:443–447.
7. Eisenberg DM, Kessler RC, Foster C, Norlock FE, Calkins DR, Delbanco TL. Unconventional medicine in the United States. N Engl J Med 1993; 328: 246–252.
8. Chang ZG, Kennedy DT, Holdford DA, Small RE. Pharmacists' knowledge and attitudes toward herbal medicine. Ann Pharmacother 2000; 34:710–715.
9. Wang J, Xu R, Jin R, Chen Z, Fidler JM. Immunosuppressive activity of the Chinese medicinal plant *Tripterygium wilfordi*. I. Prolongation of rat cardiac and renal allograft survival by the PG27 extract and immunosuppressive synergy in combination therapy with cyclosporine. Transplantation 2000; 70: 447–455.
10. Zhu M, Wong PYK, Li RC. Effect of oral administration of fennel (*Foeniculum vulgare*) on ciprofloxacin absorption and disposition in the rat. J Pharm Pharmacol 1999; 51:1391–1396.
11. Mustapha A, Yakasai IA, Aguye IA. Effect of *Tamarindus indica* L. on the bioavailability of aspirin in healthy human volunteers. Eur J Drug Metab Pharmacokinet 1996; 21:223–226.
12. Juliano RL, Ling V. A surface glycoprotein modulating drug permeability in Chinese hamster ovary cell mutants. Biochim Biophys Acta 1976; 455:152–162.
13. Van Asperen J, Van Tellingen O, Beijnen JH. The pharmacological role of P-glycoprotein in the intestinal epithelium. Pharmacol Res 1998; 37:429–435.
14. Ruschitzka F, Meier PJ, Turina M, Luscher TF, Noll G. Acute heart transplant rejection due to Saint John's wort. Lancet 2000; 355(9203):548–549.
15. Kronbach T, Fischer V, Meyer UA. Cyclosporine metabolism in human liver: identification of a cytochrome P450III gene family as the major cyclosporine metabolizing enzyme explains interactions of cyclosporine with other drugs. Clin Pharmacol Ther 1988; 43:630–635.
16. Wacher VJ, Wu CY, Benet LZ. Overlapping substrate specificities and tissue distribution of cytochrome P450 3A and P-glycoprotein: implications for drug delivery and activity in cancer chemotherapy. Mol Carcinog 1995; 13:129–134.
17. Durr D, Stieger B, Kullak-Ublick GA, et al. St. John's wort induces intestinal P-glycoprotein/MDR1 and intestinal and hepatic CYP3A4. Clin Pharmacol Ther 2000; 68:598–604.

18. Lown KS, Mayo RR, Leichtman AB, et al. Role of intestinal P-glycoprotein (mdr1) in interpatient variation in the oral bioavailability of cyclosporine. Clin Pharmacol Ther 1997; 62:248–260.
19. Johne A, Brockmoller J, Bauer S, Maurer A, Langheinrich M, Roots I. Pharmacokinetic interaction of digoxin with an herbal extract from St. John's wort (Hypericum perforatum). Clin Pharmacol Ther 1999; 66:338–345.
20. Fromm MF, Kim RB, Stein CM, Wilkinson GR, Roden DM. Inhibition of p-glycoprotein-mediated drug transport: a unifying mechanism to explain the interaction between digoxin and quinidine. Circulation 1999; 99:552–557.
21. Wang Z, Gorski JC, Hamman MA, Huang SM, Lesko LJ, Hall SD. The effects of St. John's wort (Hypericum perforatum) on human cytochrome P450 activity. Clin Pharmacol Ther 2001; 70:317–326.
22. Wang Z, Hamman MA, Huang SM, Lesko LJ, Hall SD. Effect of St. John's wort on the pharmacokinetics of fexofenadine. Clin Pharmacol Ther 2002; 71: 414–420.
23. Moore LB, Goodwin B, Jones SA, et al. St. John's wort induces hepatic drug metabolism through activation of the pregnane X receptor. Proc Natl Acad Sci USA 2000; 97:7500–7502.
24. Huang MT, Ho CT, Wang ZY, et al. Inhibition of skin tumorigenesis by rosemary and its constituents carnosal and ursolic acid. Cancer Res 1994; 54:701–708.
25. Plouzek CA, Ciolino HP, Clarke R, Yeh GC. Inhibition of P-glycoprotein activity and reversal of multidrug resistance in vitro by rosemary extract. Eur J Cancer 1999; 35:1541–1545.
26. Jodoin J, Demeule M, Beliveau R. Inhibition of the multidrug resistance P-glycoprotein activity by green tea polyphenols. Biochem Biophys Acta 2002; 1542:149–159.
27. Sadzuka Y, Sugiyama T, Sonobe T. Efficacies of tea components on doxorubicin induced antitumor activity and reversal of multidrug resistance. Toxicol Lett 2000; 114:155–162.
28. Zhou S, Koh H-L, Gao Y, Gong Z-Y, Lee EJD. Herbal bioactivation. Life Sci 2004; 74:935–968.
29. Greenblatt DJ, von Moltke LL, Harmatz JS, et al. Time course of recovery of cytochrome P450 3A function after single doses of grapefruit juice. Clin Pharmacol Ther 2003; 74:121–129.
30. Roby CA, Anderson GD, Kantor E, Dryer DA, Burstein AH. St. John's wort: effect on CYP3A4 activity. Clin Pharmacol Ther 2000; 67:451–457.
31. Piscitelli SC, Burstein AH, Chaitt D, Alfaro RM, Falloon J. Indinavir concentrations and St. John's wort. Lancet 2000; 355:547–548.
32. Hall SD, Wang Z, Huang SM, et al. The interaction between St. John's wort and an oral contraceptive. Clin Pharmacol Ther 2003; 74:525–535.
33. Ernst E. Second thoughts about the safety of St. John's wort. Lancet 1999; 354:2014–2016.
34. Rey JM, Walter G. *Hypericum perforatum* (St. John's wort) in depression: pest or blessing? Med J Aust 1998; 169:583–586.
35. Rosenberg M, Waugh M. Oral contraceptive discontinuance: a prospective evaluation of frequency and reasons. Am J Obstet Gynecol 1998; 179:577–582.

36. Schwartz U, Bschel B, Kirch W. Unwanted pregnancy on self-medication with St. John's wort despite hormonal contraception. Br J Clin Pharmacol 2003; 55:112–113.
37. Foster BC, Foster MS, Vandenhoek S, et al. An in vitro evaluation of human cytochrome P450-3A4 and P-glycoprotein inhibition by garlic. J Pharm Pharmaceut Sci 2001; 4:176–184.
38. Dalvi RR. Alteration in hepatic phase I and phase II biotransformation enzymes by garlic oil in rats. Toxicol Lett 1992; 60:299–305.
39. Gurley BJ, Gardner SF, Hubbard MA, et al. Cytochrome P450 phenotypic ratios for predicting herb-drug interactions in humans. Clin Pharmacol Ther 2002; 72:276–287.
40. Lin MC, Wang EJ, Patten C, et al. Protective effect of diallyl sulfone against acetaminophen-induced hepatotoxicity in mice. J Biochem Toxicol 1996; 11: 11–20.
41. Piscitelli SC, Burstein AH, Welden N, Gallicano KD, Falloon J. The effect of garlic supplements on the pharmacokinetics of saquinavir. Clin Infect Dis 2002; 34:234–238.
42. Gorski JC, Huang SM, Pinto A, et al. The effect of Echinacea (*Echinacea purpurea* root) on cytochrome P450 activity in vivo. Clin Pharmacol Ther 2004; 75:89–100.
43. Markowitz JS, Donovan JL, DeVane CL, et al. Multiple doses of Saw Palmetto (*Serenoa repens*) did not alter cytochrome P450 2D6 and 3A4 activity in normal volunteers. Clin Pharmacol Ther 2003; 74:536–542.
44. Dresser GK, Wacher V, Wong S, Wong HT, Bailey DG. Evaluation of peppermint oil and ascorbyl palmitate as inhibitors of cytochrome P4503A4 activity in vitro and in vivo. Clin Pharmacol Ther 2002; 72:247–255.
45. Yue QY, Jansson K. Herbal drug Curbicin and anticoagulant effect with and without warfarin: possibly related to the vitamin E component. J Am Geriatr Soc 2001; 49:838.
46. Cheema P, El-Mefty O, Jazieh AR. Intraoperative hemorrhage associated with the use of extract of Saw Palmetto herb: a case report and review of literature. J Intern Med 2001; 250:167–169.
47. Brue W, Hagenlocer M, Redl K, Tittel G, Stadler F, Wagner H. Anti-inflammatory activity of sabal fruit extracts prepared with supercritical carbon dioxide. In vitro antagonists of cyclooxygenase and 5-lipoxygenase metabolism. Arzneimittel Forsch 1992; 42:547–551.
48. Pyevich D, Bogenschutz MP. Herbal diuretics and lithium toxicity. Am J Psychiatr 2001; 158:1329.
49. Gordon JB. SSRIs and St. John's wort: possible toxicity? Am Fam Physician 1998; 57:950, 953.
50. Legnani C, Frascaro M, Guazzaloca G, Ludovici S, Cesarano G, Coccheri G. Effects of a dried garlic preparation on fibrinolysis and platelet aggregation in healthy subjects. Arzneimittel Forsch 1993; 43:119–122.
51. Rose KD, Croissant PD, Parliament CF, Levin MB. Spontaneous spinal epidural hematoma with associated platelet dysfunction from excessive garlic ingestion: a case report. Neurosurgery 1990; 26:880–882.

52. Burham BE. Garlic as a possible risk for postoperative bleeding. Plast Reconstr Surg 1995; 95:213.
53. German K, Kumar U, Blackford HN. Garlic and the risk of TURP bleeding. Br J Urol 1995; 76:518.
54. Matthews MK Jr. Association of Ginkgo biloba with intracerebral hemorrhage. Neurology 1998; 50:1933–1934.
55. Mohutsky MA, Elmer GW. Inhibition of cytochrome P450 in vitro by the herbal product Ginkgo biloba. Paper presented at the 41st Annual Meeting of the American Society of Pharmacognosy, Seattle, WA, 2000.
56. Page RL II, Lawerence JD. Potentiation of warfarin by dong quai. Pharmacotherapy 1999; 19:870–878.
57. Rosenblatt M, Mindel J. Spontaneous hyphema associated with ingestion of Ginkgo biloba extract. N Engl J Med 1997; 338:1108.
58. Barbenel DM, Yusufi B, O'Shea D, Bench CJ. Mania in a patient receiving testosterone replacement postorchidectomy taking St. John's wort and sertraline. J Psychopharmacol 2000; 14:84–86.
59. Almeida JC, Grimsley EW. Coma from the health food store: interaction between kava and alprazolam. Ann Intern Med 1996; 125:940–941.
60. Matthews JM, Etheridge AS, Black SR. Inhibition of human cytochrome P450 activities by kava extract and kavalactones. Drug Metab Dispos 2002; 30: 1153–1157.
61. Zou L, Harkey MR, Henderson GL. Effects of herbal components on cDNA-expressed cytochrome P450 enzyme catalytic activity. Life Sci 2002; 71: 1579–1589.
62. Theoharides TC. Sudden death of a healthy college student related to ephedrine toxicity from a ma huang containing drink. J Clin Psychopharmacol 1997; 17: 437–439.
63. Haller CA, Benowitz NL. Adverse cardiovascular and central nervous system events associated with dietary supplements containing ephedra alkaloids. N Engl J Med 2000; 343:1833–1838.
64. Final rule declaring dietary supplements containing ephedrine alkaloids adulterated because they present an unreasonable risk. Federal Register 2004; 69:6787–6854.
65. Galluzi S, Zanetti O, Binetti G, Trabucchi M, Frisoni GB. Coma in a patient with Alzheimer's disease taking low dose trazodone and *Gingko biloba*. J Neurol Neurosurg Psychiatr 2000; 68:679–680.
66. Sasaki K, Hatta S, Haga M, Ohshika H. Effects of bilobalide on gamma-aminobutyric acid levels and glutamic acid decarboxylase in mouse brain. Eur J Pharmacol 1999; 367:165–173.
67. Rotzinger S, Fang J, Baker GB. Trazodone is metabolized to *m*-chlorophenyl-piperazine by CYP3A4 from human sources. Drug Metab Dispos 1988; 26: 572–575.
68. Chow L, Johnson M, Wells A, Dasgupta A. Effect of the traditional Chinese medicines Chan Su, Lu-Shen-Wan, Dan Shen, and Asian Ginseng on serum digoxin measurement by Tina-quant (Roche) and Synchron LX system (Beckman) digoxin immunoassays. J Clin Lab Anal 2003; 17:22–27.

69. McRae S. Elevated serum digoxin levels in a patient taking digoxin and Siberian ginseng. Can Med Assoc J 1996; 155:293–295.
70. Aslam M, Stockley IH. Interaction between curry ingredient (karela) and drug (chlorpropamide). Lancet 1979; 313(8116):607.
71. Spigset O. Reduced effect of warfarin caused by ubidecarenone. Lancet 1994; 344:1372–1373.
72. Combs AB, Porter TH, Folkers K. Anticoagulant activity of a naphthoquinone analog of vitamin K and an inhibitor of coenzyme Q_{10}-enzyme systems. Res Commun Chem Pathol Pharmacol 1976; 13:109–114.
73. Dandekar UP, Chandra RS, Dalvi SS, et al. Analysis of clinically important interaction between phenytoin and shankhapushpi, an ayurvedic preparation. J Ethnopharmacol 1992; 35:285–288.
74. Rininger JA, Kickner S, Chigurupati P, Mclean A, Franck Z. Immunopharmacological activity of Echinacea preparations following simulated digestion on murine macrophages and human peripheral blood mononuclear cells. J Leukocyte Biol 2000; 68:503–510.
75. Piscitelli SC, Formentini E, Burstein AH, Alfaro R, Jagannatha S, Falloon J. Effect of milk thistle on the pharmacokinetics of indinavir in healthy volunteers. Pharmacotherapy 2002; 22:551–556.
76. DiCenzo R, Shelton M, Jordan K, et al. Coadministration of milk thistle and indinavir in healthy subjects. Pharmacotherapy 2003; 23:866–870.
77. Borek C. Garlic supplements and saquinavir. Clin Infect Dis 2002; 35:343.
78. Gilroy CM, Steiner JF, Byers T, Shapiro H, Georgian W. Echinacea and truth in labeling. Arch Intern Med 2003; 163:699–704.
79. Ginseng: Much ado about nothing? Consumer Reports, Nov. 1995; 699.
80. Obach RS. Inhibition of human cytochrome P450 enzymes by constituents of St. John's wort's, an herbal preparation used in the treatment of depression. J Pharmacol Expl Ther 2000; 294:88–95.
81. Budzinski JW, Foster BC, Vandenhoek S, Amason JT. An in vitro evaluation of human cytochrome P450 3A4 inhibition by selected commercial herbal extracts and tinctures. Phytomedicine 2000; 7:273–282.
82. Dresser GK, Schwartz UI, Wilkinson GR, Kim RB. Coordinate induction of both cytochrome P4503A and MDR1 by St. John's wort in healthy subjects. Clin Pharmacol Ther 2003; 73:41–50.
83. Greenblatt DJ, von Moltke LL, Daily JP, Harmatz JS, Shader RI. Extensive impairment of triazolam and alprazolam clearance by short-term low dose ritonavir: the clinical dilemma of concurrent inhibition and induction. J Clin Psychopharmacol 1999; 19:293–296.

3

In Vitro Inhibition with Botanical Products

Brian C. Foster

Therapeutic Products Directorate, Health Canada and Centre for Research in Biopharmaceuticals and Biotechnology, University of Ottawa, Ottawa, Ontario, Canada

John T. Arnason

Centre for Research in Biopharmaceuticals and Biotechnology, University of Ottawa, Ottawa, Ontario, Canada

Colin J. Briggs

Faculty of Pharmacy, University of Manitoba, Winnipeg, Manitoba, Canada

BACKGROUND

The nature of plants having secondary metabolites as defensive agents greatly increases the expectation that there will be interactions with other botanical products and drugs. If well-established traditional botanical products are used according to directions, they are likely a "low risk." Risk increases when botanical products are combined with conventional drug therapies and lies in the possibility of unknown natural product–drug interactions. Other risks include product deviation due to misidentification of species, the lack of standardization, or adulteration. Most of the interactions have been reported with cytochrome P-450 (CYP) 3A4, but there are interactions with other metabolism enzymes and transport proteins.

The intent of this review is to provide an understanding of what constitutes a representative product, experimental test conditions, and the presence of contaminants that can affect the interpretation of these interactions using an in vitro assay system. Zou et al. (1) evaluated the effects of 25 purified components of commonly used botanical products and found that many significantly inhibited one or more of the cDNA human P450 isoforms at concentrations of less than $10\,\mu M$. These findings are consistent with that of many other botanical components and suggest that there may be a potential for botanical products to affect drug disposition. However, negative findings with such purified biomarkers do not preclude the possibility that the combined total of the plant constituents could have an effect on drug safety and efficacy. This review will be limited to the complex botanical products used by various populations.

NATURAL PRODUCT VARIATION

Unlike conventional drugs, botanical products are complex mixtures that have inherent variation due to environmental and genetic factors affecting the fresh product, processing and manufacturing conditions, and the possible presence of nonactive components, which need to be converted to the active moiety. In addition, there are individual variations in the amount taken, form, manner of preparation, length of use, combination with other products, genetic characteristics, and health status of the user. Botanical products can be used either fresh or as a formulated single entity or in the blended dosage form. These forms include powder or soft gel liquid–filled capsules, cosmetics, liquids, ointments, tablets, tinctures, or suppositories. Exposure to botanical products may be intentional or fortuitous through their use in beverages, cosmetics, and foodstuffs.

Botanical bulk products may be sourced from several regions or countries and may have unique genotypic and phenotypic characteristics, which can confound interpretation of adverse event reports and product selection for clinical examination. The examination of one or even a few samples may inadvertently lead to the testing of a single chemotype. A chemotype is a variety or population of plants belonging to one particular species, which differ chemically from others of that species. These differences are genetic not phenotypic. Examples include *Melaleuca alternifolia* (2), volatile oils from single plants of *Thymus serpylloides* ssp. *gadorensis* (3), and peel and leaf oils of 43 taxa of lemons and limes obtained from fruits and leaves collected from trees under the same climatic and cultural conditions (4) where there are multiple chemotypes. Together, these factors can compromise the testing process.

An interesting example is the report from Fukuda et al. (5) who determined the amounts of three furanocoumarins in 28 white grapefruit juices, and orange, apple, lemon, grape, and tangerine beverages. Considerable differences were observed on the contents among commercial brands and also batches. The contents were determined to be $321.4 \pm 95.2\,ng/mL$ GF-I-1, $5641.2 \pm 1538.1\,ng/mL$ GF-I-2, and $296.3 \pm 84.9\,ng/mL$ GF-I-4 in white grapefruit juices. None was detected in beverages from orange, apple, grape, and tangerine, although trace amounts of GF-I-2 and GF-I-4 were found in lemon juice. The average levels of these furanocoumarins were lower in the juice from red grapefruit than in that from white fruit. This variation may reflect both genetic chemotype and phenotypic differences. The highest level of these components was found in the fruit meat. Sources of variation include the distribution of the constituents into various compartments within the fruit and procedures used in extracting juice from the whole fruit. Grapefruits exposed to freezing temperatures produce more naringin and less limonin (6). It was reported that even under stable conditions, temperature and humidity could modulate naringin concentrations. Naringin, limonin, and nomolin reach peak levels in the early development stage of the fruit and decline as the fruit matures. Processing factors can include the pressure used to extract the juice, removal of bitter components, and the balancing of the final juice product by adding back the volatile essential oils and pulp (6). The clinical effects of the products containing any of the above chemotypes may vary; hence, it is difficult to attribute an effect without additional studies or set limitations on how the data can be extrapolated.

Labeling Information

Currently, there is little consistency in the information provided on botanical product labels in Canada. Some labels are clear as to the amount of botanical product and excipients, stated indications, contraindications, and warnings. In some cases, the information is confusing or difficult to understand, confounding the comparison of products. Examples of confusing or potentially misleading information on some valerian, milk thistle, St. John's wort (SJW), and echinacea product labels are provided. Three of these examples demonstrate the confusion created by or within the industry on chemical names. Information printed on some valerian root product labels stated that the products were standardized to valerenic acid and valeric acid. Although the names are similar, valeric acid is a five-carbon molecule that is not related chemically or pharmacologically to the larger C15 valerenic acids.

Silymarin is considered the active constituent of the milk thistle seed, but it is not a single compound but a descriptive term for several flavonolignans. Constituent analysis of five milk thistle products identified six constituents (representative amount): taxifolin (3.3%), silichristin (23.6%), silidianin (5.3%), silybin A (20%), silybin B (30.7%), and isosilybin (17.3%). The total amounts of silybin A and B in the five different products analyzed ranged from 45.7% to 61%. The biological effect of each constituent is not known; hence, spectrophotometric analysis would not provide sufficient information for a critical comparison of these products.

Many SJW products are standardized to either 0.3% hypericin or 4% hyperforin. Some product labels stated standardization to hypericins.

Together hypericin and pseudohypericin have been referred to as total hypericins (7). Other biosynthetic precursors such as isohypericin, protohypericin, and protopseudohypericin may also be present, which are indistinguishable when analyzed spectrophotometrically. The perceived message from this standardization is that the remaining 96% to 99.7% of the botanical material has no pharmacological effect. This is particularly disturbing with regard to SJW where pharmacological activity has been attributed to at least two dozen constituents or groups of compounds present in *Hypericum* extracts (8,9), including quinones such as hypericin and pseudohypericin, flavonoids such as hyperoside, and phloroglucinols such as hyperforin (about 8%), and water-soluble components such as organic acids. Hence, standardization to one or two SJW constituents and testing of one to two products should be viewed as a starting point but not the end of the comparative process. In the end, simple unit weight was used to prepare solutions to determine the potential of each sample to inhibit metabolism of the test substrate. There are confounding issues with such an approach, but it does provide a simple quantitative basis for comparison of products. Hypericin, pseudohypericin, and hyperforin levels in the products examined varied widely within and between products (Table 1) (10). The results obtained from this study showed wide variation in inhibitory potential of teas (Table 2) and tablets (Table 3), which does not correlate with the constituent levels (Table 1).

The final example of potentially misleading or confusing product labels is *Echinacea* (Asteraceae). The taxonomy has been revised by morphometric analysis to four species with distinct varieties (11). Two *Echinacea* species are widely used as botanical medicines: *Echinacea angustifolia* (*syn Echinacea pallida* var. *angustifolia*) and *Echinacea purpurea* (11). A third species, *E. pallida* (*E. pallida* var. *pallida*), has been widely used in Europe. Over 70 compounds were identified in the headspace volatile components of roots, stems, leaves, and flowers of *E. angustifolia*, *E. pallida*, and *E. purpurea* analyzed by gas chromatography/mass spectrometry (MS) (12). The constituents of echinacea include alkamides, caffeic acid, glycoproteins/polysaccharides, and ketoalkenynes (11,13,14). In our study, label information indicated that two products [Neutroceutical Research Program (NRP) 10 and 58] contained 4% phenols and three products (NRP 70, 71, 73) were standardized to contain 4% echinacoside. Echinacoside is not, however, a good marker for the genus *Echinacea*. This is also indicative of the confusion in the botanical product industry, because echinacoside is a marker only for *E. angustifolia*. Echinacoside was not detected in a number of products. Where detectable, the level ranged from above detection up to 32.4 mg/g. *Echinacea* Special tea is an example of a blended tea, which is not readily evident from the label. The Special tea tested contained multiple ingredients such as lemon grass, peppermint leaf, spearmint leaf, triple echinacea root (*E. angustifolia*, *E. purpurea*, and *E. pallida*), liquorice root, ginger root, wild cherry bark, cinnamon bark, fennel seed, astragalus root, cardamom seed,

Table 1 Quantity of Active Compounds Found by HPLC Analysis in the SJW Test Products

NRP	Dry weight (mg)			% Combined hypericins
	% hyperforin	% hypericin	% pseudohypericin	
8b	0.67	0.018	0.02	0.038
8c	0.144	0.022	0.038	0.06
105a	0.32	0.03	0.064	0.094
105b	0.354	0.028	0.056	0.084
105c	0.122	0.02	0.034	0.054
118a	0.08	0.008	0.016	0.024[a]
118b	0.068	0.01	0.016	0.026[a]
119b	0.036	0.008	0.014	0.022
94	0.682	0.045	0.083	0.128
95	0.479	0.059	0.111	0.17[a]
97	2.642[b]	0.065	0.097	0.162
98	0.039	0.046	0.13	0.176[a]
99	4.198	0.08	0.133	0.263[a]
102	0.068	0.052	0.083	0.135[a]
103	1.207	0.077	0.139	0.216[a]
128	0.006	0.018	0.143	0.161[a]
129	2.013	0.057	0.132	0.189[a]
93	0.502	0.063	0.12	0.183[a]
96	2.699	0.051	0.187	0.238[a]
100	0.039	0.008	0.017	0.025[a]
104	0.589	0.039	0.069	0.108[a]
101	2[c]	3.2	1.4	4.6

[a]Product reportedly standardized to 0.3% hypericin.
[b]Product reportedly standardized to at least 3% hyperforin.
[c]Expressed in μg/mL.
Abbreviations: HPLC, high performance liquid chromatography; SJW, St. John's wort.

rose hips, elder berry, burdock root, mullein leaf, clove bud, black pepper, and standardized *E. purpurea* root extract (4% phenols).

All echinacea extracts markedly inhibited CYP-mediated metabolism. The findings with aliquots of the soft gel product extracts were variable (Table 4). Inhibition was moderate to high toward CYP2D6 and 3A4, but only NRP 69 and 72 had an inhibitory effect against CYP2C9. In addition, NRP 71 did not inhibit CYP2C19-mediated metabolism.

Manufacturing and Storage

Echinacea products provide an example of the large variation in manufactured products. The whole plant has been used for therapeutic purposes, but single-entity product can consist of *E. purpurea* herb extracts, combination

Table 2 Inhibition of Human Cytochrome P450 3A4–, P450 3A5–, and P450 3A7–Mediated Metabolism of the Marker Substrate 7-Benzyloxyresorufin by Aqueous Extractions of SJW Teas in the Fluorescence Plate Assay and Testosterone HPLC Assay (in Brackets) ($n = 3$; 25 mg/mL Stock Solutions; % Inhibition ± SD)

NRP	3A4[a]	3A4	3A5	3A7
8a	60.9 ± 0.60	62.6 ± 2.19	49.9 ± 23.71	84.0 ± 1.79
8b	58.6 ± 1.68	69.3 ± 4.76 (93.6)	51.2 ± 8.99	83.4 ± 2.26
105	70.9 ± 1.08	42.9 ± 2.41 (69.6 ± 0.06)	88.9 ± 14.31	75.8 ± 2.91
118	60.8 ± 1.35	93.0 ± 1.08 (65.2 ± 0.002)	67.6 ± 5.03	94.1 ± 2.42
119	60.1 ± 0.33	31.0 ± 1.11 (45.7 ± 0.24)	66.3 ± 6.91	91.7 ± 0.80

[a]Infusion of one bag in 200 mL deionized water.
Abbreviations: HPLC, high performance liquid chromatography; SJW, St. John's wort.

root and herb extracts, and teas, or they could be blended as root extracts of the three species, herbal teas with other botanicals, and blends of *E. purpurea* and *E. angustifolia* leaves, stems, and flowers plus a dry extract of *E. purpurea* root. The relative amounts of aerial and root stock materials in formulated products vary widely in composition. All plant tissues, irrespective of the species, contained acetaldehyde, dimethyl sulfide, camphene, hexanal, β-pinene, and limonene (12). The main headspace constituents of the aerial parts of the plant are β-myrcene, α-pinene, limonene, camphene, β-pinene, *trans*-ocimene, 3-hexen-1-ol, and 2-methyl-4-pentenal. The major headspace components of the root tissue are α-phellandrene (present only in the roots of *E. purpurea* and *E. angustifolia*), dimethyl sulfide, 2-methylbutanal, 3-methylbutanal, 2-methylpropanal, acetaldehyde, camphene, 2-propanal, and limonene. Aldehydes, particularly butanals and propanals, make up 41% to 57% of the headspace of the root tissue, 19% to 29% of the headspace of the leaf tissue, and only 6% to 14% of the headspace of flower and stem tissues. Terpenoids including α- and β-pinene, β-myrcene, ocimene, limonene, camphene, and terpinene make up 81% to 91% of the

Table 3 Inhibition of Human Cytochrome P450-Mediated Metabolism by Aliquots of Aqueous Extracts of SJW Tablets (% Inhibition ± SD; 5 mg/mL Stock Solutions Except Where Noted; $n = 3$–6)

NRP	2C9*1	2C9*2	2C19	2D6[a]	3A4[a]
93	90.0 ± 10.64	72.6 ± 3.09	78.5 ± 13.64	78.2 ± 1.29	51.1 ± 9.95
96	101.8 ± 2.98	84.0 ± 1.03	88.5 ± 13.00	84.1 ± 0.72	70.7 ± 7.50
97	61.0 ± 16.77	74.3 ± 1.45	90.8 ± 11.98	88.6 ± 2.17	80.1 ± 4.20
104	77.7 ± 11.72	70.7 ± 1.76	78.8 ± 22.24	76.5 ± 1.16	73.3 ± 18.46

[a]25 mg/mL stock solution.
Abbreviation: SJW, St. John's wort.

Table 4 Inhibition of Human Cytochrome P450-Mediated Metabolism by Aliquots of Extracts from Soft Liquid–Filled Capsule Products Containing *Echinacea* ($n \geq 6 \pm$ SD; 1.25 mg/mL Stock Solution Unless Otherwise Stated)

#	2C9	2C19	2D6	3A4
69	52.5 ± 7.73	49.4 ± 6.88	49.8 ± 0.75	68.5 ± 0.75
70[a]	ND[b]	100.0 ± 9.85	94.8 ± 0.78	100.0 ± 2.26
71[b]	ND	ND	98.2 ± 0.55	91.4 ± 2.22
72	39.5 ± 5.93	71.9 ± 3.27	75.5 ± 1.95	86.6 ± 1.03

[a]Standardized to 4% echinacosides.
[b]ND, no inhibitory activity detected.

headspace of flowers and stems, 46% to 58% of the headspace of the leaf tissue, and only 6% to 21% of the roots. The relative amounts of these products will vary greatly in the manufactured and fresh product, making it difficult to choose a representative product.

A second example is garlic products. As with other botanicals, garlic can be processed by different procedures including drying or dehydration without enzyme deactivation, aqueous or oil extraction, distillation, and heating, including frying and boiling (15), processes that contribute to the variability of the extracts and complex nature of these products. These garlic preparations can then be formulated into single and blended products as oils of steam-distilled garlic, aged garlic, garlic macerated in vegetable oils, garlic powder, and gelatinous suspensions. Lawson et al. (16) conducted an extensive phytochemical analysis of organic sulfur compounds of representative fresh and commercially available garlic products and found a wide variation in composition and chemical profile of sulfur compounds. Garlic powders suspended in a gel did not contain detectable amounts of nonionic sulfur compounds. Thiosulfinates were only recovered from garlic cloves and powders. Vinyldithiins and ajoenes were only detected in garlic macerated in vegetable oil. Diallyl, methyl allyl, and dimethyl sulfides were exclusively found in oil of steam-distilled garlic. Typical steam-distilled garlic oil products contained similar amounts of total sulfur compounds as the total thiosulfinates released from freshly homogenized cloves; however, oil-macerated products contained about 20% whereas the garlic powders varied from 0% to 100%. Garlic is aged to reduce the content of sulfur compounds, such as alliin and the odor commonly associated with garlic. Gel and aged garlic in aqueous ethanol products did not have detectable levels of these nonionic sulfur compounds. Analysis of thiosulfinates from various *Allium* sp. revealed a threefold order of magnitude variation among species (17). Common garlic (*Allium sativum*) and wild garlic had the highest levels, while Chinese chives and the leek known as elephant garlic (*Allium ampeloprasum*) had intermediary levels. Environmental conditions were also found to influence the total thiosulfinate levels. As would be expected, storage conditions affect constituent content (15). Fresh garlic stored at 4EC for two months was found to have decreased levels of γ-glutamly-*S*-allylcysteine with increased levels of alliin and allicin. Lawson et al. (16) considered the increase in alliin and allicin contents in stored garlic to be a result of sprouting. In a study considering four product classes, there were marked differences in how the various extracts inhibited CYP-mediated metabolism (18). The effect was lowest against CYP2D6. Extracts from common garlic exhibited a similar inhibitory effect on all CYP3A isoforms. Chinese and elephant garlic had a lesser inhibitory effect on 3A7; Chinese garlic extracts also had a lesser inhibitory effect on CYP3A5-mediated metabolism. These findings were confirmed in a broader study with more products (Ruddick et al., unpublished data).

Extracts from three fresh garlic varieties were screened for their effect on CYP 2C9∗1–, 2C9∗2–, 2C19–, 2D6–, and 3A4– mediated metabolism. All three varieties had a slight inhibitory effect on 2C9∗1-mediated metabolism, but highly stimulated metabolism of the marker substrate with the 2C9∗2 isoform. The extracts had negligible to no effect on 2C19- and 2D6-mediated metabolism. However, all extracts strongly inhibited 3A4-mediated metabolism. The effects of aqueous extracts from aged garlic capsules and the three fresh varieties were examined for their ability to interact with human P-glycoprotein membranes. Relative to 20 μM verapamil as the positive control, the aged, common, and Chinese phosphate buffer extracts had moderate levels of product-stimulated, vanadate-sensitive adenosine triphosphatase activity. Elephant garlic was inactive.

Spices (Table 5) were analyzed for their capacity to inhibit in vitro metabolism of drug marker substrates by human CYP isoforms (19). Aliquots and infusions of all natural product categories inhibited 3A4 metabolism to some extent. Of the spices tested with 2C9, 2C19, and 2D6, most demonstrated significant inhibitory activity. Spices showed species-specific isoform inhibition with cloves, sage, and thyme having the highest activity against the four isoforms examined.

Blended and single-entity herbal teas, and some bulk spices (Table 5), were analyzed for their capacity to inhibit in vitro metabolism of marker substrates (19). Aliquots and infusions of all natural product categories inhibited 3A4 metabolism to some extent. Of the aliquots tested with 2C9, 2C19, and 2D6, many demonstrated significant inhibitory activity on the metabolism mediated by these isoforms. Herbal tea mixtures were generally more inhibitory than single-entity herbal teas. Single-entity herbal teas showed species-specific isoform inhibition with SJW and goldenseal having the highest activity against several isoforms.

Traditional Chinese medicine (TCM) includes both crude Chinese medicinal materials (plants, animal parts, and minerals) and Chinese proprietary medicine (CPM). The quality of TCM, as with other products,

Table 5 Inhibition of Human Cytochrome P450-Mediated Metabolism by Aliquots of Aqueous Extracts of Herbal Tea and Bulk Spice (Country of Origin) (25 mg/mL Stock Solutions)

	2C9	2C19	2D6	3A4
Single-entity herbal teas				
Cat's Claw bark	11.4 ± 4.35	5.2 ± 9.03	13.4 ± 0.91	56.8 ± 0.72
Chamomile herb	60.7 ± 4.38	63.7 ± 4.36	53.6 ± 1.59	56.5 ± 0.52
Feverfew leaf	51.1 ± 10.81	46.2 ± 5.27	54.1 ± 1.10	64.7 ± 1.69
Goldenseal herb	72.9 ± 4.83	80.3 ± 4.85	77.4 ± 1.60	88.3 ± 0.45
Gotu Kola herb	24.8 ± 3.99	42.2 ± 11.34	23.9 ± 1.74	51.5 ± 0.99
Kava Kava	57.0 ± 2.87	48.9 ± 6.13	24.5 ± 2.39	49.5 ± 2.57
Siberian ginseng	25.2 ± 2.88	30.9 ± 2.75	59.6 ± 0.78	24.0 ± 2.49
SJW	68.7 ± 0.83	84.6 ± 2.77	33.0 ± 1.05	64.1 ± 1.35
Botanical mixtures				
Echinacea plus	65.0 ± 2.01	61.2 ± 6.13	66.8 ± 1.46	66.1 ± 0.73
Echinacea special	74.7 ± 3.23	81.5 ± 1.85	85.7 ± 0.58	59.2 ± 1.35[a]
Echinacea and Goldenseal	52.4 ± 6.42	77.1 ± 7.35	80.0 ± 0.61	79.9 ± 0.49
Ginger	67.6 ± 2.74	51.9 ± 16.43	57.0 ± 1.57	85.6 ± 0.80
Ginkgo biloba special	79.3 ± 5.50	61.6 ± 7.87	60.9 ± 0.98	69.4 ± 1.71[a]
Green tea with triple *Echinacea* and Kombucha	73.1 ± 1.39	68.8 ± 7.64	66.5 ± 1.34	73.0 ± 1.62[b]
Green tea with Kombucha and Chinese herbs	80.6 ± 5.77[a]	94.0 ± 6.07	65.2 ± 1.29	72.6 ± 2.69[b]
Spices				
Cloves, ground (Sri Lanka)	99.0 ± 0.76	98.6 ± 0.85	97.9 ± 1.41	94.0 ± 2.21
Ginger, ground (China or India)	53.2 ± 2.60	83.3 ± 4.43	69.8 ± 2.05	88.4 ± 3.42
Oregano leaves (Turkey)	35.4 ± 2.59	80.2 ± 7.69	94.6 ± 4.26	98.6 ± 0.46

(Continued)

Table 5 Inhibition of Human Cytochrome P450-Mediated Metabolism by Aliquots of Aqueous Extracts of Herbal Tea and Bulk Spice (Country of Origin) (25 mg/mL Stock Solutions) (*Continued*)

	2C9	2C19	2D6	3A4
Sage, ground (Turkey)	97.2 ± 1.42	99.9 ± 0.34	99.8 ± 0.59	97.0 ± 3.73
Thyme leaves (Spain)	93.1 ± 5.86	91.1 ± 5.65	96.1 ± 1.57	96.9 ± 1.67
Tumeric, ground (India)	82.3 ± 6.05	92.7 ± 4.83	48.6 ± 6.42	92.8 ± 2.28

[a]625 μg/mL.
[b]156 μg/mL.
Abbreviation: SJW, St. John's wort.

can vary (20) emphasizing that there can be broad differences in these products. In a study undertaken with 12 purported TCM products, one was found to be a CPM containing three drugs (21). Extracts from most products inhibited at least three of the four CYP450 isozymes examined in a range from 25% to 100%. All liquid samples markedly inhibited the metabolism of all four isozymes. De le ke chuan kang and Rensheng dao were the strongest CYP450 inhibitors. These in vitro findings helped demonstrate that TCMs can inhibit CYP450 2C9–, 2C19–, 2D6–, and 3A4– mediated metabolism. TCMs need to be examined further under clinical settings to determine if potential interactions occur, which affect the safety and efficacy of conventional therapeutic products.

Experimental Factors

Many of the reported interaction studies with botanical products have used a single aqueous or organic extract. However, botanical products contain several major classes of biologically active constituents, with differing chemical characteristics that can directly or indirectly affect drug disposition. A series of solvents ranging from hexane, with high lipophilicity, down to water have been used to sequentially extract different botanical products (18). In this representative example, capsule material from aged garlic extract, and the two fresh varieties of garlic and one leek were extracted sequentially (Table 6). Extracts were reduced to dryness and reconstituted into methanol prior to testing for their effect on 3A4-mediated metabolism. Most extract fractions exhibited a high inhibitory activity against the isoforms studied. There was varietal variation. Inhibition results with hexane (136%) and chloroform (116%) extracts suggest the presence of botanical fluorescent quenching substances. This observation is consistent with the

Table 6 Inhibition of Cytochrome P450 3A4–Mediated Metabolism by Sequential Solvent Extracts of a Commercially Available Product and Fresh Garlic ($n \geq 6$; Mean Percent Inhibition $\pm$ SD)

	Hexane	Chloroform	Methylene chloride	Ethyl acetate	Methanol
Aged	37.2 ± 59.6	67.8 ± 31.8	67.9 ± 5.2	83.2 ± 2.8	54.0 ± 7.3
Chinese	91.3 ± 9.8	116.1 ± 18.9	90.7 ± 5.2	85.1 ± 5.86	48.2 ± 9.0
Common	135.8 ± 36.1	92.9 ± 23.3	65.0 ± 8.0	72.9 ± 5.0	58.6 ± 14.3
Elephant	87.0 ± 6.2	72.0 ± 24.8	93.4 ± 5.0	93.3 ± 3.3	92.0 ± 5.6

concerns for intrinsic fluorescence and quenching as confounding variables in these assays noted by Zou et al. (22). As was determined with other botanical products, several 100% inhibitions were evident with this simple extraction sequence. A series of nonsequential extracts with these solvents (data not reported) also revealed high inhibitory activity in all extracts. Selective pH extraction of the Chinese garlic bulb showed significant (50–80%) inhibitory activity in the strong acid, weak acid, neutral, and basic fractions (data not shown) against CYP3A4. Because differences in the inhibitory effects of aqueous and methanolic extracts of fresh and aged garlic cloves on CYP3A4-mediated metabolism were previously noted, the three varieties were extracted under four different conditions. Results varied with variety, but in general, the distilled water and phosphate buffer extracts gave the strongest overall inhibitory effect on CYP450-mediated metabolism of the marker substrates.

Many plant constituents are conjugates, the main form being glucosides. Seven soybean varieties were analyzed by high-performance liquid chromatography (HPLC) for the isoflavones, daidzein and genistein, and their respective glycoside derivatives (Table 7) to determine if the amounts of these compounds could reliably predict the activity of the variety or year of harvest (19). Genistein levels ranged from 5.8 to 28.7 µg/g and daidzein levels from 0 to 42.6 µg/g. The glycosides daidzin and genistin were present in much larger amounts ranging from 198 to 792 µg/g and from 458 to 1261 µg/g, respectively. The free aglycones accounted for less than 7% of the total in these samples. Neither the concentration of the individual compounds nor their total correlated with the inhibition of CYP3A4-mediated metabolism across genotypes and years. In a comparative inhibition test, the glycones were inactive relative to the corresponding aglycones.

Dissolution

As with formulated pharmaceuticals, dissolution of constituents from teas is an important consideration. Visual examination of the contents from

Table 7 Concentration of Daidzein and Genistein and Their Conjugates in Five Soybean Varieties (μg/g of Seed)

Variety	Daidzin	Genistin	Daidzein	Genistein	Total	Free[a]	CYP3A4 inhibition
Bayfield							
1996	440.6	800.3	21.4	19.1	1281.4	3.2	17
1997	416.2	776.6	18.1	19.5	1230.4	3.1	74
Beck							
1997	423.4	865.8	13.5	16.7	1319.4	2.3	18
Bravor							
1996	792.4	1261.3	39.1	28.7	2121.5	3.2	19
1997	680	1106.2	20	18	1824.2	2.1	22
Korada							
1997	340.4	594.8	15.2	11.2	961.6	2.7	24
Micron							
1997	450.9	599.3	42.6	31.1	1123.9	6.6	25
Secord							
1996	358.9	796	18	20.1	1193	3.2	25
1997	198.8	458.8		5.8	663.4	<1	26
York							
1997	355.3	534.8	20.1	16	926.2	3.9	33

Note: The inhibition of cytochrome P450 3A4–mediated metabolism is given as a percentage.
[a]Percent free aglycone relative to total amounts of these flavonoids analyzed.
Abbreviation: CYP, cytochrome P-450.

tea bags from several botanical products showed that there were inter- and intraproduct differences in particulate size. Particle sizes ranged from fine powder to substantially intact leaves and stems. Under controlled tea-brewing conditions, there were marked differences in the dissolution of constituents relative to the amount and temperature of the water, degree of agitation, and time. Many of these factors are individualistic, so one individual may be exposed to different amounts of constituents relative to another person. In a representative study, several botanical products were examined as tea bag infusions at different temperatures. In this example, three different patterns were noted. The initial 10-minute values for the echinacea special tea were markedly higher than that for the other botanical products, but the inhibition curve only increased slightly with time. Two products, goldenseal herb, and echinacea and goldenseal, had low initial values, which nearly doubled after a second 10-minute incubation. The third pattern with feverfew showed a linear increase throughout the incubation period.

Westerhoff et al. (23) studied the dissolution characteristics of several SJW products under biorelevant conditions. Components of SJW have a broad spectrum of polarity and solubility, and representative compounds from each group were examined. Although labelling indicates that several of the products studied should be pharmaceutically equivalent, dissolution under biorelevant conditions revealed that they have quite different release profiles and cannot be considered interchangeable. It was concluded that biorelevant dissolution testing can be a powerful tool for comparing botanical products as well as synthetically produced drug products. Jurgenliemk and Nahrstedt (24) examined the dissolution of water-soluble phenolic constituents of *Hypericum perforatum* from a medicinal tea and a coated tablet formulation and found different dissolution profiles. In general, the flavonoid glycosides were well dissolved, followed by flavonoid aglycones and hypericin, while hyperforin was only detectable at a very low level. Interestingly, hypericin exhibited much better extraction and dissolution rates than the similarly lipophilic hyperforin. When determining the octanol–water partition coefficient, it became obvious that the solubility of pure hypericin in water increased upon addition of some phenolic constituents typical for *Hypericum* extracts. Most effective in solubilizing hypericin was hyperoside, which increased the concentration of hypericin in the water phase up to 400-fold in this model.

Stability

As with drugs and purified biomarkers, thermal- and photostability of botanical products are the factors that must be considered. Commercial dried extract and capsules of SJW were evaluated under harmonized test conditions (25). Photostability testing showed all the constituents to be photosensitive in the tested conditions. However, different opacity agents and pigments influenced the stability of the constituents. Amber containers had little effect on the photostability of the investigated constituents. Long-term thermal stability testing showed a shelf life of less than four months for hyperforins and hypericins, even when ascorbic and citric acids were added to the formulation.

Photostability affected several botanical products. To overcome this confounding factor, samples of all products were extracted and tested under reduced lighting conditions, frequently under F40 gold fluorescence lighting (18).

Marked variations in the stability of 21 tinctures and 13 related single-entity plant compounds were noted (26). Bilia et al. (27) investigated the stability of 40% and 60% v/v tinctures of artichoke, SJW, calendula flower, milk thistle fruit, and passionflower. The investigation showed a very low thermal stability of the constituents from accelerated and long-term testing as determined by HPLC–diode array detector and –MS analyses. Stability was related both to the class of flavonoids and water content of the investigated tinctures. Shelf life at 25°C of the most stable tincture (passionflower 60% v/v) was about six months, whereas that of the milk thistle tinctures was only about three months. The stability of artichoke and

SJW tinctures also were shown to be variable and seem to be related to the water content of the preparations.

TEST CONDITIONS

The first step with all botanical products is authentication to confirm identity. Bulk single-entity products can occasionally be inspected visually and authenticated by comparison to reference materials. However, most products require authentication through phytochemical analysis with comparison against authentic marker substances, preferably with a chromatographic stage to separate constituents for individual assessment. Authentication generally confirms the presence of a botanical product but does not exclude the possibility of the presence of other botanical products, adulterants, or contaminants. In some cases, historical information may suggest that samples be examined in depth for potential contaminants. Ideally, test samples of a product should be prepared from a minimum of five units mixed together to provide a representative sample of a particular product or lot. Test samples should be reduced to a consistent size using a mortar and pestle, ball mill, or blender. In our studies, we routinely begin with either a 100 mg/mL aqueous suspension or a 25 mg/mL ethanolic suspension that is then reduced further to constant particle size in a polytron to facilitate reproducible extraction for one minute. Standardization of this phase of testing is critical to ensure intra- and interday reproducibility in testing. Soft liquid–filled gel capsules are cut open, and the contents emptied into a 1.5 mL microfuge tube and extracted. The mixtures are centrifuged for 18 minutes in a microcentrifuge at a high setting to give a particulate-free stock solution.

Aliquots of aqueous or organic extracts are screened for their ability to inhibit the major human cDNA–metabolizing CYP isozyme CYP 2C9, 2C19, 2D6, and 3A marker substrates using an in vitro fluorometric micro-titer plate assay (4), modified from the one reported by Crespi et al. (28), with balanced amounts of specific activity and protein content. Despite the inherent limitations of these test substrates, these probes provide a quantitative basis for additional studies (29,30). Briefly, assays are performed with either a 2 to 4 µL of an organic extract or up to 10 µL of an aqueous extract in a total volume of 200 µL in 96-well, clear-bottom, opaque-walled microtiter plates. The complex nature of the extracts requires blank and test controls to evaluate the effects of intrinsic fluorescence and quenching as confounding variables in these assays (22). We include controls for both the blank and test product using denatured enzyme with the extraction solvent. Where possible, studies should include one or more test substrates representative of the isozyme as positive control(s).

The effect of botanical products on the expression of drug-metabolizing enzymes or transport proteins can be examined in cell culture with established cell lines or primary human hepatocytes. The cells are incubated under standard conditions and treated with the blank, positive, or negative controls and the botanical extracts. Vehicle use should be consistent in all cultures. Multiple time points should examine the immediate and prolonged effect of these treatments. After treatment, total RNA and/or microsomes are prepared from the harvested cells using standard methodologies.

All assays should be performed under reduced or F40 gold fluorescence lighting to minimize the potential for photodecomposition or activation. Assays are run in triplicate to determine percent inhibition. The tests are repeated at least once with a freshly prepared sample. If there is greater than 15% coefficiency of variation, the samples are run at least one additional time. When the reaction mixture is incubated within the plate reader, readings are taken immediately and at set times throughout the prescribed incubation period as established by the microsome supplier. For assays incubated outside of the plate reader, reactions were stopped in accordance with the product test procedure.

In studies where either intrinsic fluorescence or quenching is a confounding variable, the botanical product should be examined in an assay using a chromatographic separation step with a representative probe substance for the isozyme (29) being examined.

PRODUCT SELECTION FOR CLINICAL STUDIES

In vitro testing with cell-free systems can provide only qualitative information on the inhibitory potential of the particular extract from a specific sample to affect the isozyme-mediated metabolism of a test substrate. There is no a priori basis to extrapolate either positive or negative in vitro inhibitory results to acute or chronic clinical exposure. Despite this caveat, there were, however, clinical reports with echinacea (31), garlic (32,33), and SJW (34,35) that these botanical products can affect drug pharmacokinetics. The explanation being that in some cases, prolonged exposure to an inhibitory product led to reduced plasma levels of a probe substance presumably due to induction of a transport protein or metabolic enzyme. Negative in vitro findings are limited to the extract and the inherent weakness of these probes' substrates; only further testing with additional extracts and test products can truly demonstrate the potential of these botanical products to cause interactions. In addition, there is no a priori basis to extrapolate in vitro findings from an single active ingredient (SAI) to the complex botanical product.

The number of fresh varieties, dosage forms, and formulations in combination with the variability in botanical material make it impossible to evaluate all of these products in animal models or clinical trials. As a minimum, several products used by the patient community should be obtained and authenticated. The testing and selection criteria should include multiple-lot testing, cost, and product availability, and take into consideration how these products are used. Drug combinations are being examined increasingly in comparative clinical trials with a goal of enhancing efficacy with the same or fewer adverse events (36). In many instances, the amount of drug exposure, the total drug load, is a major contributing factor to the safety of the combinations.

Four SJW products with similar CYP3A-inhibitory activity were evaluated for their effects on cell viability, the potential of such preparations to modulate induction of nitric oxide and CYP1A1/2-mediated ethoxy-resorufin *O*-deethylase (EROD) activity in glial cell cultures (37). SJW A, B, and D had little effect on EROD activity. SJW C had the highest inductive effect on EROD activity. SJW B and C treatment resulted in the highest nitric oxide levels, raising concern for potential central nervous system toxicity. SJW A and D produced significant lactic dehydrogenase–released cell toxicity. Which product should be studied? The difficult decision is whether to choose an average or a superior product because the results of the study will subsequently be viewed as representative of all related products.

CONCLUSION

Synergistic interactions are of vital importance in phytomedicines and underpin the philosophy of herbal medicine (38). Spinella (39) emphasizes that, in addition to searching for more potent mechanisms, one must consider the additive and supra-additive effects of a plant's multiple constituents. Synergy may occur through pharmacokinetic and/or pharmacodynamic interactions. Synergistic interactions are documented for constituents within a total extract of a single botanical product, as well as between different botanical products in a formulation (38). Thus interactions with pharmacologically active secondary metabolites are not unexpected because these constituents are part of the plant defensive mechanisms. In vitro studies can help determine the potential for adverse effects associated with botanical product–drug interactions.

Accumulated findings from many studies have confirmed our earlier observations that there is seldom a direct correlation between levels of the purported active ingredient biomarkers and the potential for these extracts to affect P450-mediated metabolism. At best, in vitro studies with an inhibitory finding in these cell-free extracts can only provide a qualitative basis for further studies. A negative finding, particularly with an SAI, can only be interpreted to mean that there is no activity under the stated test conditions. Unfortunately, some negative findings have been erroneously taken to mean that related botanical products containing this SAI would not affect drug disposition. The dilemma for all health care professionals and consumers is that what is apparently safe with one botanical product and pharmaceutical, or another botanical product, may be neither safe nor effective in another combination or patient population.

REFERENCES

1. Zou L, Harkey MR, Henderson GL. Effects of herbal components on cDNA-expressed cytochrome P450 enzyme catalytic activity. Life Sci 2002; 71:1579–1589.
2. Russell MF, Southwell IA. Monoterpenoid accumulation in 1,8-cineole, terpinolene and terpinen-4-ol chemotypes of *Melaleuca alternifolia* seedlings. Phytochemistry 2003; 62:683–689.
3. Saez F. Volatile oil variability in *Thymus serpylloides* ssp. gadorensis growing wild in Southeastern Spain. Bio Chem Syst Ecol 2001; 29:189–198.
4. Lota ML, de Rocca Serra D, Tomi F, Jacquemond C, Casanova J. Volatile components of peel and leaf oils of lemon and lime species. J Agric Food Chem 2002; 50:796–805.
5. Fukuda K, Guo L, Ohashi N, Yoshikawa M, Yamazoe Y. Amounts and variation in grapefruit juice of the main components causing grapefruit-drug interactions. J Chromatogr 2000; 741(B):195–203.
6. Ameer B, Weintraub RA. Drug interactions with grapefruit juice. Clin Pharmacokinet 1887; 33:103–121.
7. Barnes J, Anderson LA, Phillipson JD. St John's wort (*Hypericum perforatum* L.): a review of its chemistry, pharmacology and clinical properties. J Pharm Pharmacol 2001; 53:583–600.
8. Moore LB, Goodwin B, Jones SA, et al. St. John's wort induces hepatic drug metabolism through activation of the pregnane X receptor. Proc Natl Acad Sci USA 2000; 97:7500–7502.
9. Wagner H, Bladt S. Pharmaceutical quality of hypericum extracts. Psych Neurol 1994(suppl 1):S65–S68.
10. Foster BC, Sockovie ER, Bellefeuille NC, et al. Effect of St. John's wort on cytochrome P-450 and flavin monooxygenase enzymes and on P-glycoprotein. Can J Infect Dis 2001; 12(suppl B):132P.
11. Binns SE, Livesey JF, Arnason JT, Baum BR. Phytochemical variation in Echinacea from roots and flowerheads of wild and cultivated populations. J Agric Food Chem 2002; 50:3673–3687.
12. Mazza G, Cottrell T. Volatile components of roots, stems, leaves, and flowers of Echinacea species. J Agric Food Chem 1999; 47:3081–3085.
13. Bauer R, Foster S. Analysis of alkamides and caffeic acid derivatives from *Echinacea simulata* and *E. paradoxa* roots. Planta Med 1991; 57:447–449.
14. Bauer R. Echinacea drugs-effects and active ingredients. Z Arztl Fortbild (Jena) 1996; 90:111–115.
15. Matsuura H. Phytochemistry of garlic horticulture and processing procedures. In: Lanchance PP, ed. Nutraceuticals, Designer Foods III: Garlic, Soy and Licorice. Trumbell, CT: Food & Nutrition Press, 1997:55–69.
16. Lawson LD, Wang Z-YJ, Hughes BG. Identification and HPLC quantification of the sulfides and dialk(en)yl thiosulfinates in commercial garlic products. Planta Med 1991; 57:363–370.
17. Block E, Naganathan S, Putman D, Zhao S-H. Allium chemistry: HPLC analysis of thiosulfinates from onion, garlic, wild garlic (Ransoms): leek, scallion, shallot, elephant (great-headed) garlic, chive, and Chinese chive. Uniquely high

allyl to methyl ratios in some garlic samples. J Agric Food Chem 1992; 40:2418–2430.

18. Foster BC, Foster MS, Vandenhoek S, et al. An in vitro evaluation of human cytochrome P450 3A4 and P-glycoprotein inhibition by garlic. J Pharm Pharmaceut Sci 2001; 4:176–184.

19. Foster BC, Vandenhoek S, Hanna J, et al. Effects of natural health products on cytochrome P-450 drug metabolism. Phytomedicine 2003; 10:334–342.

20. Su W, Feng Y, Wu Z, Zhang R, Ye W, Peng D. Study on quality evaluation of Chinese traditional patent medicine with chemical pattern recognition. Zhong Yao Cai 1998; 21:311–314.

21. Foster BC, Vandenhoek S, Li KY, Tang R, Krantis A. Effect of Chinese herbal products on cytochrome P-450 drug metabolism. J Pharm Pharmaceut Sci 2002; 5:185–189.

22. Zou L, Harkey MR, Henderson GL. Effects of intrinsic fluorescence and quenching on fluorescence-based screening of natural products. Phytomedicine 2002; 9:263–267.

23. Westerhoff K, Kaunzinger A, Wurglics M, Dressman J, Schubert-Zsilavecz M. Biorelevant dissolution testing of St. John's wort products. J Pharm Pharmacol 2002; 54:1615–1621.

24. Jurgenliemk G, Nahrstedt A. Dissolution, solubility and cooperativity of phenolic compounds from *Hypericum perforatum* L. in aqueous systems. Pharmazie 2003; 58:200–203.

25. Bilia AR, Bergonzi MC, Morgenni F, Mazzi G, Vincieri FF. Evaluation of chemical stability of St. John's wort commercial extract and some preparations. Int J Pharm 2001; 213:199–208.

26. Budzinski J, Foster BC, Vandenhoek S, Arnason JT. An in vitro evaluation of human cytochrome CYP450 3A4 inhibition by selected commercial herbal extracts and tinctures. Phytomedicine 2000; 7:273–282.

27. Bilia AR, Bergonzi MC, Gallori S, Mazzi G, Vincieri FF. Stability of the constituents of Calendula, milk-thistle and Passionflower tinctures by LC-DAD and LC-MS. J Pharm Biomed Anal 2002; 30:613–624.

28. Crespi CL, Miller VP, Penman BW. Microtiter plate assays for inhibition of human, drug-metabolizing cytochromes P450. Anal Biochem 1997; 248:188–190.

29. Tucker GT, Houston JB, Huang SM. Optimizing drug development: strategies to assess drug metabolism/transporter interaction potential—toward a consensus. Pharmaceut Res 2001; 18:1071–1080.

30. Ghosal A, Hapangama N, Yuan Y, et al. Rapid determination of enzyme activities of recombinant human cytochromes P450, human liver microsomes and hepatocytes. Biopharm Drug Dispos 2003; 24:375–384.

31. Gorski JC, Huang SM, Pinto A, et al. The effect of Echinacea (*Echinacea purpurea* root) on cytochrome P450 activity in vivo. Clin Pharmacol Ther 2004; 75:89–100.

32. Gallicano K, Choudhri S, Leclaire T, Foster BC. Effect of short-term administration of garlic supplements on single-dose ritonavir pharmacokinetics in healthy volunteers. Br J Clin Pharmacol 2003; 55:199–202.

33. Piscitelli SC, Burstein AH, Welden N, Gallicano KD, Falloon J. The effect of garlic supplements on the pharmacokinetics of saquinavir. Clin Infect Dis 2002; 34:234–238.
34. Piscitelli SC, Burstein AH, Chaitt D, Alfaro RM, Falloon J. Indinavir concentrations and St. John's wort. Lancet 2000; 355:547–548.
35. Markowitz JS, Donovan JL, DeVane CL, et al. Effect of St. John's wort on drug metabolism by induction of cytochrome P450 3A4 enzyme. J Am Med Assoc 2003; 290:1500–1504.
36. Deckers CL, Hekster YA, Keyser A, Meinardi H, Renier WO. Drug load in clinical trials: a neglected factor. Clin Pharmacol Ther 1997; 62:592–595.
37. Grenier M, Sun P, Drobitch R. Effect of St. John's wort preparations on cell viability, induction of nitric oxide and ethoxyresorufin O-deethylase activity in glial cell culture. Proceedings of the 5th Annual Symposium on Pharmaceutical Sciences. J Pharm Pharmaceut Sci 2002; 5:106.
38. Williamson EM. Synergy and other interactions in phytomedicines. Phytomedicine 2001; 8:401–409.
39. Spinella M. The importance of pharmacological synergy in psychoactive herbal medicines. Altern Med Rev 2002; 7:130–137.

4

Drug Interactions with St. John's Wort and *Echinacea*

J. Christopher Gorski

*Division of Clinical Pharmacology, Department of Medicine,
Indiana University School of Medicine, Indianapolis,
Indiana, U.S.A.*

INTRODUCTION

Botanical use is prevalent throughout the world with between 10% and 30% of individuals residing in the United States using complementary and alternative medicines routinely. Of particular concern is the finding that up to 30% of individuals taking prescription medicines have also used botanical remedies concurrently within the past year (1–3). The number of individuals consuming St. John's wort on a daily basis has been estimated at more than 11 million and approximately one-third of these are using St. John's wort to treat self-diagnosed depression. In the United States, St. John's wort is one of the top-selling botanical preparations with sales ranking second in 1999 and seventh in 2002 (4,5). Although botanical preparations are widely considered by the public to be without adverse effect or a source of drug interactions, this is not the case. The report of Ruschitzka et al. (6) clearly illustrates the danger of coadministering botanical products (i.e., St. John's wort) with prescription products and demonstrates that, despite popular belief, the indiscriminant use of botanical products does involve risk. This chapter will review the historical indications, formulations, pharmacology, and interactions between St. John's wort, *echinacea*, and other medicines.

ST. JOHN'S WORT

Indications

St. John's wort (*Hypericum perforatum*) is a perennial wildflower indigenous to Europe, North Africa, and western Asia (Fig. 1) and has been used for medicinal purposes for over two millennia. As far back as the early 16th century, St. John's wort was used primarily to treat anxiety, depression, and sleep disorders. In the late 20th and early 21st century, St. John's wort has been recommended for the treatment of mild to moderate depression (7). In support of its use for the treatment of mild to moderate depression, a number of clinical trials have demonstrated that St. John's wort has comparable efficacy to the tricyclic antidepressants (i.e., imipramine) and selective serotonin reuptake inhibitors (e.g., fluoxetine and paroxetine) (8–13).

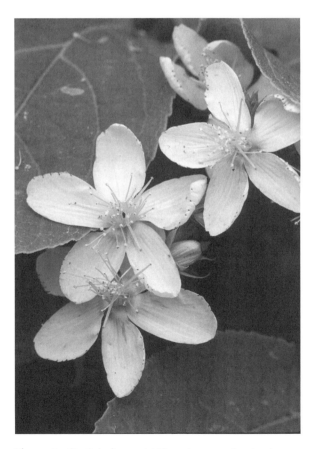

Figure 1 St. John's wort (*Hypericum perforatum*).

It should be noted that these clinical trials are typically conducted within a short time period and thus may not reflect long-term outcomes. The utility of St. John's wort in the treatment of moderate to severe depression has been investigated (14–17) in large randomized placebo-controlled multi-institutional studies. Some such studies demonstrated efficacy (16), but others failed to detect a clinically significant effect on the symptoms of the moderate to severely depressed individuals (15,17). Gelenberg et al. demonstrated a relapse rate of approximately 30% in moderate to severely depressed individuals who initially responded to St. John's wort therapy as would be expected from experience with prescription antidepressants (14).

Other conditions in which St. John's wort has been advocated include neuralgia, anxiety, neurosis, dyspepsia, and external treatment of wounds, bruises, sprains, myalgia, and first-degree burns. In vitro studies conducted in the late 1980s and early 1990s suggested that components of St. John's wort (e.g., hypericin) may have antiviral properties (18–20). However, an open-label clinical trial demonstrated that the intravenous or oral administration of the St. John's wort constituent, hypericin, provided no clinical benefit, as reflected by increasing CD4 counts or decreasing viral load in a group of HIV-infected individuals and resulted in significant adverse events necessitating discontinuation of therapy (21).

Dosage Forms

St. John's wort and some individual constituents of the preparations have been administered orally, topically, and intravenously in various pharmaceutical formulations, including tinctures, teas, capsules, purified components, and tablets. These botanical preparations of St. John's wort are prepared from plant components (i.e., flowers, buds, and stalk) whose content of the wide array of structurally diverse bioactive constituents may differ (Table 1 and Fig. 2). Many commercial tablet and capsule formulations of St. John's wort are standardized using the ultraviolet absorbance of the naphthodianthrones, hypericin, and pseudohypericin, to contain 0.3% "hypericin" content. Thus, a 300 mg dose of St. John's wort contains approximately 900 µg "hypericin" per dose. Despite the standardization of dosage forms

Table 1 Bioactive Constituents of St. John's Wort

Biochemical class	Plant source	Active constituent
Naphthodianthrones	Flowers, buds	Hypericin, pseudohypericin
Phloroglucinols	Flowers, buds	Hyperforin, adhyperforin
Flavonoids	Leaves, stalk, buds	Quercetin, hyperoside, quercitrin, isoquercitrin, I3, II8 biapigenin
Essential oils	Flowers, leaves	Terpenes, alcohols

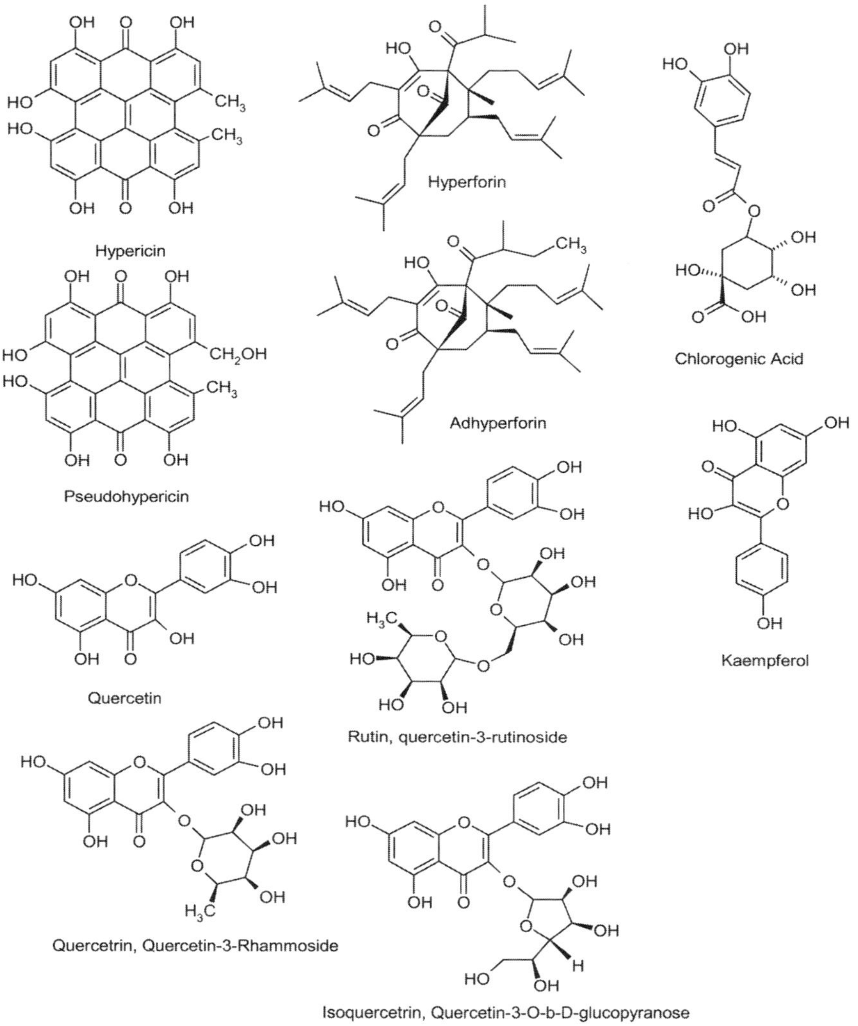

Figure 2 Chemical structures of common phytochemicals found in SJW. *Abbreviation*: SJW, St. John's wort.

on hypericin content, the principal active ingredient is thought to be a phloroglucinol, hyperforin. As a result of inappropriate standardization on an ingredient that has limited pharmacological activity, the concentration of hyperforin varies greatly among commercial preparations (Fig. 3). Draves and Walker assessed the hypericin and pseudohypericin (naphthodianthrones) content in 54 commercially available St. John's wort products (United States and Canada) and determined that only two of the

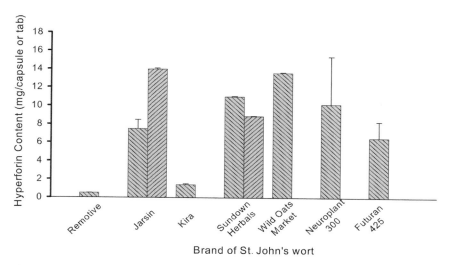

Figure 3 Variability in hyperforin content among commercially available SJW products. Data taken from published studies assessing hyperfortin content of SJW tablets or capsules. *Abbreviation*: SJW, St. John's wort. *Source*: From Refs. 22–26.

products were within 10% of the labeled claims for "hypericin" content (27). Likewise, Wurglics et al. assessed hypericin and hyperforin content and interbatch variability in eight German St. John's wort products (22). Pronounced interbatch variability was observed for some products whereas others demonstrated consistent hyperforin and hypericin content (Fig. 3). In addition, the expected naphthodianthrone (hypericin) content in the preparations also demonstrated considerable variability. It is clear from the reports of a number of investigators that there is wide inter- and intraproduct variability in hyperforin and hypericin content (22,23,28,29). The lack of consistent phytomedicinal (hypericin and hyperforin) content across and within products is not limited to St. John's wort preparations but is seen with many other botanical medicines (30). The administration of St. John's wort via tea is no longer recommended because the efficacy of this preparation is questionable; however, the drug interaction potential of St. John's wort in this formulation appears to be maintained (7,31).

The preparation used in many of the described interactions between St. John's wort and conventional pharmaceutical products is the product manufactured by Lichtwer Pharma GmbH (Berlin, Germany). This product is marketed under the trade name, Jarsin^{TM} (LI 160) in Germany and marketed in the United States under the trade name Kira^{TM}. St. John's wort may also be sold in combination products with vitamins and other botanical preparations (32). The drug interaction potential between these combination products and cytochrome P450 (CYP) 3A and P-glycoprotein substrates has not been investigated, but should be assumed to be no different than single-agent St. John's wort products.

Adverse Effects and Pharmacodynamic Interactions

It is a reasonable expectation that, as observed with other pharmacotherapies, the administration of St. John's wort will result in adverse effects. In a study examining the efficacy of St. John's wort for mild to moderate depression, dry mouth was the most common adverse effect occurring in 8% of patients (13/157), and other adverse events including headache, sweating, asthenia, and nausea occurred in 3% or less of the participants (13). In addition, only four individuals withdrew from the trial compared to 26 individuals who withdrew while taking the comparator drug, imipramine (13). Likewise, Woelk et al. reported a low incidence of adverse events in a group of 3250 (76% women) patients receiving St. John's wort three times daily (LI 160) for the treatment of depression (33). The most frequently recorded adverse events were gastrointestinal irritation (0.6%), allergic reactions (0.5%), tiredness (0.4%), and restlessness (0.3%) (33). Other adverse effects associated with St. John's wort intake include sedation, anxiety, and dizziness. It is clear from these reports that St. John's wort is well tolerated.

Dean et al. described a 58-year-old postmenopausal woman who experienced nausea, anorexia, retching, dry mouth, dizziness, thirst, cold chills, weight loss, and extreme fatigue following the discontinuation of St. John's wort (1800 mg three times daily for 32 days) (34). The symptoms peaked three days after cessation of St. John's wort for suspected photosensitivity reaction and resolved within eight days. The reported symptoms and the temporal relationship to the discontinuation of the St. John's wort dosing were considered by Dean et al. to be consistent with "withdrawal syndrome." Additionally, the high dose of St. John's wort administered was considered to be a contributing factor in the patient adverse-event profiles.

In studies examining the antiviral activity of synthetic hypericin following oral and intravenous administration for the treatment of HIV infection, a dose-limiting toxicity was moderate to severe photosensitivity, including the erythema, numbness, pain, and temperature sensitivity (21). There is a case report of hypertensive crisis in a 41-year-old male, following the ingestion of St. John's wort for approximately one week, and the consumption of tyramine-rich foods (aged cheese and red wine) (35). Although the interaction between monoamine oxidase inhibitors and the eating of tyramine-rich foods is well recognized, alcoholic extracts of St. John's wort have been shown to weakly interact with monoamine oxidase receptors A and B (36,37). Thus, the mechanism of the observed hypertensive crisis is unclear. Other serious adverse effects attributed to St. John's wort due to drug–drug pharmacokinetic or pharmacodynamic interactions include cardiovascular collapse (38), mania in patients with bipolar depression (39), and photosensitivity (40).

Mechanisms of St. John's Wort–Mediated Drug Interactions

In Vitro

Using crude extracts and isolated constituents, Obach demonstrated that St. John's wort was capable of inhibiting cDNA-expressed CYP-mediated metabolism (Table 2) (41). cDNA-expressed CYP2C9-, CYP2D6-, and CYP3A4-mediated biotransformations were inhibited by purified hyperforin. Likewise, I3, II8 biapigenin was shown to competitively inhibit CYP1A2-, CYP2C9-, and CYP3A4-mediated phenacetin *O*-deethylation, diclofenac 4-hydroxylation, and testosterone 6β-hydroxylation, respectively. The results demonstrated that constituents of *H. perforatum* were capable of inhibiting biotransformations mediated by both CYPs, CYP2D6 and CYP3A (Table 2) (41). Likewise, Budzinski et al. demonstrated that commercial tinctures of St. John's wort and hypericin, a principal component of these tinctures, were capable of inhibiting cDNA-expressed CYP3A4-mediated metabolism of 7-benzyloxyresorufin (43). Although the crude extracts and purified constituents of St. John's wort were relatively good inhibitors of CYP3A in vitro, the subsequent in vivo studies failed to confirm these observations. It is clear from the current body of literature that the coadministration of St. John's wort with many therapeutic agents, especially those that are CYP3A substrates, results in reduced serum

Table 2 Inhibition Constants and Fold Induction of CYP3A4 for the Principal Constituents of St. John's Wort on Human CYP Activities

St. John's wort constituent	CYP enzyme	K_i (μm)	Mode of inhibition	Approximate fold induction of CYP3A4 mRNA
Hyperforin	CYP2C9	1.8 ± 0.9	Competitive	7-fold
	CYP2D6	1.5 ± 0.9	Noncompetitive	
	CYP3A4	0.49 ± 0.24	Competitive	
I3, II8biapigenin	CYP1A2	0.95 ± 0.22	Competitive	n.d.
	CYP2C9	0.32 ± 0.14	Competitive	
	CYP2D6	2.3 ± 1.8	Competitive	
	CYP3A4	0.038 ± 0.006	Competitive	
Hypericin	CYP2C9	1.4 ± 1.1	Competitive	1.5-fold
	CYP2D6	2.6 ± 0.9	Competitive	
	CYP3A4	4.2 ± 2.2	Competitive	
Quercetin	CYP1A2	3.3 ± 0.6	Noncompetitive	2-fold
Kampferol	n.d.	n.d.		1.1-fold

Abbreviations: CYP, cytochrome P450; n.d., not done.
Source: From Refs. 41, 42.

concentration and diminished drug efficacy. These observations are consistent with increased drug elimination.

CYP3A4 and P-glycoprotein are transcriptionally regulated by an orphan nuclear receptor designated as the pregnane X receptor (PXR). Small molecule ligands such as rifampicin bind to PXR and encourage heterodimerization of PXR with the retinoid X receptor. mRNA synthesis of numerous target genes is stimulated after this complex undergoes translocation to complimentary sequences in the regulatory region of the genes. Moore et al. examined the effect of extracts of commercial St. John's wort preparations (i.e., Nature's way, Springville, Utah, U.S.; Nature's Plus, Melville, New York, U.S.; and Neutraceutical for Solaray, Park City, Utah, U.S.) on CYP3A4 mRNA expression in cultures of human hepatocytes (42). CYP3A4 mRNA expression was induced in human hepatocytes treated for 30 hours with either extracts of commercial St. John's wort preparations or purified hyperforin (Fig. 4) (42). Additional experiments conducted by this group employing CV-1 cells transiently transfected with both a PXR expression vector and a human chloramphenicol acetyltransferase reporter system containing a PXR-binding site demonstrated that hypericum extract and hyperforin, but not hypericin, induced CYP3A4 mRNA expression via activation of the PXR (42). Hyperforin has an EC_{50} for the activation of PXR

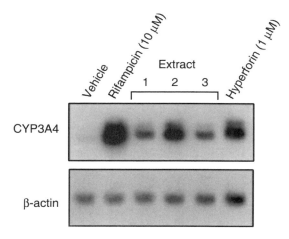

Figure 4 SJW extracts and hyperforin induce CYP3A4 expression in human hepatocytes. Northern blot analysis was performed with total RNA (10 μg) prepared from primary cultures of human hepatocytes treated for 30 hours with extracts prepared from three different commercial preparations of SJW [extract 1, Nature's Way (9 μg/mL); extract 2, Nature's Plus (75 μg/mL); extract 3, Solaray (7 μg/mL)], 1 μM hyperforin, or vehicle alone (0.1% ethanol). The blot was probed sequentially with ^{32}P-labeled fragments of CYP3A4 and β-actin. *Abbreviations*: SJW, St. John's wort; CYP, cytochrome P450. *Source*: From Ref. 42.

of around 20 nM and is one of the most potent inducers discovered to date (42). In vitro studies indicate that other constituents of St. John's wort, such as hypericin, kampferol, pseudohypericin, and hyperoside, are not PXR ligands and thus do not contribute to the enhanced CYP3A4 mRNA expression (Table 2) (42). Likewise, Wentworth et al., using a reporter gene construct containing the ligand-binding domain of the CYP3A promoter, determined that hyperforin but not hypericin was capable of activating CYP3A transcription when coexpressed with the steroid X receptor, which is synonymous with PXR. Hyperforin but not hypericin interacts directly with the receptor ligand–binding domain of PXR and contributes to the recruitment of steroid receptor coactivator-1 with an efficiency that is comparable to that of rifampicin (44). In addition, hyperforin has been shown to induce other PXR-responsive genes, such as CYP2C9, CYP2C19, CYP2B6, and p-glycoprotein (MDR-1), by mechanisms that may involve both the PXR- and the constitutive androstane receptor (CAR)-responsive elements, but the extent of induction of these genes is modest compared to that of CYP3A (45–48). In the case of the CYP2C9 gene, a PXR-responsive element was identified –1839/–1824 base pairs upstream from translation start site at the same location as the CAR-responsive element (46). Komoroski et al. reported increased mRNA and protein expression and catalytic activity following exposure of human hepatocytes to hyperforin, confirming the in vivo observations (*vide infra*) concerning CYP2C9 and CYP3A4 induction by St. John's wort (49). The treatment of human hepatocytes with hyperforin did not alter CYP1A2 expression (mRNA and protein) or catalytic activity (49). In vitro, studies using LS-180 cells have demonstrated that hyperforin was capable of inducing the PXR-dependent expression of P-glycoprotein by western blot analysis, and functionally reduced the cellular uptake of the P-glycoprotein substrate, rhodamine 123 (50).

The Role of CYP3A in Drug Interactions

The most abundant CYPs in humans belong to the CYP3A subfamily, which accounts for up to 60% of total hepatic and up to 90% of total intestinal CYP (51–53). Like other CYPs, CYP3A family members are heme-containing proteins that along with the conjugating enzymes, such as the sulfotransferases (SULTs) and glucuronosyltransferases (UGTs), are instrumental in metabolizing a wide variety of endogenous and exogenous agents (52,54). The human CYP3A subfamily includes four members, namely CYP3A4, CYP3A5, CYP3A7, and CYP3A43 (54–57). CYP3A4 is abundantly expressed in all adults and is responsible for the metabolism of a wide variety of structurally diverse chemicals including macrolide antibiotics, 3-hydroxy-3-methylgluatryl coenzyme A (HMG-CoA)–reductase inhibitors, HIV protease inhibitors, benzodiazepines, and immunosuppressants. It has been estimated that approximately 40% to 50% of drugs requiring metabolism for elimination undergo biotransformation by CYP3A4 (58–60). The CYP3A5*1 gene product is detected in about 30% of Caucasian and 70% of African-American human livers and intestines and has comparable catalytic activity and substrate selectivity to CYP3A4, although there are important exceptions to this generalization (61,62). CYP3A7 is expressed only in fetal tissue and the level of expression and catalytic activity of CYP3A43 are extremely low and consequently, an important role for these enzymes in drug metabolism is not anticipated (52,57,63).

The expression of CYP3A4 and CYP3A5 at both the intestine and liver results in a greater first-pass removal of CYP3A substrates than would be predicted if the liver was the sole organ of removal. For example, the CYP3A substrates cyclosporine, nifedipine, midazolam, and verapamil exhibit low oral bioavailability because of the substantial contribution of both intestinal wall and hepatic metabolism to their first-pass elimination in man (64–70). In view of the broad substrate selectivity, along with expression in both the enterocyte and hepatocyte, it is not surprising that modulation of CYP3A expression and activity by environment, disease, and other drugs, such as St. John's wort, is a significant public health issue with implications in regard to drug safety and efficacy. The remaining portion of the chapter will review the reported interactions between St. John's wort and prescription medications.

Interactions with CYP3A Substrates

Anticancer Agents

Irinotecan is a topoisomerase-I inhibitor, which is used in the treatment of colorectal and non–small cell lung cancer. Individuals diagnosed with cancer routinely become depressed and may require pharmacotherapy with prescription or botanical antidepressants. Mathijssen et al. reported that the disposition of 7-ethyl-10-hydroxycamptothecin (SN-38), the active metabolite of irinotecan, was altered following coadministration of St. John's wort to five individuals (71). SN-38 levels were reduced 43%, while plasma concentrations of irinotecan remained unaltered (71). The formation of a CYP3A-mediated metabolite of SN-38, 7-ethyl-10-[4-*N*-(5-aminopentanoic acid)-1-piperidino]-carbonyl-oxy-camptothecin (APC), did not appear to be significantly altered, although the APC/irinotecan serum ratio was reduced by 28% (71). Likewise, SN-38 glucuronidation was not altered by St. John's wort (71). The investigators concluded that St. John's wort and irinotecan should not be coadministered.

Imatinib is an inhibitor of the protein tyrosine kinase involved with platelet-derived growth factor (Bcr-ABL). A loss of cellular control of this tyrosine kinase has been identified as a key mechanism for malignant cell growth. The ability of imatinib to inhibit Bcr-ABL provides a rationale for its use in the treatment of human cancers such as Philadelphia chromosome–positive chronic myologenous leukemia. CYP3A4 plays a principal role in the biotransformation of imatinib (72). The effect of St. John's wort on imatinib disposition was investigated in 12 healthy volunteers using a two-period, open-labeled, fixed-sequence study by Frye et al. (73). Imatinib (400 mg) was administered before and after the administration of St. John's wort [300 mg; Kira (LI 160), Lichtwer Pharma AG, Berlin, Germany] three times a day for 14 days. The administration of St. John's wort resulted in 30% reduction in imatinib exposure from 34.5 ± 9.5 to $24.2 \pm 7.0 \, \mu g \, hr/mL$ (73). A corresponding 43% increase in the oral clearance of imatinib was observed following St. John's wort dosing. Frye et al. concluded that the imatinib–St. John's wort (drug–botanical product) interaction is clinically significant and may result in a loss of imatinib efficacy.

Anticonvulsants

Carbamazepine is a dibenzazepine carboxamide derivative that is used to treat epilepsy and other neurologic conditions. A substrate of CYP3A, carbamazepine, is also recognized as a potent in vivo and in vitro inducer of CYP3A4 (74–77). Induction of CYP3A4 by carbamazepine is mediated at least in part through activation of PXR, although other mechanisms such as glucocorticoid receptor–activation have been proposed (78,79). The effect of St. John's wort administration (300 mg t.i.d. × 14 days) on carbamazepine disposition at steady state was examined in eight healthy adults (80). The oral clearance of carbamazepine ($2.8 \pm 0.3 \, L/hr$) was not significantly altered by St. John's wort ($2.9 \pm 0.6 \, L/hr$) administration. Likewise, the area under the plasma concentration–time curve (AUC) at steady state of the CYP3A4-mediated metabolite carbamazepine 10,11-epoxide was not altered by St. John's wort dosing (37.5 ± 7.4 vs. $41.9 \pm 10.9 \, mg \, hr/L$) (80). These data indicate that a 14-day course of therapy with St. John's wort does not enhance the elimination of carbamazepine. This may reflect a lack of influence of intestinal CYP3A4 on carbamazepine disposition, given that the oral availability of carbamazepine approaches unity. In addition, the product used in this study may have lacked sufficient quantities of hyperforin to induce hepatic CYP3A4 activity. Also, many anticonvulsants (phenobarbital, carbamazepine, and phenytoin) are CYP3A inducers and modulate their own pharmacokinetics via enzyme induction. The lack of effect of St. John's wort on carbamazepine disposition may therefore reflect the possibility that the enzyme system (CYP3A4) is already close to maximal induction.

Antihypertensives

Nifedipine is a dihydropyridine calcium channel modulator, often used in the treatment of hypertension and angina. CYP3A4, with a minor contribution from CYP3A5, is the principal enzyme involved in the metabolism of nifedipine (81). Smith et al. examined the effect of St. John's wort (900 mg/day for 18 days) on nifedipine disposition by examining changes in C_{MAX} in 22 healthy volunteers (82). St. John's wort coadministration reduced the maximum nifedipine plasma concentration obtained by approximately 50%, following a 10 mg oral dose (82). It is to be expected that other dihydropyridine calcium channel blockers that rely on CYP3A for their metabolism (e.g., isradapine and nimodipine) will be similarly affected by St. John's wort administration.

Verapamil is a diphenylalkylamine calcium channel modulator that is widely used in the treatment of hypertension, angina, and cardiac arrhythmias. Verapamil is extensively metabolized by the CYP3A enzymes. Tannergren et al. examined the effect of St. John's wort on the jejunal transport and presystemic extraction of single-dose verapamil in eight healthy male volunteers using a fixed-order design (control–treatment) (83). St. John's wort (Movina™, Boehringer Ingelheim, Germany) 300 mg was administered three times daily for 14 days. The administration of St. John's wort did not alter the cellular permeability of verapamil, but did increase the excretion of the CYP3A-mediated metabolite norverapamil into the intestine. Furthermore, jejunal transport of the verapamil enantiomers was not altered by St. John's wort pretreatment. St. John's wort administration resulted in an 89% reduction in *R*- and *S*-verapamil plasma concentrations. Verapamil has also been shown to inactivate CYP3A4 through the formation of a metabolic intermediate complex and is also a modest inducer of CYP3A4 (84). The effect of St. John's wort on the disposition of verapamil at steady state has not been assessed and is not readily predictable from single-dose data. Unless proven otherwise, it would be prudent to expect that the coadministration of St. John's wort with verapamil will result in decreased verapamil concentrations and possibly efficacy.

Antiretroviral Agents

Indinavir is a protease inhibitor used in the management of HIV infection. CYP3A4 mediates the biotransformation of indinavir in vitro (85,86), and in vivo, indinavir has been shown to be a potent competitive and mechanism-based inhibitor of CYP3A4 (85,87). Piscitelli and coworkers (80) examined the effect of St. John's wort (300 mg t.i.d. × 14 days) administration on indinavir (800 mg q.i.d. × 8 hr × four doses) exposure in eight healthy volunteers (two females). The administration of St. John's wort for 14 days resulted in a significant 54% reduction in the indinavir eight-hour area under the concentration–time curve, from 35.8 ± 13.0 to $15.6 \pm 5.8 \, \mu g \times hr/mL$. The authors conclude that the magnitude in the reduction in indinavir concentrations may result in the development of antiretroviral resistance and subsequent treatment failure.

Nevirapine is a non-nucleoside reverse transcriptase inhibitor used in the treatment of AIDS. Elimination of nevirapine from the body occurs via P-glycoprotein, and it is extensively metabolized by the CYPs (88). In addition, nevirapine dosing is known to increase CYP3A and CYP2B6 enzymes by approximately 25%. This induction appears to be mediated by the orphan nuclear factor PXR. de Maat et al. reported data from five HIV-1–infected individuals who were treated with nevirapine and coadministered St. John's wort for several months (89). The median oral clearance of nevirapine for all patients (n = 171) was 3.2 L/hr (range 2.7–3.9); for the five individuals taking St. John's wort, the median oral clearance of nevirapine on St. John's wort was 4.3 (range 3.8–4.7 L/hr), whereas the median oral clearance without St. John's wort coadministration was 3.3 L/hr (range 3.2–4.2 L/hr) (89). The authors concluded that the coadministration of St. John's wort resulted in a 35% increase in median oral clearance of nevirapine and that dose adjustment is indicated (89).

Benzodiazepines

Midazolam: Midazolam is a 1,4-imidazobenzodiazepine that is widely employed therapeutically as a sedative/hypnotic in major and minor surgical procedures. In humans, midazolam is primarily eliminated from the body by CYP3A-mediated metabolism to the major primary metabolite, 1-hydroxymidazolam, and to a much lesser extent to 4-hydroxymidazolam (90,91). Midazolam is widely used as a selective metabolic probe for assessing CYP3A activity in vivo, because it is not a substrate for the P-glycoprotein efflux transporter (92,93). Following intravenous administration, less than 1% of the dose is excreted unchanged in the urine (94). Consequently, the clearance of midazolam following intravenous administration has proven to be an effective index of hepatic CYP3A activity in vivo. Up to 75% of the first-pass loss of midazolam following oral administration occurs in the intestinal wall using the simultaneous administration of oral and intravenous drug (69,70,95,96). Additionally, approximately 90% of the variability in oral availability was accounted for by variations in intestinal availability alone (70,95–97).

Wang et al. demonstrated that multiple-dose St. John's wort dosing resulted in a 50% reduction in the midazolam oral AUC and maximum serum drug concentration and a corresponding doubling of the oral clearance, from 122 ± 71 to 255 ± 128 L/hr (Table 3) (24). In contrast, the systemic clearance of midazolam increased from 34.3 ± 10.8 to 43.6 ± 15.8 L/hr, but this change was not significant (Table 3) (24). The oral bioavailability demonstrated a significant decrease from 0.28 ± 0.15 to 0.17 ± 0.06, but changes in hepatic and intestinal availability were not significant. Similar results were observed following St. John's wort administration for eight weeks in a group of 12 women (Table 3). Figure 5 illustrates the relationship between the changes in midazolam disposition observed by Wang et al. and Hall et al. and the hepatic and intestinal CYP3A expression (24,25). These changes are in good agreement with the observation of Dürr et al. who

Table 3 The Effect of SJW on the Disposition of the Prototypic CYP3A Substrate Midazolam

Study	Study phase	Midazolam systemic clearance (L/hr)	Midazolam oral clearance (L/hr)	Midazolam bioavailability (%)
Dresser et al. (98)	Control	22.9 ± 6.1	70.9 ± 20.8	33 ± 6
	SJW	32.4 ± 6.8^a	183.8 ± 48.5^a	18 ± 5^a
Wang et al. (24)	Control	34.3 ± 10.8	121.8 ± 70.7	28 ± 15
	SJW	43.6 ± 15.8	254.5 ± 127.8^a	17 ± 6^a
Hall et al. (25)	Control	37.7 ± 11.3	109.2 ± 47.8	43 ± 28
	SJW	39.0 ± 10.3	166.7 ± 81.3^a	28 ± 15^a

[a]Significantly different to control value as reported by the investigators.
Abbreviations: CYP, cytochrome P450; SJW, St. John's wort.

reported a 1.5-fold increase in intestinal CYP3A4 expression and a 1.4-fold increase in erythromycin breath test (99).

Dresser et al. administered St. John's wort (LI 160 300 mg t.i.d.) to 20 ethnically diverse individuals and observed a 44% increase in the systemic clearance of midazolam (Table 3) (98). In contrast, the oral clearance of midazolam was increased 1.7-fold (Table 3). The combined changes in midazolam disposition resulted in a significant reduction in the oral bioavailability of midazolam (Table 3). Gurley et al. examined the one-hour 1-hydroxymidazolam-to-midazolam serum ratio and concluded that St. John's wort administration for 28 days resulted in a significant increase in the ratio, which is indicative of CYP3A4 induction (100).

Alprazolam: Markowitz et al. initially reported that St. John's wort administration did not alter the disposition of alprazolam following oral dosing (101). It was subsequently determined that the duration of St. John's wort administration (three days) was insufficient to demonstrate the inductive effects of this botanical medicine on CYP3A4. In a follow-up study in which St. John's wort was administered for 14 days, there was more than a doubling of the oral clearance of alprazolam, from 3.7 ± 0.9 to 8.4 ± 3.2 L/hr (102). There was also a corresponding reduction in the elimination half-life by approximately 50%, from 12 ± 4 to 6.0 ± 2.0 hours. However, the maximum plasma concentration and the time to maximum concentration were not significantly different before and after St. John's wort dosing. The change in oral clearance is consistent with a change in the systemic elimination but not first-pass elimination of alprazolam, because the maximum serum alprazolam concentration achieved was not significantly different before and after St. John's wort administration (102). This is to be expected, considering that the oral bioavailability of alprazolam is high (≥ 0.8), which is consistent with alprazolam being a low-affinity substrate for CYP3A4 (103).

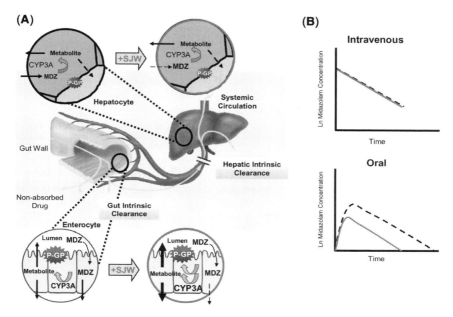

Figure 5 Schematic representation of the effect of SJW (300 mg t.i.d. × 14 days) administration on the expression of CYP3A4 at intestinal and hepatic sites and on the disposition of midazolam following intravenous and oral dosing. (**A**) Factors influencing midazolam bioavailability following oral dosing including nonadsorbed drug (negligible) and presystemic elimination (gut intrinsic clearance, $E \approx 0.5$ and hepatic intrinsic clearance, $E \approx 0.3$). Following intravenous dosing, the systemic clearance of midazolam is mediated solely by hepatic CYP3A4 (hepatic intrinsic clearance, $E \approx 0.3$). The *lower left inset* depicts the intestinal CYP3A4 biotransformation of midazolam in the absence of SJW, whereas the *upper left inset* shows the CYP3A4 metabolism of midazolam in the hepatocyte. Treatment of individuals with SJW (300 mg t.i.d. × 14 days) results in alteration of intestinal but not hepatic CYP3A4 expression and activity (see *upper* and *lower insets* outlined in *gray*). The increased expression and activity of intestinal CYP3A4 following SJW dosing results in a reduced exposure to midazolam following oral administration (**B**, *lower graph*) but not intravenous administration (**B**, *upper graph*). *Dashed black lines* represent the disposition of midazolam prior to the administration of SJW. The *solid gray lines* represent the disposition of midazolam after the administration of SJW (300 mg t.i.d. × 14 days). *Abbreviations*: SJW, St. John's wort; CYP, cytochrome P450; P-GP, P-glycoprotein; MDZ, midazolam.

HMG-CoA–Reductase Inhibitors

Sugimoto et al. examined the effect of St. John's wort administration (300 mg three times a day for 14 days) on the disposition of simvastatin and pravastatin in 16 healthy male Japanese subjects in a double-blind crossover study (104). The administration of St. John's wort significantly reduced the mean maximum plasma concentration from 3.6 ± 1.0 to 2.5 ± 0.7 after oral simvastatin (10 mg) dosing and a corresponding 48% reduction in the mean systemic exposure to simvastatin, from 11.1 ± 3.7 to 5.8 ± 1.8 ng hr/mL. The authors reported similar results for the active metabolite (simvastatin hydroxy acid) of simvastatin. In contrast to the significant changes observed with simvastatin, St. John's wort administration (300 mg three times a day for 14 days) did not significantly alter the mean maximum plasma concentration achieved following pravastatin (20 mg) administration (36.5 ± 5.7 ng/mL before vs. 30.8 ± 5.2 ng/mL after). Likewise, significant differences in the mean systemic exposure to pravastatin were not observed following placebo (109.4 ± 17.4 ng hr/mL) and St. John's wort (96.6 ± 13.4 ng hr/mL) dosing. The differences reflect the fact that simvastatin is a substrate for CYP3A4 and P-glycoprotein, whereas pravastatin is not a substrate for either CYP3A or P-glycoprotein (MDR1) (26,105,106). Similar effects are expected for other HMG-CoA–reductase inhibitors, such as lovastatin, cerivastatin, and atorvastatin, which rely on CYP3A4 and P-glycoprotein for their distribution and elimination. In the case of the CYP2C9 substrate, fluvastatin, a drug interaction between St. John's wort and fluvastatin is expected to be at most modest, even though there is evidence that St. John's wort alters CYP2C9 expression in vitro (46,49). This is because Wang et al. did not observe an alteration in the disposition of the prototypic CYP2C9 probe drug, tolbutamide, in a group of 12 healthy volunteers (24).

Immunosuppressants

Cyclosporine is a calcineurin-inhibitor immunosuppressant that is in part metabolized by CYP3A4/5 and transported by P-glycoprotein (MDR1). Coadministration of St. John's wort with cyclosporine has resulted in significant reduction in circulating cyclosporine concentrations, which has led to graft rejection (Fig. 6) (108). Breidenbach et al. reported a series of 30 renal transplant recipients who were stabilized on cyclosporine and subsequently administered St. John's wort (109). Following initiation of St. John's wort therapy, blood cyclosporine concentrations were reduced 47% (range: 33–62%) and the corresponding cyclosporine doses were increased on average 47% (15–115%), to maintain therapeutic cyclosporine blood concentrations (109). Cessation of St. John's wort dosing resulted in a 187% (84–292%) rise in blood cyclosporine concentration, which required subsequent cyclosporine dose adjustment. Figure 6 shows the fall of cyclosporine blood concentrations in two kidney transplant recipients during St. John's wort administration, despite increases in cyclosporine dose (107). These changes have been confirmed by others (110). Barone et al. reported the occurrence of acute graft rejection in two kidney transplant patients and Ruschitzka et al. reported a similar loss of immunosuppression

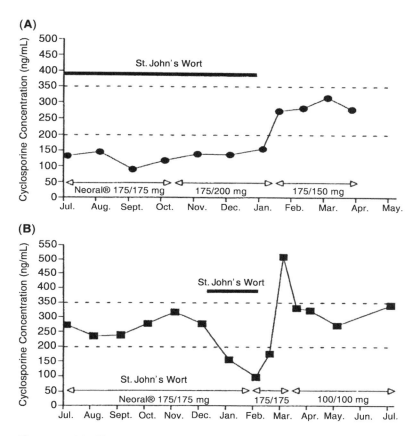

Figure 6 (**A**) Chronology (July 1999–May 2000) of CSA trough concentrations in patient 1 self-medicating with SJW (*dotted lines* = desired CSA therapeutic range). (**B**) Chronology (July 1998–July 1999) of CSA trough concentrations in patient 2 self-medicating with SJW (*dotted lines* = desired CSA therapeutic range). *Abbreviations*: SJW, St. John's wort; CSA, cyclosporine. *Source*: From Ref. 107.

in cardiac transplant patients (6,107,111). Bauer et al. also examined the effect of St. John's wort administration on the disposition of cyclosporine and its metabolites in 11 renal allograft recipients. St. John's wort was administered for 15 days and cyclosporine plasma concentrations were adjusted every four days by assessing trough concentrations. The investigators demonstrated that St. John's wort administration resulted in a 45% decrease in cyclosporine exposure compared to baseline. Likewise, metabolite exposure was altered significantly following St. John's wort administration with metabolites AM1c and AM1, demonstrating a 60% decrease after dose correction, but exposure to the metabolites AM9 and AM19 was not affected

(112). In addition, the interaction between cyclosporine and St. John's wort was confirmed by Dresser et al., with the oral clearance increasing 63% from 728 ± 195 to $1155 \pm 236 \, \text{mL/min}$ (98).

Tacrolimus is a calcineurin-inhibitor immunosuppressive used to prevent organ rejection following kidney and liver transplantation. The disposition of tacrolimus, like cyclosporine, is dependent on both CYP3A activity and P-glycoprotein activity. Circulating tacrolimus concentrations were reduced following the administration of St. John's wort (113–115). Hebert et al. examined the effect of St. John's wort (300 mg t.i.d. × 18 days; LI 160, Lichtwer Pharma AG, Berlin, Germany) coadministration on the oral disposition of tacrolimus (114). The oral clearance of tacrolimus increased from 349 ± 126 to $586 \pm 275 \, \text{mL/hr/kg}$ and a corresponding 35% decrease in the AUC from 307 ± 176 to $199 \pm 140 \, \mu\text{g hr/L}$ was observed (114). The disposition pharmacokinetics of the adjunct agent, mycophenolic acid, was not altered following coadministration with St. John's wort (115). It is clear from these reports that individuals who require immunosuppressive therapy to maintain transplanted organ function should not receive St. John's wort.

Opioids

Methadone is a long-acting opiate that is used in the treatment of opiate addiction and for analgesia. Eich-Hochli et al. described four addicts in whom St. John's wort (Jarsin) was coadministered with three daily doses of methadone (116). The administration of St. John's wort (900 mg/day) for 14 to 47 days (median 31 days) resulted in trough methadone concentrations, which were a median of 47% (range 19–60%) of the original concentration. The observed changes in methadone serum concentrations were not enantiomer selective, because both *R*- and *S*-methadone trough concentrations demonstrated reductions of similar magnitude (116). Two female patients reported symptoms suggestive of withdrawal and requested increases in their methadone dose.

Oral Contraceptives

Oral contraceptives are combination products that are typically used to prevent pregnancy. The combination of an estrogen (17-alphaethinylestradiol) and a progestin (e.g., norethindrone) is used to prevent the release of the oocyte (egg) and to alter the cervical mucous and lining of the uterus. Drugs that induce CYP3A enzymes have been associated with reduced oral contraceptive efficacy or even failure (117,118). The metabolism of the components of oral contraceptives, ethinylestradiol and norethindrone, is thought to be catalyzed at least in part by intestinal and hepatic CYP3A (119,120). A number of reports have indicated that St. John's wort may be responsible for the occurrence of breakthrough bleeding in women formerly stabilized on oral contraceptives (121). In addition, "miracle babies" have been identified in the lay press to be a result of St. John's wort consumption (122,123). Furthermore, Schwarz et al. reported oral contraceptive failure in four women after St. John's wort coadministration, which resulted in the termination of the unwanted pregnancies (124). Subsequently, Hall et al. examined the effect of St. John's wort administration on the disposition and efficacy of the oral contraceptive components, ethinylestradiol and norethindrone (Ortho-Novum 1/35), in 12 healthy females (25). St. John's wort (Sundown Herbals) was administered three times a day for eight weeks. The pharmacokinetics of ethinylestradiol and norethindrone (CYP3A substrates) were assessed before and six weeks after the start of the St. John's wort dosing. St. John's wort significantly ($P \leq 0.05$) increased the oral clearance of norethindrone from 8.2 ± 2.7 to 9.5 ± 2.4 L/hr, with a corresponding decrease in the peak serum concentration of norethindrone (from 17.4 ± 5.1 to 16.4 ± 5.2 ng/mL; $P < 0.05$) (25). Likewise, the elimination half-life of ethinylestradiol was significantly reduced from 23 ± 20 to 12 ± 7 hours (25). Furthermore, the incidence of breakthrough bleeding increased with the duration of St. John's wort administration with 7 of 12 individuals having breakthrough bleeding compared to two individuals prior to initiation of St. John's wort dosing. In good agreement with the observation of Hall et al., Pfrunder et al. reported that St. John's wort given twice daily or three times a day resulted in a greater incidence in breakthrough bleeding, 13/17 or 15/17, respectively, compared to oral contraceptive (20 µg ethinylestradiol and 150 µg desogestrel) dosing alone (125). Although, pharmacokinetic changes were not observed for ethinylestradiol, the maximum plasma concentration and the AUC of 3-ketodesogestrel decreased 18% and 44%, respectively, during twice-daily dosing of St. John's wort (125). It is clear that the combination of St. John's wort with oral contraceptive has resulted in the induction of norethindrone clearance, increased incidence of breakthrough bleeding, and reports of unplanned pregnancy and resultant termination. Thus, the coadministration of St. John's wort in women taking oral contraceptives is contraindicated and should be discouraged. To prevent this interaction, it is the author's opinion that all St. John's wort products must clearly carry warning labels concerning the potential for St. John's wort to alter the efficacy of oral contraceptives and of many other prescription products.

Interactions with Substrates of Other P450s

Theophylline

Theophylline is a bronchodilator that is commonly used to treat the symptoms of chronic asthma. The principal enzyme involved in the biotransformation of theophylline is CYP1A2 (126). In a case report, Nebel et al. described an individual who required theophylline dosage adjustment following the initiation and cessation of St. John's wort pharmacotherapy (127). The dose of theophylline (Theodur™) was increased from 300 mg twice daily to 800 mg twice daily following the initiation of St. John's wort intake. The resultant steady-state theophylline concentration was 9.2 μg/mL. Subsequently, termination of St. John's wort resulted in a twofold increase in serum theophylline concentration and necessitated dose reduction. Preliminary in vitro experiments conducted suggested that hypericin and pseudohypericin were capable of activating the xenobiotic response element, which is responsible in part for CYP1A2 induction. However, it should be noted the individual described in the case report by Nebel et al. was a smoker taking a multitude of other medications, including furosemide, morphine, zolpidem, valproic acid, ibuprofen, amitriptyline, albuterol, prednisone, and zafirlukast. Zafirlukast has been shown to be an inhibitor of theophylline both in vitro and in vivo (128,129). Thus, the observed changes in theophylline disposition may be a result of St. John's wort altering the disposition of one of the many concurrent medications. In addition, a study by Morimoto et al. failed to confirm the observation of Nebel et al. Briefly, Morimoto et al. examined the potential for St. John's wort to alter the disposition of theophylline in vivo by conducting a randomized open-label crossover study (130). The oral clearance of theophylline was determined in 12 healthy Japanese men before and after 15 days of St. John's wort administration (300 mg three times daily). St. John's wort did not alter the oral clearance of theophylline (2.3 ± 0.6 L/hr vs. 2.4 ± 0.6 L/hr) (130).

Caffeine

Caffeine is a methylxanthine that is a central nervous system stimulant found in a number of beverages such as coffee, tea, soda (Pepsi™, Coke™, Mountain Dew™, etc.), and over-the-counter products (Vivarin™, NoDoz™, etc.). Caffeine is principally metabolized to paraxanthine by CYP1A2 and the six-hour plasma ratio (paraxanthine to caffeine) has been used as an index of in vivo CYP1A2 activity (131–133). The administration of St. John's wort (300 mg three times daily) for two weeks did not alter the disposition of caffeine (24). In the same study, Wang et al. reported that a single dose of St. John's wort (900 mg) did not affect the oral clearance of caffeine (24). Likewise, Wenk et al. examined the effect of 14 days of St. John's wort administration (300 mg t.i.d., $n = 16$) on the in vivo activities of CYP3A4, CYP1A2, and CYP2D6 using 6β-hydroxycortisol-to-cortisol urinary ratio, paraxanthine-to-caffeine salivary ratio, and dextromethorphan-to-dextrorphan urinary metabolic ratio, respectively (134). The mean values for the salivary estimates of CYP1A2 were not significantly altered by treatment with St. John's wort (134). This observation is in good agreement with the observation of Morimoto et al. with St. John's wort and theophylline (*supra vide*) (130). In addition, Komoroski et al. noted that hyperforin did not alter the mRNA expression, protein expression, or catalytic activity of CYP1A2 in human hepatocytes (49). These observations taken together suggest that interactions between CYP1A2 substrates and St. John's wort are unlikely.

Omeprazole

H. perforatum II 300 mg (Hypericum Buyer's club) was used in assessing the effect of St. John's wort on the pharmacokinetics of a single dose of omeprazole (135). A placebo-controlled randomized crossover study was conducted over a five-week period in 12 individuals. Six individuals had CYP2C19 $*1/*1$ and six individuals had either $*2/*2$ ($n = 4$) or $*2/*3$ ($n = 2$) genotypes. The sulfoxidation of omeprazole is mediated primarily by CYP3A4 and the 5-hydroxylation of omeprazole is mediated principally by CYP2C19. Administration of St. John's wort 300 mg three times a day for 14 days resulted in a significant reduction in the AUC of omeprazole in both homozygous wild-type individuals and homozygous variant individuals. A corresponding increase in the principal metabolites for both CYP2C19 (5-hydroxyomeprazole) and CYP3A4 (omeprazole sulfone)-mediated biotransformations demonstrated increased AUCs following St. John's wort administration. The authors suggest that the study provides evidence for in vivo CYP2C19 induction by St. John's wort (47).

Warfarin

Warfarin is an anticoagulant that is administered as a racemic mixture with the *S*-enantiomer having most of the pharmacologic activity. Warfarin is extensively metabolized in the liver by CYP2C9 with 7-hydroxylation being the principal route of metabolism for the *S*-enantiomer. *R*-warfarin is 8-hydroxylated, 6-hydroxylated, and 10-hydroxylated by CYP2C19, CYP1A2, and CYP3A4, respectively. Likewise, additional enzymes are involved in the metabolism of the *S*-warfarin, namely CYP3A4 and CYP1A2. In light of the overlap between the P450s involved in warfarin metabolism and those affected by St. John's wort, namely CYP2C9, CYP2C19, and CYP3A4, it is clear that an interaction between St. John's wort and warfarin is possible. To determine the potential for interaction, Jiang et al. examined the effect of St. John's wort administration on the pharmacokinetics and pharmacodynamics of warfarin (25 mg) administered to 12 healthy male volunteers (136). The oral clearance of *S*- and *R*-warfarin was increased 36% and 29%, from 198 ± 38 to 270 ± 44 mL/min and from 110 ± 25 to 142 ± 29 mL/min, respectively. A corresponding reduction in the pharmacodynamic effect was observed with St. John's wort (one tablet three times a day for two weeks) dosing, significantly reducing the area under the effect curve of the international normalized ratio of prothrombin time by approximately 20% from 111 ± 49.3 to 88.3 ± 30.7 (136). Although the data quite clearly indicate that St. John's wort and warfarin should not be coadministered, the enzyme(s) responsible for the increased clearance of *S*- and *R*-warfarin in vivo cannot be determined, because changes in metabolite formation were not assessed. Thus, it is possible that the observed changes in *S*- and *R*-warfarin clearance were a result of a St. John's wort–mediated induction of CYP2C9, CYP2C19, CYP3A4, or some combination of these enzymes.

The Role of P-Glycoprotein in St. Johns's Wort Interaction

Fexofenadine

Fexofenadine is a nonsedating antihistamine that has been shown to be transported by P-glycoprotein (MDR1) and organic anion transport polypeptide in vitro using cell culture models and MDR1 knockout animals (137). Wang et al. demonstrated that the administration of St. John's wort for 14 days resulted in a significant increase in the oral clearance of fexofenadine observed after a single 900 mg dose of St. John's wort, from 62 ± 26 L/hr to 91 ± 32 L/hr (138). In good agreement with the observations of Wang et al., Dresser et al. observed a significant reduction in the maximum plasma concentration and a 94% increase in the oral clearance of fexofenadine following the administration of St. John's wort (Jarsin 300 three times daily for two weeks) (98). The increase in the oral clearance of fexofenadine reported by these two groups is consistent with PXR-mediated induction of P-glycoprotein (MDR1) by St. John's wort.

Digoxin

Digoxin is a cardiac glycoside that is used traditionally in the treatment of congestive heart failure and is a substrate of the transporter P-glycoprotein. Johne et al. conducted a single-blind, placebo-controlled parallel study in 25 healthy volunteers (12 women). Volunteers were given a 0.25 mg loading dose of digoxin followed by 0.125 mg daily for 10 days. On day 6 of digoxin dosing, a single 900 mg (three tablet) dose of St. John's wort (LI 160) or placebo was administered and on day 15 of digoxin dosing (10 days of St. John's wort or placebo), the pharmacokinetic study was repeated. Single dose of St. John's wort had no effect on the pharmacokinetics of digoxin (139). In contrast, 10 days of St. John's wort dosing resulted in significant 25% decrease in the AUC from 0 to 24 hours and a corresponding 24% decrease in the maximum plasma concentration. Treatment with placebo did not alter the pharmacokinetic parameters of digoxin. Likewise, Dürr et al. demonstrated an 18% reduction in digoxin exposure with a corresponding increase in intestinal P-glycoprotein/MDR1 and CYP3A4 (99). In agreement with the above results, Mueller et al. reported that hyperforin-rich St. John's wort products (i.e., LI 160) resulted in a significant 25%

reduction in the 24-hour area under the digoxin concentration–time curve (140). The observation with fexofenadine and digoxin are in good agreement. It is clear that P-glycoprotein, along with CYP3A4, provides a competent barrier to the absorption of xenobiotics. The administration of St. John's wort for a period of two weeks results in a reduction in drug exposure due to the increased efflux activity of P-glycoprotein at the brush border membrane of enterocytes. For drugs that are not substrates of CYP3A, the increased expression of P-glycoprotein results in a reduced bioavailability

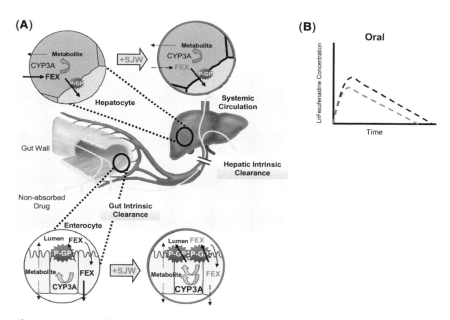

Figure 7 The effect of SJW administration on the expression and activity of P-glycoprotein and the disposition of fexofenadine following oral dosing. (**A**) Factors influencing fexofenadine bioavailability following oral dosing, including nonadsorbed drug and presystemic elimination and hepatic intrinsic clearance. Following oral dosing, the oral clearance of fexofenadine is controlled in part by intestinal and hepatic P-glycoprotein. The *lower left inset* depicts intestinal P-glycoprotein transport of fexofenadine in the absence of SJW whereas the *upper left inset* shows hepatic P-glycoprotein transport of fexofenadine. Treatment of individuals with SJW (300 mg t.i.d. × 14 days) results in alteration of intestinal but not hepatic P-glycoprotein expression and activity (see *upper* and *lower insets* outlined in *gray*). (**B**) The increased expression and activity of intestinal P-glycoprotein following SJW dosing results in a reduced exposure to fexofenadine following oral administration. *Dashed black lines* represent the disposition of fexofenadine prior to the administration of SJW. The *solid gray lines* represent the disposition of fexofenadine after the administration of SJW (300 mg t.i.d. × 14 days). *Abbreviations*: P-GP, P-glycoprotein; SJW, St. John's wort; CYP, cytochrome P450; FEX, fexofenadine.

but no change in the elimination half-life. This pattern of interaction is suggestive of an alteration in first-pass elimination but not systemic clearance. Figure 7 illustrates the relationship between changes in intestinal and hepatic P-glycoprotein expression and the disposition of fexofenadine (138).

ECHINACEA

Echinacea is a widely available over-the-counter botanical remedy used for the treatment of the common cold, coughs, bronchitis, "flu," and inflammation of the mouth and pharynx (141–144). It is one of the more popular botanical remedies with a sales ranking of 5 and sales of US $70 million (4). About 10% to 20% of the adult and child botanical users consume *echinacea* routinely (145–149). Three species of *echinacea* (*Echinacea purpurea*, *E. angustinfolia*, and *E. pallida*) have been used medicinally (141). However, only the aboveground parts of *E. purpura* and the root of *E. pallida* have been approved for oral administration by the German E Commission (7).

The beneficial effect of *echinacea* in the treatment of infections appears to be a result of its ability to stimulate the host's immune system. Following exposure to *echinacea*, macrophages and T-lymphocytes demonstrate increased phagocytic activity and release of immunomodulators such as tumor necrosis factor-α and interferons (150,151). Although the exact mechanism of *echinacea* immunostimulatory effect is unknown, controlled studies suggest that the oral administration of *echinacea* is beneficial in the early treatment of upper respiratory infections (152). However, this observation is still controversial and the usefulness of long-term *echinacea* administration to prevent illness appears to be limited (153). Although *echinacea* appears to be well tolerated following acute and chronic dosing, the unsupervised self-medication by patients in an effort to cure, ameliorate, and/or prevent sickness provides the potential for a multitude of drug–botanical product interactions.

Budzinski et al. examined the capability of 5% to 10% (v/v) dilutions of marketed *echinacea* tinctures to inhibit the metabolism of 7-benzyloxyresorufin by cDNA-expressed CYP3A4 (43). The relative inhibitory concentration, in relation to the full-strength product for *E. angustifolia* roots, *E. purpurea* roots, *E. angustifolia/purpurea* mixture (1:1), and *E. purpurea* tops was 1.1%, 4.0%, 6.7%, and 8.6%, respectively (43). The effect of these *echinacea* extracts on the in vitro catalytic activity of other drug-metabolizing enzymes (e.g., CYP1A2, CYP2C9, and CYP2D6) has not been assessed. However, extracts of teas prepared from combination products containing *echinacea* plus other botanical products (e.g., goldenseal, lemon grass leaf, spearmint leaf, and wild cherry bark) have inhibited drug metabolism mediated by cDNA-expressed CYP2C9, CYP2C19, and CYP2D6 (154). The effect of extracts of *E. purpurea* on other hepatic and intestinal enzyme systems such as UGTs and SULTs has not been reported.

Although in vitro data suggest that *echinacea* products may be inhibitory, Gorski et al. observed a mixed effect in vivo. The effect of *E. purpurea* (Nature's Bounty 400 mg q.i.d. for eight days) on the in vivo activity of CYP1A2, CYP2C9, CYP2D6, and CYP3A4 was investigated in 12 healthy volunteers (six males). This two-period, open-label, fixed-order study involved the administration of a cocktail of probes (caffeine, dextromethorphan, tolbutamide, and intravenous and oral midazolam) that were administered before and after eight days of *echinacea* (400 mg four times daily) dosing. The results of the study are shown in Table 4 (155). Briefly, *echinacea* reduced the oral clearance of caffeine and tolbutamide by 27% and 11%, respectively (Table 4) (155). Although the change in tolbutamide clearance was statistically significant, the clinical relevance of the observed change is unclear. It appears from this study that *echinacea* does not alter the in vivo catalytic activity of CYP2D6, as reflected by the absence of change in the oral clearance of dextromethorphan (Table 4) (155). In contrast to the activity of these enzymes, hepatic and intestinal CYP3A alterations are a little less clear. The systemic clearance of midazolam, a reflection of hepatic CYP3A activity, was increased significantly (Table 4). In light of the enhanced systemic elimination of midazolam and considering the "well-stirred" model of hepatic elimination, it is predicted that the oral clearance of midazolam should be increased and midazolam exposure reduced. Or in other words, the oral clearance reflects the contribution of both intestinal and hepatic CYP3A to first-pass elimination and hepatic CYP3A to the systemic elimination of midazolam. However, the oral clearance of midazolam was not significantly altered by *echinacea* dosing (Table 4) (155). In

Table 4 The Effect of *echinacea* (400 mg q.i.d. × 8 days) on the Disposition of Prototypic CYP Substrates In Vivo

CYP and substrate	Parameter (L/hr)	*N*	Before *echinacea*	After *echinacea*
CYP1A2				
Caffeine	CL_{PO}	11	6.6 ± 3.8	4.9 ± 2.3[a]
CYP2C9				
Tolbutamide	CL_{PO}	12	0.81 ± 0.18	0.72 ± 0.19[a]
CYP2D6 EMs				
Dextromethorphan	CL_{PO}	11	1289 ± 414	1281 ± 483
CYP3A				
Midazolam	CL_{IV}	12	32 ± 7	43 ± 16
Midazolam	CL_{PO}	12	137 ± 19	146 ± 71

[a]Significantly different to control value as reported by the investigators.
Abbreviations: EMs, extensive metabolizers; CL_{PO}, oral clearance; CL_{IV}, systemic clearance; CYP, cytochrome P450.
Source: From Ref. 155.

addition, the oral availability of midazolam (F_{PO}) was significantly increased from 0.23 ± 0.06 to 0.33 ± 0.13 (155). Given the relationship between hepatic (F_H) and intestinal (F_G) availabilities and oral bioavailability ($F_{PO} = F_H \times F_G$), it is possible to examine the effect of *echinacea* on these

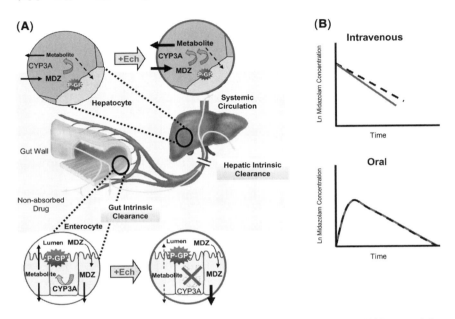

Figure 8 Schematic representation of the effect of *echinacea* (400 mg q.i.d. × 8 days) administration on the expression of CYP3A4 at intestinal and hepatic sites and on the disposition of midazolam following intravenous and oral dosing. (**A**) Factors influencing midazolam bioavailability following oral dosing including nonadsorbed drug (negligible) and presystemic elimination (gut intrinsic clearance, $E \approx 0.7$ and hepatic intrinsic clearance, $E \approx 0.3$). Following intravenous dosing, the systemic clearance of midazolam is mediated solely by hepatic CYP3A4 (hepatic intrinsic clearance, $E \approx 0.3$). The *lower left inset* depicts the intestinal CYP3A4 biotransformation of midazolam in the absence of *echinacea* whereas the *upper left inset* shows the CYP3A4 metabolism of midazolam in the hepatocyte. Treatment of individuals with *echinacea* (400 mg q.i.d. × 8 days) results in induction of hepatic CYP3A4 expression and activity (see *upper insets* outlined in *gray*) and inhibition of intestinal CYP3A4 activity or expression (see *lower inset* outlined in *gray*). The increased expression and activity of hepatic CYP3A4 following *echinacea* dosing results in a reduced exposure to midazolam following intravenous administration (**B**, *upper graph*). However, the effect of *echinacea* on intestinal CYP3A4 results in no change in midazolam exposure following oral midazolam dosing (**B**, *lower graph*). *Dashed black lines* represent the disposition of midazolam prior to the administration of *echinacea*. The *solid gray* lines represent the disposition of midazolam after the administration of *echinacea*. *Abbreviations*: CYP, cytochrome P450; MDZ, midazolam; Ech, *echinacea*; P-GP, P-glycoprotein.

independent sites of CYP3A expression. As expected from the change in the systemic clearance, the hepatic availability was reduced significantly from 0.72 ± 0.08 to 0.61 ± 0.016 (155). In contrast to the observed enhanced hepatic extraction ($F = 1-E$) of midazolam caused by *echinacea* dosing, the intestinal availability of midazolam was enhanced 85% from 0.33 ± 0.11 to 0.61 ± 38, resulting in an unchanged midazolam exposure (AUC) following oral midazolam administration. This observation suggests that intestinal CYP3A is inhibited (155). Figure 8 illustrates the relationship between alteration in hepatic and intestinal CYP3A activity and expression and the disposition of midazolam following intravenous and oral adminis-tration. The mechanism(s) of the differential effects of *echinacea* on intest-inal and hepatic CYP3A could be due to one or more of the following: (i) intestinal and hepatic CYP3A induction is mediated by tissue-specific acti-vators; (ii) the inducing component is rapidly absorbed and thus the intes-tine has limited exposure; (iii) hepatic and intestinal CYP3A are induced, but there is a potent inhibitor of CYP3A which is not systemically available; and (iv) a metabolite of a constituent of the *echinacea* preparation is respon-sible for the induction of hepatic CYP3A but not intestinal CYP3A. It is interesting that Gurley et al. reported no effect of *echinacea* on CYP3A; however, midazolam was only administered as an oral dose (156). The dif-ferential effect of *echinacea* on intestinal and hepatic CYP3A complicates the predication of drug interactions with other CYP3A substrates. For instance, drugs that undergo minimal first-pass elimination by the intestine and liver may demonstrate an increased oral clearance as expected due to the induction of hepatic CYP3A. However, substrates that undergo high first-pass elimination by the intestine may demonstrate increased serum con-centrations due to the inhibitory effect of *echinacea* on intestinal CYP3A. It is clear from the data presented that caution should be used when *echinacea* and CYP3A substrates are coadministered (40).

REFERENCES

1. Eisenberg DM, Davis RB, Ettner SL, et al. Trends in alternative medicine use in the United States, 1990–1997: results of a follow-up national survey [see comments]. JAMA 1998; 280(18):1569–1575.
2. O'Hara M, Kiefer D, Farrell K, Kemper K. A review of 12 commonly used medicinal herbs. Arch Fam Med 1998; 7(6):523–536.
3. Fairfield KM, Eisenberg DM, Davis RB, Libman H, Phillips RS. Patterns of use, expenditures, and perceived efficacy of complementary and alternative therapies in HIV-infected patients [see comments]. Arch Intern Med 1998; 158(20):2257–2264.
4. Blumenthal M. Herb sales down 3% in mass market retail stores-sales in natural food stores still growing but at lower rata. Herbal Gram 2000; 49:68.

5. Blumenthal M. Herb sales down in mainstream market, up in natural food stores. Herbal Gram 2002; 55:60.

6. Ruschitzka F, Meier PJ, Turina M, Luscher TF, Noll G. Acute heart transplant rejection due to Saint John's wort [letter] [see comments]. Lancet 2000; 355(9203):548–549.

7. Blumenthal M. Herbal Medicine: Expanded Commission E Monographs. 1st ed. Austin, TX: American Botanical Council, 2000.

8. Behnke K, Jensen GS, Graubaum HJ, Gruenwald J. *Hypericum perforatum* versus fluoxetine in the treatment of mild to moderate depression. Adv Ther 2002; 19(1):43–52.

9. Schrader E. Equivalence of St John's wort extract (Ze 117) and fluoxetine: a randomized, controlled study in mild-moderate depression. Int Clin Psychopharmacol 2000; 15(2):61–68.

10. Brenner R, Azbel V, Madhusoodanan S, Pawlowska M. Comparison of an extract of hypericum (LI 160) and sertraline in the treatment of depression: a double-blind, randomized pilot study. Clin Ther 2000; 22(4):411–419.

11. van Gurp G, Meterissian GB, Haiek LN, McCusker J, Bellavance F. St John's wort or sertraline? Randomized controlled trial in primary care. Can Fam Physician 2002; 48:905–912.

12. Wheatley D. LI 160, an extract of St. John's wort, versus amitriptyline in mildly to moderately depressed outpatients—a controlled 6-week clinical trial. Pharmacopsychiatry 1997; 30(suppl 2):77–80.

13. Woelk H. Comparison of St John's wort and imipramine for treating depression: randomised controlled trial. BMJ 2000; 321(7260):536–539.

14. Gelenberg AJ, Shelton RC, Crits-Christoph P, et al. The effectiveness of St. John's wort in major depressive disorder: a naturalistic phase 2 follow-up in which nonresponders were provided alternate medication. J Clin Psychiatr 2004; 65(8):1114–1119.

15. Shelton RC, Keller MB, Gelenberg A, et al. Effectiveness of St John's wort in major depression: a randomized controlled trial. JAMA 2001; 285(15):1978–1986.

16. Lecrubier Y, Clerc G, Didi R, Kieser M. Efficacy of St. John's wort extract WS 5570 in major depression: a double-blind, placebo-controlled trial. Am J Psychiatr 2002; 159(8):1361–1366.

17. Davidson JRT, Gadde KM, Fairbank JA, et al. Effect of *Hypericum perforatum* (St John's wort) in major depressive disorder: a randomized controlled trial. JAMA 2002; 287(14):1807–1814.

18. Hudson JB, Lopez-Bazzocchi I, Towers GH. Antiviral activities of hypericin. Antiviral Res 1991; 15(2):101–112.

19. Tang J, Colacino JM, Larsen SH, Spitzer W. Virucidal activity of hypericin against enveloped and non-enveloped DNA and RNA viruses. Antiviral Res 1990; 13(6):313–325.

20. Degar S, Prince AM, Pascual D, et al. Inactivation of the human immunodeficiency virus by hypericin: evidence for photochemical alterations of p24 and a block in uncoating. AIDS Res Hum Retroviruses 1992; 8(11):1929–1936.

21. Gulick RM, McAuliffe V, Holden-Wiltse J, et al. Phase I studies of hypericin, the active compound in St. John's Wort, as an antiretroviral agent in

HIV-infected adults. AIDS Clinical Trials Group Protocols 150 and 258. Ann Intern Med 1999; 130(6):510–514.

22. Wurglics M, Westerhoff K, Kaunzinger A, et al. Comparison of German St. John's wort products according to hyperforin and total hypericin content. J Am Pharm Assoc (Wash) 2001; 41(4):560–566.

23. Wurglics M, Westerhoff K, Kaunzinger A, et al. Batch-to-batch reproducibility of St. John's wort preparations. Pharmacopsychiatry 2001; 34(suppl 1): S152–S156.

24. Wang Z, Gorski JC, Hamman MA, Huang SM, Lesko LJ, Hall SD. The effects of St John's wort (*Hypericum perforatum*) on human cytochrome P450 activity. Clin Pharmacol Therapeut 2001; 70(4):317–326.

25. Hall SD, Wang Z, Huang S-M, et al. The interaction between St John's wort and an oral contraceptive. Clin Pharmacol Therapeut 2003; 74(6):525–535.

26. Wang E, Casciano CN, Clement RP, Johnson WW. HMG-CoA reductase inhibitors (statins) characterized as direct inhibitors of P-glycoprotein. Pharm Res 2001; 18(6):800–806.

27. Draves AH, Walker SE. Analysis of the hypericin and pseudohypericin content of commercially available St John's Wort preparations. Can J Clin Pharmacol 2003; 10(3):114–118.

28. de los Reyes GC, Koda RT. Determining hyperforin and hypericin content in eight brands of St. John's wort. Am J Health Syst Pharm 2002; 59(6):545–547.

29. Ganzera M, Zhao J, Khan IA. *Hypericum perforatum*—chemical profiling and quantitative results of St. John's Wort products by an improved high-performance liquid chromatography method. J Pharm Sci 2002; 91(3):623–630.

30. Garrard J, Harms S, Eberly LE, Matiak A. Variations in product choices of frequently purchased herbs: caveat emptor. Arch Intern Med 2003; 163(19): 2290–2295.

31. Alscher DM, Klotz U. Drug interaction of herbal tea containing St. John's wort with cyclosporine. Transpl Int 2003; 16(7):543–544.

32. Muller D, Pfeil T, von den Driesch V. Treating depression comorbid with anxiety—results of an open, practice-oriented study with St John's wort WS 5572 and valerian extract in high doses. Phytomedicine 2003; 10(suppl 4): 25–30.

33. Woelk H, Burkard G, Grunwald J. Benefits and risks of the hypericum extract LI 160: drug monitoring study with 3250 patients. J Geriatr Psychiatr Neurol 1994; 7(suppl 1):S34–S38.

34. Dean AJ, Moses GM, Vernon JM. Suspected withdrawal syndrome after cessation of St. John's wort. Ann Pharmacother 2003; 37(1):150.

35. Patel S, Robinson R, Burk M. Hypertensive crisis associated with St. John's Wort. Am J Med 2002; 112(6):507–508.

36. Bladt S, Wagner H. Inhibition of MAO by fractions and constituents of hypericum extract. J Geriatr Psychiatr Neurol 1994; 7(suppl 1):S57–S59.

37. Thiede HM, Walper A. Inhibition of MAO and COMT by hypericum extracts and hypericin. J Geriatr Psychiatr Neurol 1994; 7(suppl 1):S54–S56.

38. Irefin S, Sprung J. A possible cause of cardiovascular collapse during anesthesia: long-term use of St. John's Wort. J Clin Anesth 2000; 12(6):498–499.

39. Nierenberg AA, Burt T, Matthews J, Weiss AP. Mania associated with St. John's wort. Biol Psychiatr 1999; 46(12):1707–1708.

40. Ernst E, Rand JI, Barnes J, Stevinson C. Adverse effects profile of the herbal antidepressant St. John's wort (Hypericum perforatum L.). Eur J Clin Pharmacol 1998; 54(8):589–594.

41. Obach RS. Inhibition of human cytochrome P450 enzymes by constituents of St. John's Wort, an herbal preparation used in the treatment of depression. J Pharmacol Exp Ther 2000; 294(1):88–95.

42. Moore LB, Goodwin B, Jones SA, et al. St. John's wort induces hepatic drug metabolism through activation of the pregnane X receptor. Proc Natl Acad Sci USA 2000; 97(13):7500–7502.

43. Budzinski JW, Foster BC, Vandenhoek S, Arnason JT. An in vitro evaluation of human cytochrome P450 3A4 inhibition by selected commercial herbal extracts and tinctures. Phytomedicine 2000; 7(4):273–282.

44. Wentworth JM, Agostini M, Love J, Schwabe JW, Chatterjee VK. St John's wort, a herbal antidepressant, activates the steroid X receptor. J Endocrinol 2000; 166(3):R11–R16.

45. Hennessy M, Kelleher D, Spiers JP, et al. St Johns wort increases expression of P-glycoprotein: implications for drug interactions. Br J Clin Pharmacol 2002; 53(1):75–82.

46. Chen Y, Ferguson SS, Negishi M, Goldstein JA. Induction of human CYP2C9 by rifampicin, hyperforin, and phenobarbital is mediated by the pregnane X receptor. J Pharmacol Exp Ther 2004; 308(2):495–501.

47. Chen Y, Ferguson SS, Negishi M, Goldstein JA. Identification of constitutive androstane receptor and glucocorticoid receptor binding sites in the CYP2C19 promoter. Mol Pharmacol 2003; 64(2):316–324.

48. Goodwin B, Moore LB, Stoltz CM, McKee DD, Kliewer SA. Regulation of the human CYP2B6 gene by the nuclear pregnane X receptor. Mol Pharmacol 2001; 60(3):427–431.

49. Komoroski BJ, Zhang S, Cai H, et al. Induction and inhibition of cytochromes p450 by the St. John's wort constituent hyperforin in human hepatocyte cultures. Drug Metab Dispos 2004; 32(5):512–518.

50. Perloff MD, von Moltke LL, Stormer E, Shader RI, Greenblatt DJ. Saint John's wort: an in vitro analysis of P-glycoprotein induction due to extended exposure. Br J Pharmacol 2001; 134(8):1601–1608.

51. Watkins PB, Wrighton SA, Schuetz EG, Molowa DT, Guzelian PS. Identification of glucocorticoid-inducible cytochromes P-450 in the intestinal mucosa of rats and man. J Clin Invest 1987; 80(4):1029–1036.

52. Wrighton SA, Stevens JC. The human hepatic cytochromes P450 involved in drug metabolism. Crit Rev Toxicol 1992; 22(1):1–21.

53. Kolars JC, Schmiedlin-Ren P, Schuetz JD, Fang C, Watkins PB. Identification of rifampin-inducible P450IIIA4 (CYP3A4) in human small bowel enterocytes. J Clin Invest 1992; 90(5):1871–1878.

54. Nelson DR, Koymans L, Kamataki T, et al. P450 superfamily: update on new sequences, gene mapping, accession numbers and nomenclature. Pharmacogenetics 1996; 6(1):1–42.

55. Domanski TL, Finta C, Halpert JR, Zaphiropoulos PG. cDNA cloning and initial characterization of CYP3A43, a novel human cytochrome P450. Mol Pharmacol 2001; 59(2):386–392.

56. Gellner K, Eiselt R, Hustert E, et al. Genomic organization of the human CYP3A locus: identification of a new, inducible CYP3A gene. Pharmacogenetics 2001; 11(2):111–121.

57. Westlind A, Malmebo S, Johansson I, et al. Cloning and tissue distribution of a novel human cytochrome p450 of the cyp3a subfamily, cyp3a43. Biochem Biophys Res Commun 2001; 281(5):1349–1355.

58. Evans WE, Relling MV. Pharmacogenomics: translating functional genomics into rational therapeutics. Science 1999; 286(5439):487–491.

59. Benet LZ, Kroetz DL, Shen DD. Pharmacokinetics: the dynamics of drug absorption, distribution, and elimination. In: Hardman JG, Limbird LE, eds. Goodman & Gilman's: The Pharmacological Basis of Therapeutics. 9th ed. New York: McGraw-Hill, 1996:3–27.

60. Li AP, Kaminski DL, Rasmussen A. Substrates of human hepatic cytochrome P450 3A4. Toxicology 1995; 104(1–3):1–8.

61. Wrighton SA, Brian WR, Sari MA, et al. Studies on the expression and metabolic capabilities of human liver cytochrome P450IIIA5 (HLp3). Mol Pharmacol 1990; 38(2):207–213.

62. Wrighton SA, Ring BJ, Watkins PB, VandenBranden M. Identification of a polymorphically expressed member of the human cytochrome P-450III family. Mol Pharmacol 1989; 36(1):97–105.

63. Finta C, Zaphiropoulos PG. The human cytochrome P450 3A locus. Gene evolution by capture of downstream exons. Gene 2000; 260(1–2):13–23.

64. Fromm MF, Busse D, Kroemer HK, Eichelbaum M. Differential induction of prehepatic and hepatic metabolism of verapamil by rifampin. Hepatology 1996; 24(4):796–801.

65. Fromm MF, Dilger K, Busse D, Kroemer HK, Eichelbaum M, Klotz U. Gut wall metabolism of verapamil in older people: effects of rifampicin-mediated enzyme induction. Br J Clin Pharmacol 1998; 45(3):247–255.

66. Hebert MF, Roberts JP, Prueksaritanont T, Benet LZ. Bioavailability of cyclosporine with concomitant rifampin administration is markedly less than predicted by hepatic enzyme induction. Clin Pharmacol Therapeut 1992; 52(5):453–457.

67. Wu CY, Benet LZ, Hebert MF, et al. Differentiation of absorption and first-pass gut and hepatic metabolism in humans: studies with cyclosporine. Clin Pharmacol Therapeut 1995; 58(5):492–497.

68. Holtbecker N, Fromm MF, Kroemer HK, Ohnhaus EE, Heidemann H. The nifedipine-rifampin interaction. Evidence for induction of gut wall metabolism. Drug Metab Dispos 1996; 24(10):1121–1123.

69. Thummel KE, O'Shea D, Paine MF, et al. Oral first-pass elimination of midazolam involves both gastrointestinal and hepatic CYP3A-mediated metabolism. Clin Pharmacol Therapeut 1996; 59(5):491–502.

70. Gorski JC, Jones DR, Haehner-Daniels BD, Hamman MA, O'Mara EM Jr, Hall SD. The contribution of intestinal and hepatic CYP3A to the interaction

between midazolam and clarithromycin. Clin Pharmacol Therapeut 1998; 64(2):133–143.

71. Mathijssen RH, Verweij J, de Bruijn P, Loos WJ, Sparreboom A. Effects of St. John's wort on irinotecan metabolism. J Natl Cancer Inst 2002; 94(16): 1247–1249.

72. Gleevec (imatinib mesylate) [full prescribing information]. East Hanover, NJ: Novartis Pharmaceuticals, 2002.

73. Frye RF, Fitzgerald SM, Lagattuta TF, Hruska MW, Egorin MJ. Effect of St John's wort on imatinib mesylate pharmacokinetics. Clin Pharmacol Therapeut 2004; 76(4):323–329.

74. Backman JT, Olkkola KT, Ojala M, Laaksovirta H, Neuvonen PJ. Concentrations and effects of oral midazolam are greatly reduced in patients treated with carbamazepine or phenytoin. Epilepsia 1996; 37(3):253–257.

75. Albani F, Riva R, Baruzzi A. Clarithromycin-carbamazepine interaction: a case report. Epilepsia 1993; 34(1):161–162.

76. Pichard L, Fabre I, Fabre G, et al. Cyclosporin A drug interactions. Screening for inducers and inhibitors of cytochrome P-450 (cyclosporin A oxidase) in primary cultures of human hepatocytes and in liver microsomes. Drug Metab Dispos 1990; 18(5):595–606.

77. Faucette SR, Wang H, Hamilton GA, et al. Regulation of CYP2B6 in primary human hepatocytes by prototypical inducers. Drug Metab Dispos 2004; 32(3):348–358.

78. Usui T, Saitoh Y, Komada F. Induction of CYP3As in HepG2 cells by several drugs. Association between induction of CYP3A4 and expression of glucocorticoid receptor. Biol Pharm Bull 2003; 26(4):510–517.

79. Luo G, Cunningham M, Kim S, et al. CYP3A4 induction by drugs: correlation between a pregnane X receptor reporter gene assay and CYP3A4 expression in human hepatocytes. Drug Metab Dispos 2002; 30(7):795–804.

80. Burstein AH, Horton RL, Dunn T, Alfaro RM, Piscitelli SC, Theodore W. Lack of effect of St John's Wort on carbamazepine pharmacokinetics in healthy volunteers. Clin Pharmacol Ther 2000; 68(6):605–612.

81. Williams JA, Ring BJ, Cantrell VE, et al. Comparative metabolic capabilities of CYP3A4, CYP3A5, and CYP3A7. Drug Metab Dispos 2002; 30(8):883–891.

82. Smith M, Lin KM, Zheng YP. An open label trial of nifedipine-herb interactions: nifedipine with St John's wort, Ginseng, or Ginkgo Biloba. Clin Pharmacol Therapeut 2001; 69(2):P86.

83. Tannergren C, Engman H, Knutson L, Hedeland M, Bondesson U, Lennernas H. St John's wort decreases the bioavailability of R- and S-verapamil through induction of the first-pass metabolism. Clin Pharmacol Therapeut 2004; 75(4):298–309.

84. Jones DR, Hall SD. Mechanism based inhibition of cytochrome P450: in vitro kinetics and in vitro-in vivo correlations. In: Rodrigues AD, ed. Drug-Drug Interactions: From Basic Pharmacokinetics Concepts to Marketing Issues. New York, NY: Marcel Dekker, 2001.

85. Chiba M, Hensleigh M, Nishime JA, Balani SK, Lin JH. Role of cytochrome P450 3A4 in human metabolism of MK-639, a potent human immunodeficiency virus protease inhibitor. Drug Metab Dispos 1996; 24(3):307–314.

86. Chiba M, Hensleigh M, Lin JH. Hepatic and intestinal metabolism of indinavir, an HIV protease inhibitor, in rat and human microsomes. Major role of CYP3A. Biochem Pharmacol 1997; 53(8):1187–1195.
87. Koudriakova T, Iatsimirskaia E, Utkin I, et al. Metabolism of the human immunodeficiency virus protease inhibitors indinavir and ritonavir by human intestinal microsomes and expressed cytochrome P4503A4/3A5: mechanism-based inactivation of cytochrome P4503A by ritonavir. Drug Metab Dispos 1998; 26(6):552–561.
88. Erickson DA, Mather G, Trager WF, Levy RH, Keirns JJ. Characterization of the in vitro biotransformation of the HIV-1 reverse transcriptase inhibitor nevirapine by human hepatic cytochromes P-450. Drug Metab Dispos 1999; 27(12):1488–1495.
89. de Maat MM, Hoetelmans RM, Math t RA, et al. Drug interaction between St John's wort and nevirapine. Aids 2001; 15(3):420–421.
90. Kronbach T, Mathys D, Umeno M, Gonzalez FJ, Meyer UA. Oxidation of midazolam and triazolam by human liver cytochrome P450IIIA4. Mol Pharmacol 1989; 36(1):89–96.
91. Gorski JC, Hall SD, Jones DR, VandenBranden M, Wrighton SA. Regioselective biotransformation of midazolam by members of the human cytochrome P450 3A (CYP3A) subfamily. Biochem Pharmacol 1994; 47(9):1643–1653.
92. Schmiedlin-Ren P, Thummel KE, Fisher JM, Paine MF, Lown KS, Watkins PB. Expression of enzymatically active CYP3A4 by Caco-2 cells grown on extracellular matrix-coated permeable supports in the presence of 1alpha, 25-dihydroxyvitamin D3. Mol Pharmacol 1997; 51(5):741–754.
93. Kim RB, Wandel C, Leake B, et al. Interrelationship between substrates and inhibitors of human CYP3A and P-glycoprotein. Pharm Res 1999; 16(3): 408–414.
94. Greenblatt DJ, Abernethy DR, Locniskar A, Harmatz JS, Limjuco RA, Shader RI. Effect of age, gender, and obesity on midazolam kinetics. Anesthesiology 1984; 61(1):27–35.
95. Gorski JC, Wang Z, Haehner-Daniels BD, Wrighton SA, Hall SD. The effect of hormone replacement therapy on CYP3A activity. Clin Pharmacol Therapeut 2000; 68(4):412–417.
96. Gorski JC, Vannaprasaht S, Hamman MA, et al. The effect of age, sex, and rifampin administration on intestinal and hepatic cytochrome P450 3A activity. Clin Pharmacol Therapeut 2003; 74(3):275–287.
97. Masica AL, Mayo G, Wilkinson GR. In vivo comparisons of constitutive cytochrome P450 3A activity assessed by alprazolam, triazolam, and midazolam. Clin Pharmacol Therapeut 2004; 76(4):341–349.
98. Dresser GK, Schwarz UI, Wilkinson GR, Kim RB. Coordinate induction of both cytochrome P4503A and MDR1 by St John's wort in healthy subjects. Clin Pharmacol Therapeut 2003; 73(1):41–50.
99. Durr D, Stieger B, Kullak-Ublick GA, et al. St John's Wort induces intestinal P-glycoprotein/MDR1 and intestinal and hepatic CYP3A4. Clin Pharmacol Therapeut 2000; 68(6):598–604.

100. Gurley BJ, Gardner SF, Hubbard MA, et al. Cytochrome P450 phenotypic ratios for predicting herb-drug interactions in humans. Clin Pharmacol Therapeut 2002; 72(3):276–287.

101. Markowitz JS, DeVane CL, Boulton DW, Carson SW, Nahas Z, Risch SC. Effect of St. John's wort (Hypericum perforatum) on cytochrome P-450 2D6 and 3A4 activity in healthy volunteers. Life Sci 2000; 66(9):PL133–PL139.

102. Markowitz JS, Donovan JL, DeVane CL, et al. Effect of St John's wort on drug metabolism by induction of cytochrome P450 3A4 enzyme. JAMA 2003; 290(11):1500–1504.

103. Gorski JC, Jones DR, Hamman MA, Wrighton SA, Hall SD. Biotransformation of alprazolam by members of the human cytochrome P4503A subfamily. Xenobiotica 1999; 29(9):931–944.

104. Sugimoto K, Ohmori M, Tsuruoka S, et al. Different effects of St John's wort on the pharmacokinetics of simvastatin and pravastatin. Clin Pharmacol Therapeut 2001; 70(6):518–524.

105. Sakaeda T, Takara K, Kakumoto M, et al. Simvastatin and lovastatin, but not pravastatin, interact with MDR1. J Pharm Pharmacol 2002; 54(3):419–423.

106. Transon C, Leemann T, Dayer P. In vitro comparative inhibition profiles of major human drug metabolising cytochrome P450 isozymes (CYP2C9, CYP2D6 and CYP3A4) by HMG-CoA reductase inhibitors. Eur J Clin Pharmacol 1996; 50(3):209–215.

107. Barone GW, Gurley BJ, Ketel BL, Abul-Ezz SR. Herbal supplements: a potential for drug interactions in transplant recipients. Transplantation 2001; 71(2):239–241.

108. Moschella C, Jaber BL. Interaction between cyclosporine and *Hypericum perforatum* (St. John's wort) after organ transplantation. Am J Kidney Dis 2001; 38(5):1105–1107.

109. Breidenbach T, Kliem V, Burg M, Radermacher J, Hoffmann MW, Klempnauer J. Profound drop of cyclosporin A whole blood trough levels caused by St. John's wort (Hypericum perforatum). Transplantation 2000; 69(10):2229–2230.

110. Ahmed SM, Banner NR, Dubrey SW. Low cyclosporin—a level due to Saint-John's-wort in heart transplant patients. J Heart Lung Transplant 2001; 20(7):795.

111. Barone GW, Gurley BJ, Ketel BL, Lightfoot ML, Abul-Ezz SR. Drug interaction between St. John's wort and cyclosporine. Ann Pharmacother 2000; 34(9):1013–1016.

112. Bauer S, Stormer E, Johne A, et al. Alterations in cyclosporin A pharmacokinetics and metabolism during treatment with St John's wort in renal transplant patients. Br J Clin Pharmacol 2003; 55(2):203–211.

113. Bolley R, Zulke C, Kammerl M, Fischereder M, Kramer BK. Tacrolimus-induced nephrotoxicity unmasked by induction of the CYP3A4 system with St John's wort. Transplantation 2002; 73(6):1009.

114. Hebert MF, Park JM, Chen YL, Akhtar S, Larson AM. Effects of St. John's Wort (Hypericum perforatum) on tacrolimus pharmacokinetics in healthy volunteers. J Clin Pharmacol 2004; 44(1):89–94.

115. Mai I, Stormer E, Bauer S, Kruger H, Budde K, Roots I. Impact of St John's wort treatment on the pharmacokinetics of tacrolimus and mycophenolic acid in renal transplant patients. Nephrol Dial Transplant 2003; 18(4):819–822.

116. Eich-Hochli D, Oppliger R, Golay KP, Baumann P, Eap CB. Methadone maintenance treatment and St. John's Wort—a case report. Pharmacopsychiatry 2003; 36(1):35–37.

117. Skolnick JL, Stoler BS, Katz DB, Anderson WH. Rifampin, oral contraceptives, and pregnancy. JAMA 1976; 236(12):1382.

118. LeBel M, Masson E, Guilbert E, et al. Effects of rifabutin and rifampicin on the pharmacokinetics of ethinylestradiol and norethindrone. J Clin Pharmacol 1998; 38(11):1042–1050.

119. Guengerich FP. Oxidation of 17 alpha-ethynylestradiol by human liver cytochrome P-450. Mol Pharmacol 1988; 33(5):500–508.

120. Back DJ, Breckenridge AM, MacIver M, et al. The gut wall metabolism of ethinyloestradiol and its contribution to the pre-systemic metabolism of ethinyloestradiol in humans. Br J Clin Pharmacol 1982; 13(3):325–330.

121. Rey JM, Walter G. *Hypericum perforatum* (St John's wort) in depression: pest or blessing? Med J Aust 1998; 169(11–12):583–586.

122. Vegano D. Study shows St. John's wort might weaken birth control. USA Today 2000; May 1.

123. Anonymous. Pregnancies prompt herb warning. BBC News 2002; February 6.

124. Schwarz UI, Buschel B, Kirch W. Unwanted pregnancy on self-medication with St John's wort despite hormonal contraception. Br J Clin Pharmacol 2003; 55(1):112–113.

125. Pfrunder A, Schiesser M, Gerber S, Haschke M, Bitzer J, Drewe J. Interaction of St John's wort with low-dose oral contraceptive therapy: a randomized controlled trial. Br J Clin Pharmacol 2003; 56(6):683–690.

126. Birkett DJ, Miners JO. Chapter 35: Methylxanthines. In: Levy RH, Thummel KE, Trager WF, Hansten PD, Eichelbaum M, eds. Metabolic Drug Interactions. 1st ed. Philadelphia: Lippincott Williams & Wilkins, 2000:469–482.

127. Nebel A, Schneider BJ, Baker RK, Kroll DJ. Potential metabolic interaction between St. John's wort and theophylline [letter]. Ann Pharmacother 1999; 33(4):502.

128. Katial RK, Stelzle RC, Bonner MW, Marino M, Cantilena LR, Smith LJ. A drug interaction between zafirlukast and theophylline. Arch Intern Med 1998; 158(15):1713–1715.

129. Shader RI, Granda BW, von Moltke LL, Giancarlo GM, Greenblatt DJ. Inhibition of human cytochrome P450 isoforms in vitro by zafirlukast. Biopharm Drug Dispos 1999; 20(8):385–388.

130. Morimoto T, Kotegawa T, Tsutsumi K, Ohtani Y, Imai H, Nakano S. Effect of St. John's Wort on the pharmacokinetics of theophylline in healthy volunteers. J Clin Pharmacol 2004; 44(1):95–101.

131. Tassaneeyakul W, Mohamed Z, Birkett DJ, et al. Caffeine as a probe for human cytochromes P450: validation using cDNA-expression, immunoinhibition and microsomal kinetic and inhibitor techniques. Pharmacogenetics 1992; 2(4):173–183.

132. Tassaneeyakul W, Birkett DJ, McManus ME, et al. Caffeine metabolism by human hepatic cytochromes P450: contributions of 1A2, 2E1 and 3A isoforms. Biochem Pharmacol 1994; 47(10):1767–1776.

133. Jeppesen U, Loft S, Poulsen HE, Brsen K. A fluvoxamine-caffeine interaction study. Pharmacogenetics 1996; 6(3):213–222.

134. Wenk M, Todesco L, Krahenbuhl S. Effect of St John's wort on the activities of CYP1A2, CYP3A4, CYP2D6, N-acetyltransferase 2, and xanthine oxidase in healthy males and females. Br J Clin Pharmacol 2004; 57(4):495–499.

135. Wang LS, Zhou G, Zhu B, et al. St John's wort induces both cytochrome P450 3A4-catalyzed sulfoxidation and 2C19-dependent hydroxylation of omeprazole. Clin Pharmacol Therapeut 2004; 75(3):191–197.

136. Jiang X, Williams KM, Liauw WS, et al. Effect of St John's wort and ginseng on the pharmacokinetics and pharmacodynamics of warfarin in healthy subjects. Br J Clin Pharmacol 2004; 57(5):592–599.

137. Cvetkovic M, Leake B, Fromm MF, Wilkinson GR, Kim RB. OATP and P-glycoprotein transporters mediate the cellular uptake and excretion of fexofenadine. Drug Metab Dispos 1999; 27(8):866–871.

138. Wang Z, Hamman MA, Huang SM, Lesko LJ, Hall SD. Effect of St John's wort on the pharmacokinetics of fexofenadine. Clin Pharmacol Therapeut 2002; 71(6):414–420.

139. Johne A, Brockmoller J, Bauer S, Maurer A, Langheinrich M, Roots I. Pharmacokinetic interaction of digoxin with an herbal extract from St John's wort (*Hypericum perforatum*). Clin Pharmacol Ther 1999; 66(4):338–345.

140. Mueller SC, Uehleke B, Woehling H, et al. Effect of St John's wort dose and preparations on the pharmacokinetics of digoxin. Clin Pharmacol Therapeut 2004; 75(6):546–557.

141. Robbers JE, Tyler VE. Tyler's Herbs of Choice. Binghamton, NY: The Hawthorne Press Inc, 1999.

142. Barrett B. Medicinal properties of Echinacea: a critical review. Phytomedicine 2003; 10(1):66–86.

143. Barrett B. Echinacea: a safety review. HerbalGram 2003; 57:36–39.

144. Barrett B, Vohmann M, Calabrese C. Echinacea for upper respiratory infection. J Fam Pract 1999; 48(8):628–635.

145. Tsen LC, Segal S, Pothier M, Bader AM. Alternative medicine use in presurgical patients. Anesthesiology 2000; 93(1):148–151.

146. Tsui B, Dennehy CE, Tsourounis C. A survey of dietary supplement use during pregnancy at an academic medical center. Am J Obstet Gynecol 2001; 185(2):433–437.

147. Planta M, Gundersen B, Petitt JC. Prevalence of the use of herbal products in a low-income population. Fam Med 2000; 32(4):252–257.

148. Cala S, Crismon ML, Baumgartner J. A survey of herbal use in children with attention-deficit-hyperactivity disorder or depression. Pharmacotherapy 2003; 23(2):222–230.

149. O'Dea JA. Consumption of nutritional supplements among adolescents: usage and perceived benefits. Health Educ Res 2003; 18(1):98–107.

150. Rininger JA, Kickner S, Chigurupati P, McLean A, Franck Z. Immunopharmacological activity of Echinacea preparations following simulated digestion

on murine macrophages and human peripheral blood mononuclear cells. J Leukoc Biol 2000; 68(4):503–510.

151. Percival SS. Use of Echinacea in medicine. Biochem Pharmacol 2000; 60(2): 155–158.

152. Lindenmuth GF, Lindenmuth EB. The efficacy of Echinacea compound herbal tea preparation on the severity and duration of upper respiratory and flu symptoms: a randomized, double-blind placebo-controlled study. J Altern Complement Med 2000; 6(4):327–334.

153. Turner RB, Riker DK, Gangemi JD. Ineffectiveness of Echinacea for prevention of experimental rhinovirus colds. Antimicrob Agents Chemother 2000; 44(6):1708–1709.

154. Foster BC, Vandenhoek S, Hana J, et al. In vitro inhibition of human cytochrome P450-mediated metabolism of marker substrates by natural products. Phytomedicine 2003; 10(4):334–342.

155. Gorski JC, Huang S-M, Pinto A, et al. The effect of Echinacea (*Echinacea purpurea* root) on cytochrome P450 activity. Clin Pharmacol Therapeut 2004; 75(1):89–100.

156. Gurley BJ, Gardner SF, Hubbard MA, et al. Assessment of botanical supplementation on human cytochrome P450 phenotype: *Citrus aurantium*, Echinacea, milk thistle, saw palmetto. Clin Pharmacol Therapeut 2004; 75(2):P35.

5

Botanical Products–Drug Interactions: Focus on Garlic, Ginkgo and Ginseng

Y. W. Francis Lam

*Departments of Pharmacology and Medicine,
University of Texas Health Science Center at
San Antonio, San Antonio, and College of Pharmacy,
University of Texas at Austin, Austin, Texas, U.S.A.*

E. Ernst

*Complementary Medicine, Peninsula Medical School,
University of Exeter, Exeter, and University of Plymouth, Plymouth, U.K.*

INTRODUCTION

Garlic, ginkgo, and ginseng are, respectively, the second, first, and fourth top-selling botanical supplements in U.S. retail outlets (1). Their retail sales are impressive, totalling US $35, $46, and $31 million, respectively. These 2002 figures look impressive but actually represent a substantial decline in comparison to those of 2001 (–17%, –35%, and –33%, respectively). Given this nevertheless huge popularity, it is important for health care professionals to advise patients responsibly about the proper use of these products. This chapter summarizes our current knowledge with an emphasis on botanical product–drug interactions.

GARLIC (*ALLIUM SATIVUM* L.)

Background

Fresh garlic bulb, dried and powdered extract, or oil extracted from the bulb have been used for medicinal purposes. The active constituents include alliin, allinase, diallyldisulfide, ajoens, and others. Alliin is enzymatically converted to allicin, the major garlic component, which is also responsible for its characteristic, sulfur-like smell. Although the best-researched pharmacological property of garlic is that of lowering total serum cholesterol levels, probably via inhibition of hepatic cholesterol synthesis (2,3), multiple additional pharmacological actions of garlic, including antibacterial, antiviral, antifungal, antihypertensive (4), hypoglycemic, antithrombotic (5), antimutagenic (6), and antiplatelet activities, have been described.

The recommended dose is about 4 g of fresh garlic daily, which is equivalent to approximately 8 mg garlic oil or 600 to 900 mg garlic powder preparations standardized to 1.3% alliin content. Adverse effects of garlic are usually mild and transient; they include breath and body odor, allergic reactions, nausea, heartburn, and flatulence.

Garlic has been reported to inhibit platelet aggregation, and patients with bleeding abnormalities should be cautioned about the uncontrolled use of garlic supplements. It is recommended that garlic supplements be discontinued before major surgery. The following section describes the available evidence of pharmacodynamic and pharmacokinetic interaction between garlic and prescription drugs.

Interactions

Pharmacodynamic Interaction

The primary garlic metabolite allicin has been shown to possess antiplatelet activity (7). Bordia (8) showed that administration of essential oil of garlic 25 mg daily for five days resulted in significant inhibition of platelet aggregation. A case report of spontaneous epidural hematoma in an 87-year-old male was attributed to excessive garlic consumption. Because the patient was not taking any prescription medications at the time of the bleeding episode, and all laboratory parameters, including clotting factor profile, were normal, the clinicians believed that the only probable explanation for the occurrence of the hematoma was the patient's daily ingestion of four cloves (approximately 2 g) of garlic for an unspecified time period (9).

Another case reporting bleeding disorders associated with garlic use described a 72-year-old male patient admitted to the hospital with acute urinary retention and scheduled to undergo a transurethral resection for benign prostrate hyperplasia. He was not taking any medications on admission except for years of garlic tablets consumption for "medicinal purposes." However, no information regarding the strength and amount of garlic was provided. The patient experienced hemostasis and hemorrhage at the site of resection during and after surgery. The patient had a full recovery with four units of blood transfusion. Platelet aggregation test was not done during the hospitalization. However, three months after resumption of garlic use, the patient returned to clinic and blood tests were reported to show abnormal platelet aggregation (10).

Therefore, this pharmacological effect suggests that use of garlic could potentially increase the effect of anticoagulants. Two brief cases described that patients who had been stabilized on warfarin experienced a doubling of international normalized ratio (INR) after they took garlic products, but there were no information provided regarding the strength of garlic preparation and the duration of use, the INR values, description of symptoms, and clinical outcomes (11). Other than these two anecdotal cases, there are no literature reports of interaction between garlic and anticoagulants such as warfarin. Despite this lack of clinical data, especially from pharmacokinetic studies, the potential for irreversible platelet function inhibition has prompted the suggestion to discontinue garlic use at least one week prior to surgery, so as to minimize the risk of postoperative bleeding.

Garlic, as a component of curry, had also been suggested to enhance the hypoglycemic effects of the oral hypoglycemic agent chlorpropamide in a 40-year-old Pakistani woman (12). The estimated amount of garlic consumed by the patient was not provided. In addition, because the food product also contains karela, another ingredient reported to also possess hypoglycemic effect (13), it is impossible to conclude from this brief report that a cause–effect relationship exists for garlic. Since the publication of this report there have been no additional evidence to confirm the clinical observation or formal study to evaluate the likely mechanism. Table 1 summarizes all reported interactions based on case reports and pharmacokinetic studies in humans.

Pharmacokinetic Interaction

Garlic is one of the most common botanical remedies used by patients with human immunodeficiency virus (HIV), probably because of to the antiviral claim associated with its consumption, as well as the possibility of lowering total serum cholesterol, which could counteract the common side effect of hypercholesterolemia associated with the use of antiretroviral drug regimens.

Conflicting results have been reported in vitro and in animals regarding the effect of garlic on drug metabolism (14,15). Piscitelli et al. (16) investigated in human volunteers the effect of garlic supplements on the pharmacokinetics of saquinavir. Because saquinavir has negligible inhibitory or induction effect on drug-metabolizing enzymes, its use as a study drug by the investigators would minimize the potential of confounding the effect of garlic.

Ten healthy volunteers participated in a three-period, single-sequence interaction study. In period 1, they received 1200 mg of saquinavir three

Table 1 Case Reports and Pharmacokinetic Study of Interactions Between Garlic and Prescription Drugs

Garlic regimen	Sex/age	Diagnosis	Interacting drug dosage/duration	Other concomitant drugs	Clinical result of interaction	Possible mechanism
Unknown	Not specified		Warfarin, dosage regimen not specified	None	None provided	Inhibition of platelet aggregation
Unspecified	Female, 40-years-old	Diabetes	Chlorpropamide, dosage regimen not specified	None mentioned	Decreased glycosuria and blood glucose	Hypoglycemic effect
GarlicPure Maximum Allicin Formula, twice daily for 20 days		Healthy volunteers	Saquinavir, 1200 mg three times daily	None	Reduced AUC, C_{max}, and C_{min} of saquinavir	Possible induction of CYP3A4
500 mg garlic oil t.i.d. × 28 days	6 male, 6 female	Healthy volunteers	Phenotypic markers: midazolam 8 mg orally	None	No change in midazolam metabolic ratio	No change in CYP3A4 activity
10 mg of natural source odorless garlic × 4 days	5 male, 5 female	Healthy volunteers	Single 400 mg dose of ritonavir	None	No change in ritonavir kinetics	No effect on enzyme activity

Abbreviations: AUC, concentration–time curve; C_{max}, maximum concentration; C_{min}, minimum concentration; CYP, cytochrome P-450.

times daily for three days, with blood sampling over eight hours after administration of the 10th dose on day 4. All subjects then entered phase 2 of the study, in which they received garlic caplets (GarliPure Maximum Allicin Formula; Natrol) twice daily for 20 days (days 5–24). In addition, saquinavir was administered concurrently for three days (days 22–24), with blood sampling over eight hours after administration of the 10th saquinavir and 25th garlic dose on day 25. Both garlic and saquinavir were discontinued for 10 days, after which saquinavir was administered in period 3 for 10 doses with blood sampling as in period 1. Adherence assessment was based on interview at each study visit and dosing calendars kept by the subjects.

Compared to baseline saquinavir pharmacokinetic parameters obtained in period 1, the use of garlic reduced the mean saquinavir area under the concentration–time curve (AUC) by 51%, and the maximum (C_{max}) and minimum (C_{min}) saquinavir concentrations by 54% and 49%, respectively. After a 10-day washout, the AUC, C_{max}, and C_{min} values were within a range of 60% to 70% of baseline values. The magnitude of the decline in concentration might result in therapeutic failure and viral rebound in patients with HIV. Based on the pharmacokinetic parameters obtained in period 3, it also appears that garlic might have a prolonged, albeit lesser, effect on saquinavir exposure. The effects of combined treatment with other protease inhibitors that are also potent cytochrome P-450 (CYP) enzymes modulators need to be further evaluated.

Although this study was not designed to address the mechanism of the interaction, the use of garlic clearly resulted in reduction of saquinavir bioavailability, possibly via induction of CYP enzymes, specifically the CYP3A4 isoform that is primarily responsible for metabolism of saquinavir. Therefore, it is likely that other drugs with significant CYP3A4-mediated metabolism could also be affected. Other mechanisms could include induction of P-glycoprotein and/or impairment of absorption. The results from this study also highlight several problems associated with interpretation of botanical product–drug interaction data from different studies. First, the study results were consistent with that of Dalvi (15), who showed a significant increase in CYP enzyme activity after five days administration of garlic in rats, and provided further evidence that in vivo studies employing short-term or single-dose administration (17) and in vitro microsomal studies (14) could provide contradictory results that might not be observed with prolonged use in clinical setting.

On the other hand, Gurley et al. showed that a four-week administration of 500 mg garlic oil three times daily resulted in no significant change in phenotypic ratios of probe drugs for several CYP enzymes, including CYP3A4 (18). While the specific constituent(s) responsible for the effect on drug metabolism is not known, Borek (19) suggested that allicin is converted to an intermediate by-product that induces production of CYP enzymes. To minimize product variability in content, investigators from both studies (16,18) used single lot of the supplement from the same manufacturer. The study of Piscitelli et al. (16) used garlic preparation (GarliPure Maximum Allicin Formula) that is supposedly standardized according to allicin content, whereas product information regarding allicin content were not provided by Gurley et al. (18). If allicin is responsible for garlic's effect on metabolism, garlic preparations that contain minimal or no allicin content might have a different metabolic effect compared to one with maximum allicin content.

Finally, even if all garlic preparations were standardized to allicin content, currently the "standardization" practices and therefore the standardized content can vary significantly from one manufacturer to another, while product inconsistency has not been demonstrated for garlic preparations, there is literature data on the disparity of constituent content among different *echinacea* products (20) and ginseng products (21) (refer to Chapter 2 for further details). As such, the choice of a specific botanical product or preparation may make a difference in the presence and magnitude of a botanical product–drug interaction.

GINKGO (*GINKGO BILOBA* L.)

Background

Medicinal ginkgo products are made from the leaves of the plant, the main pharmacological constituents of which include ginkgolides A, B, C, J, bilobalide, and flavonoids. Ginkgo leads to an increase in microcirculatory blood flow, inhibition of erythrocyte aggregation, platelet-activating factor antagonism, free radical scavenging, and edema protection. These actions suggest that there is no single mechanism of action but that a complex interaction of a multitude of effects could be responsible for its many therapeutic claims, including intermittent claudication (22), dementia (23,24), and tinnitus (25).

The recommended dosages of an oral standardized dry extract of ginkgo (24% ginkgo flavonol glycosides and 6% terpene lactones) are 120 to 240 mg daily for dementia and memory impairment, and 120 to 160 mg daily for intermittent claudication and tinnitus. Adverse effects include gastrointestinal disturbances, diarrhea, vomiting, allergic reactions, pruritus, headache, dizziness, and nose bleeds.

Interactions

Pharmacodynamic Interaction

The most frequently cited potential interaction associated with the use of ginkgo is the potentiation of anticoagulants. This is biologically plausible considering the well-documented antiplatelet effects of the various ginkgolides of ginkgo (26), which have been associated with cases of postoperative bleeding (27), spontaneous hyphema (28), and spontaneous intracranial bleeding (29–32).

While it is not known whether these case reports are just coincidence or actually have a cause–effect relationship, it does establish the bleeding potential of ginkgo and therefore the caution regarding additive pharmaco-dynamic effect with concurrent use of aspirin or anticoagulants, although currently there is little supporting data. A 78-year-old female patient who had been stabilized on warfarin for five years experienced an intracerebral hemorrhage after taking an unknown regimen of ginkgo for two months. The prothrombin time and partial thromboplastin time were 16.9 and 35.5 seconds, respectively, when the hemorrhage was discovered. Discontinuance of both warfarin and ginkgo resulted in no further bleeding episode and no vitamin K administration was required (30).

A 70-year-old man developed a spontaneous bleeding of the iris into the anterior chamber of the eye (hyphema) after ingesting concentrated ginkgo extract 40 mg twice daily for one week. His only other medication was aspirin taken for three years at a dosage of 325 mg without any adverse bleeding event. After the bleeding episode, the patient continued the aspirin regimen but not the ginkgo supplement, and there were no additional bleeding events over the next three months. The clinicians attributed the bleeding event to an interaction between aspirin and ginkgo (28). Based on these and reports of spontaneous bleeding with ginkgo alone, ginkgo has also been recommended to be discontinued before major surgery. In addition, concurrent use of ginkgo with aspirin (28) or other nonsteroidal anti-inflammatory drugs might pose an additive risk of bleeding. Further studies are necessary to confirm the potential of interaction between ginkgo and warfarin or aspirin.

An interaction between *G. biloba* administered as 80 mg leaf extract twice a day and low-dose trazodone (20 mg twice daily) was suspected in a patient with Alzheimer's disease, who took the two products together. It is postulated that a pharmacodynamic (increased gamma-aminobutyric acid-ergic activity) and pharmacokinetic mechanisms [increased metabolism of trazodone to *m*-chlorophenylpiperazine (*m*-CPP), which acts on the benzodiazepine-binding sites and releases gamma-aminobutyric acid] contribute to the observed effect (32). Table 2 provides a list of reported pharmacodynamic and pharmacokinetic interactions involving ginkgo.

Pharmacokinetic Interaction

Gurley et al. evaluated the effect of *G. biloba* standardized to contain 24% of flavone glycosides and 6% terpene lactones on phenotypic markers of CYP1A2, 2D6, 3A4 and 2E1. Twelve healthy individuals (six males and six females) received 60 mg of the standardized *G. biloba* preparation four times per day for 28 days. The four CYP phenotypes were assessed before and at the end of the 28-day study period. Although there was a trend of increased CYP2E1 activity by 23%, the effect was not statistically significant. *G. biloba* produced no significant changes in phenotypic ratios of the other three CYP isoforms. The results from this study suggested that standardized *G. biloba*

Table 2 Case Reports and Pharmacokinetic Study of Interactions Between Ginkgo and Synthetic Drugs

Ginkgo dosage/duration	Sex/age	Diagnosis	Interacting drug dosage/duration	Other concomitant drugs	Clinical result of interaction	Possible mechanism
Concentrated 50:1 extract 40 mg b.i.d. for 1 wk	Male/70	Coronary artery bypass	Aspirin 325 mg/day for 3 yrs	None	Spontaneous hyphema	Additive inhibition on platelet aggregation
(EGb716) leaf extract 80 mg b.i.d. for 3 days	Female/80	Alzheimer's disease	Trazodone 20 mg b.i.d. for 3 days	Bromazepam, donazepil, vitamin E (in the past 3 mos but not concomitantly with ginkgo)	Coma (Glasgow coma scale 6/15)	Possible increase of GABAergic activity by ginkgo flavonoids
Unknown regimen for 2 mos	Female/78	Coronary artery bypass and progressive dementia	Warfarin for 5 yrs	None mentioned	Intracerebral hemorrhage	Additive effect on coagulation mechanisms
60 mg standardized Ginkgo biloba preparation	6 males and 6 females	Healthy subjects	Phenotypic markers: midazolam 8 mg, caffeine 100 mg, debrisoquine 5 mg, chlorzoxasone 500 mg	None	No significant change in metabolic ratio of phenotypic markers	Lack of effect on CYP isoenzymes

Abbreviation: CYP, cytochrome P-450.

preparation containing 24% of flavone glycosides and 6% terpene lactones have minimal effect on the activity of the four CYP isoforms, and therefore the metabolism of drugs mediated by these enzymes (18).

In general, the study results also are consistent with that of Duche et al. (33), who reported that administration of a 13-day regimen of *G. biloba* in healthy volunteers did not affect the pharmacokinetics of antipyrine, a nonspecific marker of overall CYP enzyme activity. However, there was no evaluation of CYP2C9 activity in both studies, so it remains unknown whether any reports or concerns of interaction with warfarin could have a pharmacokinetic basis as well. Separately, Smith et al. (34) reported in an abstract that *G. biloba* administered over an 18-day period produced a 53% increase in concentration of nifedipine, a CYP3A4 substrate. However, the amount of flavone glycosides and terpene lactones in the botanical supplement were not known (34), and nifedipine might not reflect CYP3A4 activity in a manner similar to that with midazolam, which is a well-recognized, specific marker for CYP3A4. In another study, 14 patients with Alzheimer's disease received the acetycholinesterase inhibitor donepezil 5 mg per day for at least 20 weeks with steady-state donepezil concentrations of $22.7 \pm 10.3 \, \text{ng/mL}$ and a Mini-Mental Scale Examination (MMSE) score of 9.0 ± 7.8. Concurrent administration of 90 mg/day of *G. biloba* for 30 days did not alter the concentration (24.4 ± 12.6 ng/mL) and MMSE score (8.7 ± 7.7), suggesting that there is no adverse interaction between the *G. biloba* and donepezil when used together in patients with Alzheimer's disease (35). However, the amount of flavone glycosides and terpene lactones in the botanical supplement were also not known.

ASIAN GINSENG (*PANAX GINSENG* C. A. MEYER)

Background

There is considerable confusion about terminology for the different species known collectively to the consumer as ginseng; Asian ginseng is also sometimes called Chinese ginseng, Korean ginseng, ninjin (Japanese), or true ginseng. It is often confused with Siberian ginseng (*Eleutherococcus senticosus* Maxim), which belongs to the same family (*Araliaceae*) but is a different genus. Another popular ginseng product is American ginseng or Canadian ginseng (*Panax quinquefolius* L.)

The dried roots of Asian ginseng are used for medicinal purposes and its main constituents are triterpene saponins known as ginsenosides or panaxosides. The pharmacologic actions of ginseng include immunomodulatory, anti-inflammatory, antitumor, smooth muscle relaxation, stimulant, and hypoglycemic effects (36).

The recommended dosage is 200 mg daily of standardized extract (4% total ginsenosides). Reported adverse effects include insomnia, diarrhea, vaginal bleeding, mastalgia, swollen tender breasts, increased libido, manic episodes, and a possible cause of Stevens–Johnson syndrome (2). A "Ginseng abuse syndrome" (consumed dose approximately 3 g daily) has been described with symptoms such as hypertension, sleeplessness, skin eruptions, morning diarrhoea, and agitation. Doses of 15 g daily and over were associated with depersonalization, confusion, and depression (2). A recent systematic review of the totality of the safety data concluded that adverse effects associated with the use of ginseng are rare, mild, and transient (37).

Interactions

Pharmacodynamic Interactions

The most frequently reported interactions are those with monoamine oxidase inhibitors (MAOIs) (2). There were reports in the literature of a potential interaction between ginseng and the MAOI phenelzine (38,39). The symptoms described included insomnia, headache and tremulousness in a 64-year-old woman when ginseng was added to her phenelzine regimen (38). Jones and Runikis reported that the use of ginseng in a 42-year-old woman treated with phenelzine was associated with manic-like symptoms, irritability, tension headache, and occasional vague visual hallucinations. After discontinuing the ginseng, the patient's symptoms resolved with only a few headache episodes thereafter. The clinicians considered that her other medications including lorazepam and triazolam were not contributory factors and the symptoms were mostly likely associated with ginseng–phenelzine interaction (39). However, ginseng is a stimulant and one of the common side effects of the use of ginseng is insomnia (40), and MAOI can also cause insomnia and headache; it is difficult to determine whether the described symptoms in these two reports are related to the use of each product alone or are attributed to botanical product–drug interaction.

Ginseng has the potential to interfere with the coagulation cascade and therefore interact with warfarin. However, there is no literature report of increased INR with concurrent use of both drugs. Interestingly, the use of ginseng has been associated with decreased INR (41,42). Janetzky and Morreale described a 47-year-old man with a mechanical heart valve, who was stabilized on warfarin with therapeutic INR within the range of 3.0 to 4.0. Two weeks after the patient took an unknown strength of ginger (*P. ginseng*) three times daily, his INR decreased to 1.5. Upon discontinuance of the ginger preparation, his INR returned to 3.3 two weeks later. Fortunately, there were no adverse effects during the two-week period of subtherapeutic INR (41). On the other hand, a thrombosis of a prosthetic aortic valve was attributed to the use of ginseng in a patient who had been stabilized on warfarin regimen (dosage regimen and INR values not reported) (42).

Because there is no human pharmacokinetic study evaluating this potential interaction or metabolic study data showing an effect of ginseng

Table 3 Case Reports of Interactions Between Ginseng and Synthetic Drugs

Ginseng dosage/duration	Sex/age	Diagnosis	Interacting drug dosage/duration	Other concomitant drugs	Clinical result of interaction	Possible mechanism
Ginseng tea (38)	Female/64	Depression	Phenelzine 45–60 mg/d (dose and duration not reported)	None mentioned	Insomnia, headache, tremulousness	Increased cAMP levels by ginsenosides
Ginseng (39)	Female/42	Depression	Phenelzine 45 mg/d	Bee pollen, triazolam, lorazepam	Manic symptoms (irritability, hallucinations)	Increased cAMP levels by ginsenosides
Ginseng (41) (Ginsana® capsules t.i.d. for 2 wks	Male/47	Heart valve replacement	Warfarin 5 mg/d for 5 yrs; 7.5 mg each Tuesday	Diltiazem, nitroglycerin, salsalate	Decreased INR (from about 3.3 to 1.5)	Not known
Ginseng product (42)	Male/58	Coronary heart disease, diabetes	Warfarin	Several (but no details mentioned)	Decreased INR to 1.4, thrombosis	Not known

Abbreviations: INR, international normalized ratio; cAMP, cyclic adenosine monophosphate.

on CYP2C9, the primary CYP isoenzyme responsible for metabolism of the pharmacologically more potent *S*-isomer of warfarin, the reported paradoxical decrease in INR associated with ginger use is difficult to explain and evaluate. An animal study in rats demonstrated no effect of ginseng on either absorption or elimination of a single dose of warfarin. There were also no changes in prothrombin time after steady-state dosing of warfarin (43).

The confusion about ginseng terminology mentioned above extends to case reports of ginseng–drug interactions, and it is not sure that all of these pharmacodynamic interactions are related to *P. ginseng*. In particular, the intake of concomitant drugs is a potentially significant confounding factor. Any conclusions about causality seem premature at this time. Table 3 summarizes case reports of interactions between ginseng and synthetic drugs.

Pharmacokinetic Interactions

Anderson et al. evaluated the effect of *P. ginseng* on the 6-β-hydroxycortisol to cortisol ratio, a marker of CYP3A4 activity. Ten male and 10 female healthy subjects were given 100 mg of *P. ginseng* standardized to contain 4% ginsenosides (Ginsana^{TM}) twice daily for 14 days. Comparing the 6-β-hydroxycortisol-to-cortisol ratio before and after the 14-day regimen of *P. ginseng* showed no appreciable difference, suggesting that there is no enzyme induction effect on CYP3A4 (44). The result from this study confirms the data of Gurley et al. (18) who administered 500 mg of *P. ginseng* standardized to contain 5% ginsenosides (brand name not provided).

It is of note that both Asian and Siberian ginsengs contain glycosides with structural similarities to digoxin, and both ginseng products have been reported to interfere with fluorescent polarization immunoassay determination of digoxin concentrations. Even though not an in vivo interaction per se, the digoxin-like immunoreactive substances associated with the use of ginseng cause false elevation of digoxin concentrations and could result in inappropriate dosage adjustment (45).

COMMENT

There is little doubt about the therapeutic potential of some of the herbal medicines discussed in this chapter. Their safety profile is equally encouraging. The scope for botanical product–drug interactions (Table 1), however, seems considerable. This is sharply contrasted by the paucity of actual clinical reports of such interactions occurring in practice. There are at least two explanations for this overt discrepancy. Firstly, interactions could indeed be rare. Secondly, the paucity of reports could be the result of underreporting. Underreporting of adverse effects is significant and, in the realm of herbal medicine, it is likely to be even larger than with conventional drugs (46). In the absence of sufficient data it is impossible to decide which explanation is correct. What we can say, however, is that the subject of botanical product–drug interactions is potentially important and grossly under-researched. Thus it warrants further systematic study.

REFERENCES

1. Blumenthal M. Herb sales down in mainstream market, up in natural food stores. Herbalgram 2002; 55:60.
2. Ernst E, Pittler MH, Stevinson C, White AR. The Desktop Guide to Complementary and Alternative Medicine. Edinburgh: Mosby, 2001.
3. Stevinson C, Pittler MH, Ernst E. Garlic for treating hypercholesterolemia. Ann Intern Med 2000; 133:420–429.
4. Silagy C, Neil A. A meta-analysis of the effect of garlic on blood pressure. J Hypertens 1994; 12:463–468.
5. Breithaupt-Grogler K, Ling M, Boudoulas H, Belz GG. Protective effects of chronic garlic intake on elastic properties of aorta in the elderly. Circulation 1997; 96:2649–2655.
6. Ernst E. Can allium vegetables prevent cancer? Phytomed 1997; 4:79–83.
7. Makheja AN, Bailey JM. Antiplatelet constituents of garlic and onions. Agents Actions 1990; 29:360–363.
8. Bordia A. Effect of garlic on platelet aggregation in vitro. Atherosclerosis 1978; 30:355–360.
9. Rose KD, Croissant PD, Parliament CF, Levin MB. Spontaneous spinal epidural hematoma with associated platelet dysfunction from excessive garlic ingestion: a case report. Neurosurgery 1990; 26:880–882.
10. German K, Kumar U, Blackford HN. Garlic and the risk of TURP bleeding. Br J Urol 1995; 76:518.
11. Sunter WH. Warfarin and garlic. Pharmaceut J 1991; 246:722.
12. Aslam M, Stockley I. Interaction between curry ingredient (karela) and drug (chlorpropamide). Lancet 1979; 313(8116):607.
13. Leatherdale BA, Panesar RK, Singh G, Atkins TW, Bailey CJ, Bignell AH. Improvement in glucose tolerance due to *Momordica charantia* (karela). Br Med J 1981; 282:1823–1824.
14. Foster BC, Foster MS, Vandenhoek S, et al. An in vitro evaluation of human cytochrome P450-3A4 and P-glycoprotein inhibition by garlic. J Pharm Pharmaceut Sci 2001; 4:176–184.
15. Dalvi RR. Alteration in hepatic phase I and phase II biotransformation enzymes by garlic oil in rats. Toxicol Lett 1992; 60:299–305.
16. Piscitelli SC, Burstein AH, Welden N, Gallicano KD, Falloon J. The effect of garlic supplements on the pharmacokinetics of saquinavir. Clin Infect Dis 2002; 34:234–238.
17. Gallicano K, Foster B, Choudhri S. Effect of short-term administration of garlic supplements on single-dose ritonavir pharmacokinetics in healthy volunteers. Br J Clin Pharmacol 2002; 55:199–202.
18. Gurley BJ, Gardner SF, Hubbard MA, et al. Cytochrome P450 phenotypic ratios for predicting herb-drug interactions in humans. Clin Pharmacol Ther 2002; 72:276–287.

19. Borek C. Garlic supplements and saquinavir. Clin Infect Dis 2002; 35:34.
20. Gilroy CM, Steiner JF, Byers T, Shapiro H, Georgian W. Echinacea and truth in labeling. Arch Intern Med 2003; 163:699–704.
21. Consumer Reports, Nov 1995.
22. Pittler MH, Ernst E. Ginkgo biloba extract for the treatment of intermittent claudication. A meta-analysis. Am J Med 2000; 108:276–281.
23. Ernst E, Pittler MH. *Ginkgo biloba* for dementia: a systematic review of double-blind placebo-controlled trials. Clin Drug Invest 199; 17:301–308.
24. Canter PH, Ernst E. *Ginkgo biloba*: a smart drug? A systematic review of controlled trials of the cognitive effects of *Ginkgo biloba* extracts in healthy-people. Psychopharmacol Bull 2002; 36:108–123.
25. Ernst E, Stevinson C. *Ginkgo biloba* for tinnitus: a review. Clin Otolaryngol 1999; 24:164–167.
26. Chung KF, Dent G, McCuster M, Guinot P, Page CP, Barnes PJ. Effect of ginkgolide mixture (BN 52063) in antagonizing skin and platelet responses to platelet activating factor in man. Lancet 1987; 1:248–251.
27. Fessenden JM, Wittenborn W, Clarke L. *Ginkgo biloba*: a case report of herbal medicine bleeding postoperatively from a laparoscopic cholecystectomy. Ann Surg 2001; 67:33–35.
28. Rosenblatt M, Mindel J. Spontaneous hyphema associated with ingestion of *Ginkgo biloba* extract. N Engl J Med 1997; 336:1108.
29. Gilbert GJ. *Ginkgo biloba*. Neurology 1997; 48:1137.
30. Matthews MK Jr. Association of *Ginkgo biloba* with intracerebral hemorrhage. Neurology 1998; 50:1933–1934.
31. Rowin J, Lewis SL. Spontaneous bilateral subdural hematomas associated with chronic *Ginkgo biloba* ingestion. Neurology 1996; 46:1775–1776.
32. Galluzi S, Zanetti O, Binetti G, Trabucchi M, Frisoni GB. Coma in a patient with Alzheimer's disease taking low-dose trazodone and *Ginkgo biloba*. J Neurol Neurosurg Psychiat 2000; 68:679–680.
33. Duche JC, Barre J, Guinot P, et al. Effect of *Ginkgo biloba* extract on microsomal enzyme induction. Int J Clin Pharm Res 1989; 9:165–168.
34. Smith M, Lin KM, Zheng YP. An open trial of nifedipine-herb interactions: nifedipine with St. John's wort, ginseng or ginkgo biloba. Clin Pharmacol Ther 2001; 69:P86.
35. Yasui-Furukori N, Furukori H, Kaneda A, Kaneko S, Tateishi T. The effects of *Ginkgo biloba* extracts on the pharmacokinetics and pharmacodynamics of donepezil. J Clin Pharmacol 2004; 44:538–542.
36. Vogler BK, Pittler MH, Ernst E. The efficacy of ginseng. A systematic review of randomised clinical trials. Eur J Clin Pharmacol 1999; 55:567–575.
37. Thompson Coon J, Ernst E. Panax ginseng. A systematic review of adverse effects and drug interactions. Drug Saf 2002; 25:323–344.
38. Shader RJ, Greenblatt DJ. Phenelzine and the dream machine-ramblings and reflections. J Clin Psychopharmacol 1985; 5:65.
39. Jones BD, Runikis AM. Interaction of ginseng with phenelzine. J Clin Psychopharmacol 1987; 7:201–202.

40. Scaglione F, Cattaneo G, Alessandria M, Cogo R. Efficacy and safety of the standardized ginseng extract G115 for potentiating vaccination against the influenza and protection against the common cold. Drugs Exp Clin Res 1996; 22:65–72.
41. Janetzky K, Morreale AP. Probable interaction between warfarin and ginseng. Am J Health Syst Pharm 1997; 54:692–693.
42. Rosado MF. Thrombosis of a prosthetic aortic valve disclosing a hazardous interaction between warfarin and a commercial ginseng product. Cardiology 2003; 99:111.
43. Zhou M, Chan KW, Ng LS, Chang S, Li RC. Possible influences of ginseng on pharmacokinetics and pharmacodynamics of warfarin in rats. J Pharm Pharmacol 1999; 51:175–180.
44. Anderson GD, Rosito G, Mohustsy MA, Elmer GW. Drug interaction potential of soy extract and *Panax ginseng*. J Clin Pharmacol 2003; 43:643–648.
45. Dasgupta A, Wu S, Actor J, Olsen M, Wells A, Datta P. Effect of Asian and Siberian ginseng on serum digoxin measurement by five digoxin immunoassays. Significant variation in digoxin-like immunoreactivity among commercial ginsengs. Am J Clin Pathol 2003; 119:298–303.
46. Barnes J, Mills SY, Abbot NC, Willoughby M, Ernst E. Different standards for reporting ADRs to herbal remedies and conventional OTC medicines face-to-face interviews with 515 users of herbal remedies. Br J Clin Pharmacol 1998; 45:496–500.

6

A Review of Chinese Botanical Product–Drug Interactions

Y. W. Francis Lam

*Departments of Pharmacology and Medicine,
University of Texas Health Science Center at
San Antonio, San Antonio, and College of Pharmacy,
University of Texas at Austin, Austin, Texas, U.S.A.*

Ming Ou

*Guangzhou University of Traditional Chinese Medicine,
Guangzhou, P.R. China*

INTRODUCTION

Many Asian communities throughout the world have used Chinese botanical products for centuries. Recently, the usage of these botanical products has also increased in Western societies. Although the use of Chinese botanical products is on the rise, the potential and significance of interaction with Western drugs is not widely recognized and well characterized. While there are very few adequate, well-controlled clinical studies designed to investigate the potential for interaction between Chinese botanical products and drugs, in the English literature, there are examples of documented interaction between commonly used Chinese botanical products and currently available Western drugs, and these case reports will be reviewed in this chapter. In addition, issues that are more pertinent to the evaluation of the importance and clinical relevance of Chinese botanical product–drug interactions will be discussed.

In contrast to theoretical, in vitro, or animal data, the reports reviewed in this chapter provide the clinicians more relevant information, including description of the time course, the magnitude of the suspected interaction, and clinical outcome of the patient. This not only allows an evaluation of the clinical significance, but also provides a basis for further evaluation with well-designed studies. Obviously, case reports have their own inherent limitations, including the existence of potential confounding variables and limited generalizability, which in view of the known product variability of active constituents or content, could be of particular importance in botanical product–drug interactions. Finally, it should be recognized that the occurrence of one or more case reports does not necessarily imply an absolute contraindication of concurrent use of the botanical product and prescription or over-the-counter drug.

Currently, most of the literature reports of Chinese botanical product–drug interaction in humans involve warfarin (Table 1), likely a function of its narrow therapeutic index requiring close monitoring of therapy with international normalized ratio (INR) and the presence of coumarin derivatives in a number of Chinese botanical products rendering them with anticoagulant property. In addition, some Chinese botanical products also possess antiplatelet effects and have potential for adverse interactions with analgesic drugs such as aspirin or nonsteroidal anti-inflammatory drugs. Based on human, animal, and in vitro data, other Chinese botanical products such as hawthorn have also been reported to interact with a variety of drugs.

It should be noted that while the focus of most Chinese botanical product–drug interaction reports understandably is on the occurrence of adverse effects, not all interactions result in an undesirable effect. An example is *Salviae miltiorrhizae* (danshen), which has been reported by multiple clinicians to cause bleeding with the concurrent use of warfarin [section "*Salviae miltiorrhizae* (Danshen)"], whereas less is known about the potential benefits that might result from combining danshen with an aminoglycoside. Wang et al. had demonstrated in animals the potential usefulness of combining danshen with kanamycin to reduce aminoglycoside-induced free-radical generation in vitro and ototoxicity in vivo, without interfering with serum concentration or efficacy of kanamycin in mice (1). Other examples of potential beneficial botanical product–drug interaction that warrants further studies include the combined use of the Chinese medicinal plant *Tripterygium wilfordi* and cyclosporin, which is described in Chapter 2.

In addition to the more conventional nomenclature system of using the botanical name, e.g., *Angelica sinensis* [section "*Angelica sinensis* (Chinese Angelica, Dong Quai)"], Chinese botanical products also can be identified by their pinyin name, e.g., dong quai for *A. sinensis*. Although most English literature refer to Chinese botanical products by their botanical names or pharmaceutical names, the corresponding pinyin names are often used instead in most Chinese herbal literature. Therefore, searching

Table 1 Summary of Chinese Botanical Product–Warfarin Interactions Based on Case Reports

Botanical product	Known or presumed mechanism of interaction	Description of interaction outcome	Comment
Dong quai	Coumarin constituents; inhibition of platelet aggregation; possible inhibition of CYP isoenzymes	Increased INR and PT; no bleeding episode in one case; widespread bruising in another report	
Danshen	Inhibition of platelet aggregation	Increased INR ± increased PT; no bleeding episode	Fresh frozen plasma and packed red blood cells were administered in all cases
Chinese wolfberry	Unknown; possible inhibition of CYP isoenzymes	Increased INR; no bleeding episode	
Quilinggao	Antiplatelet, antithrombotic constituents	Increased INR; bruising	
Green tea	Antagonism by vitamin K constituent	Decreased INR; no signs and symptoms of suboptimal anticoagulation	
Ginseng	Unknown	Decreased INR; thrombosis of a prosthetic aortic valve	

Abbreviations: CYP, cytochrome P-450; INR, international normalized ratio; PT, prothrombin time.

for literature information regarding Chinese botanical products should ideally include the pinyin names in the search strategies, especially if the source of information is primary Chinese herbal literature.

CHINESE BOTANICAL PRODUCTS AND WARFARIN

Angelica sinensis (Chinese Angelica, Dong Quai)

Dong quai (dang gui, tang kuei) is the extract from the dried root of *Radix Angelicae sinensis* (Fig. 1), which belongs to the family Umbelliferae. It has been used for many years as a Chinese botanical remedy for management of menstrual cramps, irregular menses, and menopausal symptoms, and the

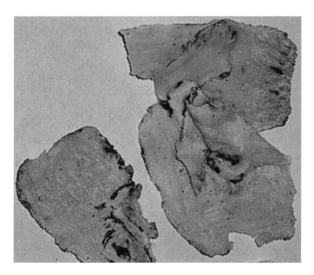

Figure 1   *Angelica sinensis* (Chinese angelica, Dong Quai).

usual dosage range is 3 to 15 g per day of raw drug prepared as a hot water decoction or alcoholic infusion. Different preparations, including alcoholic extracts, tablets, and teas, are available to the consumer. Dong quai contains coumarins and also may inhibit platelet aggregation. Therefore, this Chinese botanical product could potentially enhance the pharmacologic effect of warfarin-like compounds.

Page and Lawrence (2) reported a 46-year-old female patient with rheumatic heart disease and atrial fibrillation, who was referred to the anticoagulation clinic for warfarin therapy management. She was successfully managed with warfarin (Coumadin; Dupont Pharmaceutical Co, Wilmington, Delaware, U.S.A.) 5 mg/day, which maintained her INR within the range of 2 to 3 for about two years. At a routine clinic visit, the patient was found to have an elevated INR of 4.05 compared to 1.89 a month earlier. The prothrombin time (PT) also increased over the same time period from 16.2 to 23.5 seconds. Because she did not show any evidence of clinical bleeding, and there were no readily identifiable sources for the increased laboratory values, including dosing error and abnormal liver function, she was instructed to withhold the warfarin dose for one day. The patient missed a follow-up clinic visit and only returned after another month had passed. At that time her PT and INR were further increased to 27 seconds and 4.9, respectively. The patient also disclosed that she had been taking dong quai at a dosage of 565 mg once to twice daily for four weeks to manage her perimenopausal symptoms. She was instructed to miss a day of warfarin dosing with no additional change of warfarin dosage, and also to discontinue consumption of dong quai. Two weeks after discontinuing the dong quai regimen, her PT and INR decreased to 21.6 seconds and 3.41, respectively, with further reduction to 18.5 seconds and 2.48 after an additional two weeks. Ellis and Stephens reported similar interaction in a brief case report describing a patient with a mitral valve replacement, who had been stabilized on warfarin (dosage regimen not reported) for 10 years. After taking an unknown quantity of dong quai for a month, she presented to the clinic with an INR of 10. Although details of the report were very few, significant bruising as a result of the interaction was shown in a photographic figure published with the case (3).

Although the exact mechanism is not known, the coumarin constituent of dong quai is likely responsible for the enhanced pharmacological effect. An animal study also suggested that the basis of the interaction is likely pharmacodynamic and not pharmacokinetic in nature (4). Nevertheless, it should be noted that dong quai belongs to the family Umbelliferae, and plants within this family contain furocoumarins, which have been reported to inhibit cytochrome P-450 (CYP) activity, especially CYP3A4 (5). In this regard, it is of note that the extract of the dried root of *Radix Angelica dahurica*, another botanical product belonging to the Umbelliferae family, has been reported to increase the area under the plasma concentration–time curve (AUC) and to prolong the elimination half-life of tolbutamide in rats by 2.5- and 2.3-fold, respectively, which was likely a result of the inhibitory effect of its furocoumarin components on different CYP isoenzymes, including those belonging to the 2C subfamily (6). Based on in vitro studies, it has also been suggested that another dong quai component, sodium ferulate, might inhibit platelet aggregation and cyclooxygenase activity (7). Further studies are needed to confirm the possibility of pharmacokinetic mechanisms and identify the inhibitory components.

Salviae miltiorrhizae (Danshen)

Danshen, the dried root and rhizome of *S. miltiorrhizae* (Fig. 2), is another Chinese botanical product used for its ability to alleviate menstrual irregularities, as well as for its vasodilative and hypotensive functions in a variety of cardiovascular conditions (8). The botanical product had also been shown to inhibit platelet aggregation in vitro (9). Danshen is widely available in different preparations for oral consumption, with usual dose range of 9 to 15 g per decoction. In addition, its increasing popularity is reflected by its availability even in Chinese cigarettes (10).

Clinicians from Hong Kong reported a case of potential danshen–warfarin interaction in a 48-year-old female with a history of rheumatic heart disease, atrial fibrillation, and mitral stenosis (11). The patient underwent successful transvenous mitral valvuloplasty for management of her medical conditions, and was discharged with 1 mg warfarin, as well as

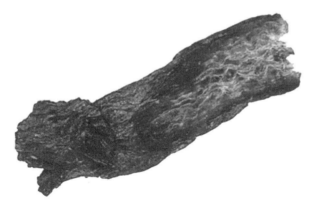

Figure 2   *Salvia miltiorrhizae* (Danshen).

furosemide and digoxin. Since discharge the patient's warfarin dosage ranged from 2.5 to 3.5 mg daily with an INR of 1.5 to 3. Her last warfarin dose adjustment was an increase in dose to 4 mg daily in response to an INR of 1.35. Since then the patient also had intermittent influenza-like symptoms, for which she took botanical products with danshen as one of the main ingredients, every other day. When the patient presented to the emergency room several weeks later because of increased flu-like symptoms, her clotting profile was noted to be significantly abnormal with an INR exceeding 5.6 and PT above 60 seconds. There was no other clinical source of clotting abnormality and the most likely cause of over-anticoagulation was believed to be an interaction between warfarin and danshen. Although the patient stopped taking both warfarin and all botanical products, and received fresh frozen plasma, her clotting abnormality persisted for more than five days. Nevertheless, the patient suffered no clinical evidence of bleeding and over the next four months, she was stable on a daily warfarin regimen of 3 mg and an INR of 2.5.

There were two additional reports of danshen–warfarin interaction in the literature. A 62-year-old man with rheumatic mitral regurgitation had been stabilized on warfarin 5 mg with INR of about 3.0 over four weeks after discharge. His other medications included captopril, furosemide, and digoxin. The patient then started taking danshen daily to help his heart condition. Two weeks later, he was admitted to the hospital with an INR of 8.4. Both the warfarin and danshen regimens were stopped. Fresh frozen plasma and packed red blood cells were administered, eventually decreasing the INR to 2.0. Over the next two weeks, he was restarted on warfarin and the dose titrated back to the previous regimen of 5 mg/day, resulting in a stable INR of 3 (12).

Another case involved a 66-year-old male patient who was stabilized on 2 to 2.5 mg of warfarin per day with INR of about 2. About nine days prior to admission to the hospital, the patient developed nonspecific chest wall pain, for which he self-treated with two to three topical applications of 15% methyl salicylate and two decoctions of danshen over the next few days. On the day of admission, his INR was found to be greater than 5.5, and his warfarin regimen was stopped, followed by administration of fresh frozen plasma and packed red blood cells. The INR was subsequently stabilized at 2.0 to 2.5 (13).

These three cases suggested that danshen might potentiate the anticoagulant effect of warfarin, although information regarding consumption of other Chinese botanical products was not available for two (11,12) of the three cases. In the report of Tam et al. (13), the patient also self-medicated with topical application of methyl salicylate, which might have initially exaggerated the anticoagulant effect of danshen. In all three reports, the absence of identifiable precipitating factors and the temporal relationship between botanical product consumption and onset of exaggerated anticoagulation effect suggested an interaction between danshen and warfarin. In addition to inhibiting platelet aggregation and interfering with extrinsic blood coagulation, danshen was also shown to affect warfarin pharmacokinetics in an animal study (14). Chan et al. reported that single-dose administration of danshen in rats increased the AUC and maximal concentration of the *R*- and *S*-isomers of warfarin. In addition, concurrent administration of warfarin and danshen for three days also increased the steady-state *R*- and *S*-warfarin concentrations, with resultant increases in PT by 11 seconds (15).

Lycium barbarum (*L. chinese*, Chinese Wolfberry, Gou Qi Zi, Fructus Lycii Chinensis)

The dried fruit of *L. barbarum* L., a common Chinese botanical product (Fig. 3) (16) belonging to the family of Solanacaea, is available in different tea formulations for its beneficial effects on the kidney and the liver. Lam et al. described a potential interaction between a concentrated Chinese herbal tea and warfarin in a 61-year-old Chinese woman (17). The patient had been stabilized on a weekly warfarin dosage regimen of 18 to 19 mg/week, with a therapeutic INR ranging between 2 and 3, for her recurring atrial fibrillation. There were no signs and symptoms of abnormal anticoagulation.

On a routine anticoagulation clinic evaluation, the patient's INR was elevated to 4.1 from 2.5 obtained at the prior monthly visit, albeit with no clinical evidence of bleeding. There was no reported change in any of her medication regimens, diet, or lifestyle. However, the patient indicated that she had been consuming one cup of a concentrated herbal tea made from dried fruits of *L. barbarum* L. several times a day, to manage blurred vision secondary to a sore eye. When she presented to the clinic, the vision problems had already resolved. The patient was advised to discontinue

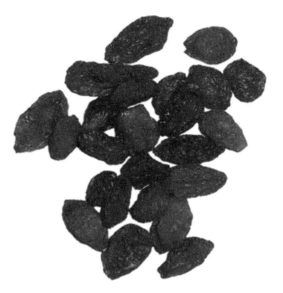

Figure 3   *Lycium barbarum* (*Lycium chinese*, Chinese wolfberry, Gou Qi Zi, Fructus Lycii Chinensis).

the herbal tea consumption, and the warfarin weekly dosage regimen was adjusted to 16 mg with a resultant INR of 2.0, followed by 18 mg/week with a resultant INR of 2.2, before resumption of the original dose of 19 mg/ week with a resultant INR of 2.5.

This case suggested that the elevated INR might be related to the consumption of the herbal tea made from the dried fruits of *L. barbarum* L. The investigators further performed an experiment using human liver microsomes to investigate the effect of the tea on warfarin metabolism. Using method provided by the patient, the investigator produced the herbal tea by adding 5 g of the fruit to 100 mL of boiling water. The hot water decoction was eventually reduced in volume to about 30 mL. The extract was then filtered and the resulting filtrate used in microsomal incubation. The investigators reported that the prepared tea inhibited the metabolism of the *S*-warfarin isomer by CYP2C9. Furthermore, based on the amount of tea ingested, the solids concentration of the prepared tea, and assumed values of bioavailability and volume of distribution, the plasma concentration of the inhibitory component was estimated to be much lower than the inhibitory concentrations calculated from the in vitro experiment. However, the investigators emphasized the lack of knowledge regarding actual measured inhibitory concentration at the active site of metabolism and the actual bioavailability and distribution volumes of the inhibitory component. In addition, whether *L. barbarum* also possesses an anticoagulant or antiplatelet effect is not known. Therefore, despite the time sequence of INR changes with the use of the herbal tea, it is not known whether the effect is related to altered CYP or non-CYP disposition variables or to an anticoagulant effect of the botanical product itself.

Chinese Botanical Product Quilinggao

It is not uncommon for Chinese botanical products to be combined in different preparations for a variety of uses. "Quilinggao," also referred to as "Essence of Tortoise Shell," is a combination Chinese botanical product produced by different manufacturers and promoted for improving general health and reducing internal "body heat." At times, consumers consider and take the product as a health food rather than an herbal medicine. Clinicians in Hong Kong recently reported a patient with clinical evidence of bleeding and over-anticoagulation after consuming different brands of quilinggao (18).

A 61-year-old man had been receiving warfarin for his atrial fibrillation and chronic rheumatic heart disease. With a warfarin regimen of 3 mg alternating with 3.5 mg every other day, his INR was mostly stabilized within the range of 1.6 to 2.8. On a routine clinic visit for INR monitoring, his INR was found to be greater than 6.0 and he had complained of gum bleeding and epistaxis over three days prior to the clinic visit. There were no reports of changes in medication adherence and dietary habit of vitamin K. Upon further questioning, the patient revealed that he had been taking the combination botanical product quilinggao daily for over three years with a change in the brand just one week prior to the clinic visit. Although he noticed bruising on his left leg five days after taking the new (second) brand of quilinggao product, he continued to consume one can per day until the clinic visit.

His warfarin therapy was withheld and his INR decreased to 2.9 and 1.9, three and five days later, respectively. His warfarin regimen was restarted at the same 3/3.5 mg on alternate days as before. The patient was later discharged with an INR of 2.5. He was consulted regarding the possible adverse consequences of taking warfarin and quilinggao concurrently. However, immediately after discharge, he began drinking one can of another (third) brand of quilinggao product daily and three days later his INR was elevated to 5.2. The patient was readmitted to the hospital and warfarin therapy withheld, resulting in decreases of INR to 4.3 and 3.4, two and three days later, respectively. The warfarin therapy was eventually restarted after an INR of 1.9 was reached.

Among the different ingredients listed on the labels, from the first and the second brands of quilinggao products, Chuanbeimu (*Fritillaria cirrhosa*) in the first brand, as well as Beimu (*Fritillaria* spp.), Chishao (*Paeoniae rubra*, Chinese peony), Jinyinhua (*Lonicera japonica*), and Jishi (*Poncirus trifoliata*) in the second brand were constituents that had antiplatelet and/or antithrombotic effects. The potential interacting constituent(s) could not be identified with the third quilinggao product because the patient could not remember its brand name. There was no readily identifiable cause for over-anticoagulation during both hospitalizations, and the temporal relationship between consumption of the last two quilinggao products and the changes in the INR values suggested that an additive interaction between the botanical product and warfarin was the likely cause of the exaggerated pharmacologic effect. The difference in interaction outcome between the first and second quilinggao products could be related to the greater number of interacting botanical constituents present in the second brand product.

Camellia sinensis (Green Tea)

Consumption of green tea is a common practice in Asian countries such as China and Japan, and its use as a dietary supplement in the United States has also increased significantly over the years, perhaps reflecting a belief that it may prevent carcinogenesis (19–21). Although it is not usually considered as a botanical product, dry green tea leaves contain as much as 1.4 mg of vitamin K per 100 g of dry leaves (22). Dietary intake of vitamin K facilitates clotting factor synthesis and is well known to antagonize the anticoagulant effect of warfarin. The following report described a probable case of interaction between warfarin and green tea (23).

A 44-year-old Caucasian male had been treated with warfarin for more than a year for prophylaxis of thromboembolic complications associated with his St. Jude mechanical valve replacement in the aortic position. The therapeutic goal was to maintain his INR within the range of 2.5 to 3.5, and a review of the patient's medication history indicated that a decrease in his INR was always associated with a reduction in warfarin dose. One month prior to clinic visit, his warfarin regimen was 7.5 mg/day and the INR was 3.2. At the clinic, the patient's INR was found to be 3.79 with the same warfarin dosage regimen. However, he was asymptomatic and there was no obvious reason for the increased INR. He was counseled on the importance of a consistent intake of vitamin K–containing foods and instructed to continue on the same dosage regimen.

About three weeks later, the patient returned to the clinic for INR monitoring, and the value reported the next day was 1.37. Multiple attempts to contact the patient failed and he was lost to follow-up for another month, at which time he returned to clinic for a recheck of INR, which was reported as 1.14. The patient reported no change in compliance, diet, medications, or disease states. Nevertheless, on further questioning about his diet, the patient indicated that a week prior to his previous INR of 1.37, he had begun drinking about one-half to one gallon of green tea each day. The patient did not show any signs and symptoms associated with suboptimal anticoagulation, and he was instructed to continue his warfarin regimen and stop the green tea consumption. One week later, the patient's INR was 2.55, and subsequent values were mostly within the target range.

The time course of green tea consumption and discontinuance suggests that the tea could partially account for the changes in the patient's INR values. Although brewed green tea was reported to only contain 0.03 μg of vitamin K per 100 g of brewed tea (24), this patient's copious consumption of the green tea would obviously provide an exogenous amount of vitamin K that exceeds the usual recommended daily dietary intake of 0.5 to 1.0 μg/kg of vitamin K. In addition, the final concentration of vitamin K in any brewed tea would be affected not only by the amount of dry tea leaves used for brewing, but also by the volume of water used to prepare the tea for consumption.

In summary, this case highlights the importance of consistent dietary intake of vitamin K for patients receiving warfarin therapy, and the fact that less well-known sources of exogenous vitamin K could provide an amount that greatly exceeds the recommended range of daily dietary intake.

Panax ginseng CA Meyer (Ginseng, Chinese Ginseng, Korean Ginseng)

Decreased INR associated with the use of *P. ginseng* was reported in a 47-year-old patient who had been stabilized on warfarin (25). Another case of inadequate anticoagulation with ginseng product resulting in thrombosis on a mechanical aortic valve prosthesis was reported in a 58-year-old patient (26). Additional details of these two case reports are discussed in Chapter 5.

CHINESE BOTANICAL PRODUCTS AND PHENPROCOUMON

Zingiber officinale (ginger) has been used for centuries by traditional medical practitioners in East Asian countries to manage symptoms of common cold and rheumatic and digestive disorders, as well as for prophylaxis in the management of nausea and vomiting. For these different purposes, ginger has been used either as fresh or dried root, or in different preparations including capsules, liquid extracts, powders, tablets, or teas. In addition, aqueous extract of ginger has been shown to inhibit thromboxane synthase in a dose-dependent manner, thereby resulting in the reduction of platelet aggregation (27). This hemostasis effect could be related to gingerols, the active ingredients of ginger (28). Therefore, the potential exists for ginger to interact pharmacologically with coumarin derivatives. While to date there has been no report of interaction between ginger and warfarin, ginger has been recently reported to interact with phenprocoumon, a coumarin derivative commonly used in most European countries.

Kruth et al. (29) reported that a 76-year-old woman who had been stabilized on long-term phenprocoumon therapy with therapeutic INR values was admitted to the hospital, secondary to elevated INR of greater than 10, prolonged partial thromboplastin time (PTT) of 84.4 seconds (normal < 35 seconds), and epistaxis. Although the patient took several concurrent medications for her medical problems, which included atrial fibrillation, hypertension, chronic heart failure, and osteoporosis, none of the drugs is known to interact with coumarin derivatives. More importantly, there have not been any changes in any of her drug regimens. However, for several weeks before the bleeding incident, the patient had regularly taken several ginger preparations, including dried ginger and tea prepared from ginger powder. Ginger intake was discontinued and with administration of several doses of vitamin K, the patient's INR and PTT eventually returned to baseline values, enabling resumption of her normal doses of phenprocoumon, with no further recurrence of bleeding episodes.

The time course of ginger administration and the absence of other potential interacting drugs suggest that ginger might be the cause of over-anticoagulation in this patient. In vitro evidence of CYP2C9 involvement in phenprocoumon metabolism (30) is not supported by human pharmacokinetic data (31). The effect of ginger on CYP activity is not known and a possible pharmacokinetic basis cannot be established at this time. Although the literature evidence of ginger's effect on hemostasis is conflicting (section "Chinese botanical products and aspirin"), this case suggests that caution needs to be exercised with ginger use in patients receiving anticoagulants. In this regard, it is noteworthy that even though abnormal clotting function as well as mild clinical bleeding in a 25-year-old woman was attributed to several natural coumarin constituents in a herbal tea product (32), the herbal tea also contains one whole ginger root that might exaggerate the anticoagulant effect of the coumarin constituents.

CHINESE BOTANICAL PRODUCTS AND ASPIRIN

As discussed above, the pharmacological action of ginger has prompted suggestion that concurrent use of ginger and aspirin or nonsteroidal anti-inflammatory drugs may exaggerate bleeding potential, especially if the amount of ginger used is larger than that found in usual food items. The following case report indicates such potential, and there are three human studies in the literature, investigating the effect of ginger on platelets.

An unspecified but potentially large amount of marmalade containing 15% raw ginger was consumed by a patient, resulting in significant inhibition of platelet aggregation, although the patient was asymptomatic. One week after discontinuation of the ginger supplement, platelet function was found to be normal. The investigator also performed an in vitro study and reported that ground raw ginger has the potential to inhibit platelet aggregation (33).

To determine the relevance of in vitro results to clinical setting, Srivastava extended his previous in vitro study (27) to seven healthy female volunteers, who received 5 g of fresh ginger daily for one week. The serum thromboxane activity (thromboxane B_2 formation) at baseline was not significantly different compared to that obtained after one week of ginger administration. There were also no evidence of ecchymosis or reports of unusual bleeding episodes (34).

Eight healthy male volunteers received a single 2 g dose of dried ginger (Schwartz spice) or placebo in a randomized, double-blind, crossover study. Three blood samples were obtained before, and at 3 and 24 hours after dose administration. Ginger intake resulted in no significant effect on bleeding time, platelet count, and platelet aggregation compared to administration of placebo capsules (35).

In another study, 18 healthy subjects (nine men and nine women) received an extemporaneous formulation of vanilla custard containing 15 g of raw Brazilian ginger root, 40 g of cooked stem ginger, or placebo once daily for 14 days in a randomized crossover manner. Blood sampling was performed on days 12 and 14 of each treatment for determination of platelet thromboxane B_2 production ex vivo. There were no significant changes with either of the ginger preparations when compared to placebo. In addition, no treatment order effects were noted, although there were no washout periods between the three treatment phases (36).

The effect of ginger on platelet aggregation and the potential for increased bleeding have been cited as reasons to exercise caution in the use of ginger in patients receiving aspirin and nonsteroidal anti-inflammatory drugs (37). Although the three clinical investigations reviewed above are associated with the usual study limitations, including extrapolation of observed effects from healthy volunteers to patients, relevance of negative findings in a small number of subjects, variable range of ginger doses and preparations used in the subjects, as well as whether the doses studied represent equivalent doses found in dietary supplements or botanical preparations, there is insufficient evidence at this time to conclude an unequivocal significant antiplatelet effect associated with the use of ginger. Additional human studies similar to those conducted for St. John's wort would clarify the interaction potential of ginger.

Angelica sinensis (Chinese Angelica, Dong Quai)

In addition to the presence of natural coumarin derivatives, phytochemical analysis found that dong quai also contains ferulic acid and osthole as ingredients. Ferulic acid was reported to have antithrombotic activity (38). Similarly, study using the closely related *Angelica pubescens* also found osthole to be antithrombotic (39). These two chemical constituents exert their antithrombotic effects by interfering with different pathways responsible for platelet activation. Ferulic acid inhibits the release of serotonin and adenosine diphosphate from platelets, as well as reduces the thromboxane A_2 production, resulting in impaired platelet aggregation. Osthole directly inhibits the conversion of arachidonic acid to thromboxane A_2. Therefore, even though currently there is no report of an interaction available in the English literature, dong quai may potentiate the risk of bleeding if used concurrently with aspirin or nonsteroidal anti-inflammatory drugs.

CHINESE BOTANICAL PRODUCTS AND DIGOXIN

Crataegus pinnatifida (Hawthorn Fruit, Shanzha)

Hawthorn has long been used as a medicinal substance, and an extract such as WS 1442, a formulation of hawthorn leaves with flowers, has been evaluated in different studies for treatment of heart failure (40–42). Patients with New York Heart Association class II heart failure participated in a placebo-controlled, randomized, multicenter trial. They received 30 drops of the extract three times daily for eight weeks. At the end of the study, heart failure condition was improved (41). A meta-analysis of available clinical trials suggests that the extract is useful as an adjunct treatment for patients with mild to moderate heart failure (42). Therefore, it is likely that hawthorn products would be administered together with digoxin in clinical management of patients (Fig. 4).

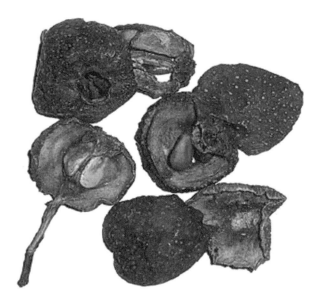

Figure 4 *Crataegus pinnatifida* (Hawthorn fruit, Shanzha).

Although a synergistic interaction between hawthorn and digoxin has been reported in Chinese herbal literature (43), until recently, there has been no case report or pharmacokinetic/pharmacodynamic data available in the English literature. A recent study evaluated the interaction potential between hawthorn and digoxin. Eight healthy volunteers participating in the study received, in a randomized crossover manner, digoxin 0.25 mg daily for 10 days and digoxin 0.25 mg daily concurrent with 450 mg twice daily of Crataegus extract WS 1442 (Dr. Willmar Schwabe Pharmaceuticals) for 21 days, with a three-week wash-out period between the two treatment phases. Based on pharmacokinetic analysis of digoxin concentration–time profiles from both the treatment periods, administration of the hawthorn preparation produced a slight and statistically insignificant change in any of the pharmacokinetic parameters. There were also no statistically significant differences in blood pressure, heart rate, and PR interval (44). The pharmacological results from this study appear to contradict the Chinese literature of synergism between hawthorn fruit and cardiac glycoside. However, hawthorn may increase digoxin's effect on myocardial contractility, although that was not measured in the study. Future studies confirming the lack of pharmacokinetic interaction and adverse additive effect would provide additional evidence that hawthorn and digoxin can be administered safely together.

CHINESE BOTANICAL PRODUCTS AND DIGOXIN-LIKE IMMUNOREACTIVITY

As discussed earlier, many patients use danshen for a variety of cardiovascular uses (8). Currently, there is no literature report of interaction between danshen and digoxin. However, Chinese botanical products can interfere with clinical laboratory monitoring of digoxin serum concentrations via their digoxin-like immunoreactive components (45). For example, danshen contains more than 20 diterpene quinines with chemical structures similar to digoxin. Depending on the type of immunoassay used, both falsely elevated and falsely decreased concentrations have been reported (46). Similarly, the bufadienolide constituents of the Chinese botanical product lu-shen-wan also bear structural similarity with digoxin, resulting in serum digoxin concentration of about 0.9 ng/mL in patients who took lu-shen-wan pills (47). Even though it is not necessarily considered to be a real botanical product–drug interaction, it would be prudent to check for potential interference by serum digoxin concentration determination, when these Chinese botanical products are used together with digoxin.

LIMITATIONS OF CURRENT LITERATURE

Although literature publications on the use of herbal medicine have increased over the years, there are relatively few retrievable literature reports regarding concurrent use of Chinese botanical products and prescription and/or over-the-counter medications, when compared to drug interaction reports associated with concurrent use of two or more Western prescription drugs. While this may simply reflect a lack of reporting system for the consumers, another likely reason could be that pertinent information is not readily available in the English literature. Pharmacodynamic and pharmacokinetic interaction cases have been published in Chinese herbal literature, including *Herb-Drug Interaction and Combined Medication*, *Chinese Herbal Medicine*, and *Pharmacology and Application of Herbal Medicine*, and attempts are currently undertaken to provide this information in the mainstream literature.

Most of the Chinese botanical product–drug interaction cases involving warfarin and/or salicylate described above did not result in clinical bleeding episodes. Nevertheless, these and other botanical product–drug interaction reports discussed in this chapter underscore the limitation of available evidence based on case reports and extrapolation of relevance to other botanical products, which could be confounded by patient-specific variables, details of individual report, as well as variability in the content of active constituents among different botanical products. These limitations of interpretation and extrapolation are further challenged by unique ways of prescribing and preparing Chinese botanical products by Traditional Chinese Medicine (TCM) practitioners and patients, respectively. These will be discussed in the following sections.

SPECIFIC ISSUES REGARDING EVALUATION OF CHINESE BOTANICAL PRODUCT–DRUG INTERACTIONS

Prescribing vs. Over-the-Counter Use of Chinese Botanical Product

Using traditional and acceptable ways of reviewing and analyzing the drug–drug interaction literature, it is tempting for clinicians to report a case and/or review the literature of botanical product–drug interaction based on the available information for an individual botanical product. However, many herbal remedies used by consumers contain multiple herbs, e.g., the Chinese botanical product quilinggao reviewed above (18), Ping Wei San, the Chinese medicine used for the management of gastrointestinal disorders (48), and the different Kampo medicine (traditional Chinese botanical prescriptions) available in Japan (Table 2) (49). Different constituents within a botanical formula or remedy could have multiple effects on an individual constituent that range from augmenting to antagonizing its intended effect, thereby posing limitation on the usefulness of research or report pertaining to an individual botanical constituent.

In contrast to over-the-counter use by consumers, Chinese botanical products prescribed by TCM practitioners or herbalists are usually in the

Table 2 Selected Examples of Variable Botanical Constituents from Different Chinese Botanical Products

Botanical product	Botanical constituents	Composition (% w/w) or comment	Reference
Shosaiko	*Bupleuri radix*	29.2	(49)
	Pinelliae tuber	20.8	
	Scutellariae radix	12.5	
	Ginseng radix	12.5	
	Glycyrrhiza radix	8.3	
	Zingberis rhizoma	4.2	
	Zizyphi fructus	12.5	
Sairei	*Bupleuri radix*	17.5	(49)
	Pinelliae tuber	12.5	
	Scutellariae radix	7.5	
	Ginseng radix	7.5	
	Glycyrrhiza radix	5.0	
	Zingberis rhizoma	2.5	
	Zizyphi fructus	7.5	
	Atractylodis lanceae rhizoma	7.5	
	Alismatis rhizoma	12.5	
	Polyporous	7.5	
	Cinnamomi cortex	5.0	
	Rehmanniae radix	7.5	
Quilinggao brand #1	*Fritillaria cirrhosa*	Not associated with change in INR in patient	(13)
	Glycyrrhiza uralensis		
	Land tortoise shell		
	Ganoderma lucidum		
	Similax glabra		
Quilinggao brand #2	*Fritillaria* spp.	Increased INR in patient	(13)
	Glycyrrhiza uralensis		
	Land tortoise shell		
	Similax glabra		
	Baihuasheshecao		
	Dictamnus dasycarpus		
	Fragrant angelica		
	Scutellaria barbata		
	Mentha haplocalyx		
	Atractylodes chinensis		
	Paeonia rubra, Kochia scoparia		
	Ledebouriella seseloides		
	Poria cocos, Arbus cantoniensis		
	Fructus tribuli		
	Schizonepeta tenuifolia		

(*Continued*)

Table 2   Selected Examples of Variable Botanical Constituents from
Different Chinese Botanical Products (*Continued*)

Botanical product	Botanical constituents	Composition (% w/w) or comment	Reference
Ping Wei San	*Lonicera japonica*		(48)
	Poncirus trifoliate		
	Forsythia suspense		
	Taraxacum mongolicum		
	Rehemannia glutinosa		
	Trichosanthes kirilowii		
	Scrophularia ningpoensis		
	Geditsia sinensis		
	Altractylodes lancea		
	Magnolia officinalis		
	Citrus reticulata		
	Glycyrrhiza uralensis		
	Zingiber officinale		
	Zyzyphus jujube		

form of a formula combination, designed to enhance or reduce the effects of different botanical products. Indeed, it is a common knowledge that TCM practitioners and herbalists prefer prescribing Chinese botanical products in the form of "raw herbs" or raw plant materials rather than fixed-formula products, so that modification to a formula can be used to achieve the desirable therapeutic effect with minimal adverse outcome for a specific patient. TCM practitioners and herbalists have contended that by using a balanced combination of Chinese botanical products and by taking a therapeutic approach that tailor to a patient's holistic needs, i.e., his or her physical and psychological loss of balance, the Chinese botanical products have minimal potential to interact with Western drugs. Obviously, this knowledge of appropriate combination of Chinese botanical products would not play a role in the consumer's choice of botanical remedies purchased over the counter. In addition, the TCM practitioner usually assesses the patient on a regular basis, and adjustment is then made to the ingredient within the formulation. In this regard, it is not much different from warfarin dose adjustment by a clinician based on the patient's INR and clinical status.

By the same token, not all Chinese botanical products are compatible with each other. Classic Chinese herbal texts have mentioned 18 Incompatibles (Shi Ba Fan) and 19 Counteractions (Shi Jiu Wei). The 18 Incompatibles refer to a classic list of 18 botanical product–botanical product interactions, whereas the 19 Counteractions list 19 botanical product combinations in which the effect of one botanical product counteracts that of the other. Given this complexity of modified effect, self-administration of Chinese botanical products without consultation with health care providers or TCM practitioners likely poses more risk than benefit. In addition, for conventional drugs, the magnitude of interaction is mostly dose related or concentration related. Undoubtedly, the dosage of the interacting constituent, whether known or yet to be identified, could vary from one manufacturer to another. Therefore patients switching between different Chinese botanical products might have different outcomes, according to the botanical product–drug interaction, as discussed above for the patient who experienced an apparent interaction between quilinggao products and warfarin.

Preparation of Chinese Herbal Medicine for Consumption

After the prescription is filled and taken home, the Chinese botanical products or formula are usually prepared prior to consumption. In contrast to an oral dosage form of a synthetic drug taken orally in its entirety, the raw botanical products can be ground and taken directly. More commonly, the botanical product or formula of multiple botanical products can be prepared either as a hot water decoction (extraction) or as a 35% to 45% alcoholic infusion. The decoction method of preparation involves boiling the botanical products in about 500 to 600 mL of water until the volume is reduced to one-half and drinking the supernatant of the resulting concentrate or "soup." The infusion method of preparation involves immersing the botanical products in liquor (usually ethanol) for a period of time and then drinking the supernatant. Because it is known that allicin, the major component of garlic, is destroyed when garlic is cooked in oil, how the boiling process would affect the metabolic activity of major constituents has not been studied systematically. Interestingly, Guo et al. (50) had shown that in vitro CYP3A4 inhibition by seven botanical products was consistently greater with the infusion method of preparation. This was true regardless of the lots or geographic locations of the source of the botanical products. Therefore, this represents an additional complexity in evaluating the botanical product–drug or botanical product–botanical product interaction and the need for inquiring the method of preparation during interview of patients regarding their use of botanical products.

Chinese Fixed-Botanical Formulations

Commercial Chinese fixed-botanical formulations are manufactured and marketed in various dosage forms. It is usually not known to what extent individual botanical constituent(s) would be chemically altered during the manufacturing process, regardless of whether the final formulation contains a standardized amount of an active constituent. In addition, commercially available products might differ in their formulation of constituents. The case report by Page and Lawrence (2) listed different over-the-counter dong quai–containing botanical supplements that are available in the United States. Some of these supplements contain not only dong quai, but also multiple botanical products such as ginger, licorice root, or Siberian ginseng. The patient described in their report took Nature's Way PMS formula, which contains dong quai, cramping bark, chaste tree berry, licorice root, and ginger, in addition to folic acid and several vitamins. Although specific ingredient information may not be easily available or apparent in case report or literature review, it is important to take into consideration the multiple ingredients within a commercially available product or a Chinese botanical formula, when reporting cases of botanical product–drug interaction, so that clinicians can come to appropriate conclusions regarding the significance of the interaction and/or extrapolation of the result to other products. Another good example of this attempt to report constituents within a botanical product or formulation is the case of the quilinggao–warfarin interaction discussed above (18).

Similar to the challenges outlined in Chapter 2, the fact that most Chinese herbal medicines are complex mixtures of multiple active constituents further complicates the interpretation of study data, as well as extrapolation to other botanical products. Japanese Kampo (traditional Chinese herbal mixtures) prescriptions have been used for many years to treat different chronic conditions and are presently manufactured in Japan as drugs with standardized quantities and qualities of constituents. Homma et al. (51) evaluated the effect of three commonly used Japanese Kampo prescriptions, Sho-saiko-to (Xiao Chai Hu Tang), Saiboku-to, and Sairei-to, on prednisolone pharmacokinetics in humans. All three botanical prescriptions contain glycyrrhizin, a strong inhibitor of 11-β-hydroxysteroid dehydrogenase. Chen et al. (52) had shown that glycyrrhizin decreased plasma clearance and increased AUC and concentration of prednisolone.

However, even though glycyrrhizin was present in all three Kampo prescriptions, Homma et al. (51) reported differential effect with respect to changes in prednisolone pharmacokinetics. Concurrent administration of Sho-saiko-to resulted in a 17% decrease in prednisolone AUC. On the other hand, coadministration of Saiboku-to resulted in a 15% increase in prednisolone AUC. Sairei-to administration resulted in no appreciable change in prednisolone pharmacokinetics. Similarly, Sho-saiko-to increased the prednisone to prednisolone ratio, which reflects 11-β-hydroxysteroid dehydrogenase activity, whereas the ratio was decreased in the presence of Saiboku-to and not changed by administration of Sairei-to. Sho-saiko-to contains seven botanical products with glycyrrhizin being one of them, whereas a total of 12 botanical products including glycyrrhizin are present in Sairei-to, although the relative amount of glycyrrhizin differs between these two botanical products (Table 2). These results suggest that botanical prescriptions containing higher glycyrrhizin content or constituents other than glycyrrhizin might be responsible for this differential effect on predni-solone pharmacokinetics and 11-β-hydroxysteroid dehydrogenase activity. The report by Wong and Chan (18) on warfarin–quilinggao interaction also illustrates these two limitations: the presence of multiple active or interacting constituents and the often present variation in the composition of the constituents between different manufacturers (Table 2). In this regard, although Sho-saiko-to and Sairei-to were shown to not alter the pharmacokinetics of the quinolone ofloxacin in seven healthy volunteers (53), it remains to be determined whether other Kampo prescriptions such as Saiboku-to would produce the same negligible effect.

CONCLUSION

With an increasing number of consumers using traditional Chinese herbal medicines, mostly without the advice of health professionals or TCM practitioners, the likelihood of Chinese botanical product–drug interactions is potentially high. To date, the number of interaction reports remain relatively low and, fortunately, few cases reported adverse clinical outcome in patients. However, the low prevalence of interaction simply might reflect a lack of recognition of the interaction potential, scant information from the primary Chinese literature, insufficient number of patients taking Chinese botanical products and potent Western drugs at the same time, or a combination of these factors. As demonstrated by the numerous interaction reports involving warfarin, it is important for clinicians to inquire patients specifically about their use of botanical products, which most do not necessarily disclose during patient interview or medication review. Likewise, to understand further the magnitude and clinical significance of potential or reported interactions, it is important to have more pharmacokinetic and pharmacodynamic studies conducted with quality botanical products in healthy volunteers and/or patients.

REFERENCES

1. Wang AM, Sha SH, Lesniak W, Schacht J. Tanshinone (*Salviae miltiorrhizae* extract) preparations attenuate aminoglycosides-induced free radical formation in vitro and ototoxicity in vivo. Antimicrob Agents Chemother 2003; 47:1836–1841.
2. Page RL II, Lawrence JD. Potentiation of warfarin by dong quai. Pharmacotherapy 1999; 19:870–876.
3. Ellis GR, Stephens MR. Minerva (photograph and brief case report). Br Med J 1999; 319:650.
4. Lo ACT, Chan K, Yeung JHK, Woo KS. Dang gui (*Angelica sinensis*) affects the pharmacodynamics but not the pharmacokinetics of warfarin in rabbits. Eur J Drug Metab Pharmacokinet 1995; 20:53–60.

5. Fukuda K, Ohta T, Oshima Y, Ohashi N, Yoshikawa M, Yamazoe Y. Specific CYP3A4 inhibitors in grapefruit juice: furocoumarin dimmers as components of drug interaction. Pharmacogenetics 1997; 7:391–396.
6. Ishihara K, Kashida H, Yuzurihara M, et al. Interaction of drugs and Chinese herbs: pharmacokinetic changes of tolbutamide and diazepam caused by extract of *Angelica dahurica*. J Pharm Pharmacol 2000; 52:1023–1029.
7. Mei QB, Tao JY, Cui B. Advances in the pharmacological studies of radix *Angelica sinensis* (Oliv) Diels (Chinese dang gui). Chin Med J 1991; 104:776–781.
8. Mashour NH, Lin GI, Frishman WH. Herbal medicines for the treatment of cardiovascular disease: clinical considerations. Arch Intern Med 1998; 158: 2225–2234.
9. Wang Z, Roberts JM, Grant PG, Colman RW, Schreiber AD. The effect of a medicinal Chinese herb on platelet function. Thromb Haemost 1982; 48: 301–306.
10. Cheng TO. Warfarin danshen interaction. Ann Thorac Surg 1999; 67:894.
11. Yu CM, Chan JCN, Sanderson JE. Chinese herbs and warfarin potentiation by 'Danshen.' J Intern Med 1997; 241:337–339.
12. Izzat MB, Yim APC, El-Zufari MH. A taste of Chinese medicine. Ann Thorac Surg 1998; 66:941–942.
13. Tam LS, Chan TYK, Leung WK, Critchley JAJH. Warfarin interactions with Chinese traditional medicines: danshen and methyl salicylate medicated oil. Aust NZ J Med 1995; 25:258.
14. Lo ACT, Chan K, Yeung JHK, Woo KS. The effects of danshen (*Salvia miltiorrhiza*) on pharmacokinetics and dynamics of warfarin in rats. Eur J Drug Metab Pharmacokinet 1992; 17:257–262.
15. Chan K, Lo AC, Yeung JH, Woo KS. The effects of danshen (*Salvia miltiorrhiza*) on pharmacodynamics and pharmacokinetics of warfarin enantiomers in rats. J Pharm Pharmacol 1995; 47:402–406.
16. Ou M. Chinese-English Manual of Common Herbs Used in Traditional Chinese Medicine. Hong Kong: Guangdong Science and technology Publishing House, Joint Publishing (HK), 1999:357.
17. Lam AY, Elmer GW, Mohutsky MA. Possible interaction between warfarin and *Lycium barbarum* L. Ann Pharmacother 2001; 35:1199–1201.
18. Wong ALN, Chan TYK. Interaction between warfarin and the herbal product Quilinggao. Ann Pharmacother 2003; 37:836–838.
19. Gao YT, McLaughlin JK, Blot WJ, Ji BT, Dai Q, Fraumeni JF. Reduced risk of esophageal cancer associated with green tea consumption. J Natl Cancer Inst 1994; 86:855–858.
20. Lambert JD, Yang CS. Cancer chemopreventive activity and bioavailability of tea and tea polyphenols. Mutat Res 2003; 523–524:201–208.
21. Yang CS, Maliakal P, Meng XF. Inhibition of carcinogenesis by tea. Ann Rev Pharmacol Toxicol 2002; 42:25–54.
22. Booth SL, Sadowski JA, Pennington JAT. Phylloquinone (vitamin K1) content of foods in the U.S. Food and Drug Administration's total diet study. J Agric Food Chem 1995; 43:1574–1579.
23. Taylor JR, Wilt VM. Probable antagonism of warfarin by green tea. Ann Pharmacother 1999; 33:426–428.

24. Booth SL, Madabushi HT, Davidson KW. Tea and coffee brews are not significant dietary sources of vitamin K (phylloquinone). J Am Diet Assoc 1995; 95:82–83.

25. Janetzky K, Morreale AP. Probable interaction between warfarin and ginseng. Am J Health Syst Pharm 1997; 54:692–693.

26. Rosado MF. Thrombosis of a prosthetic aortic valve disclosing a hazardous interaction between warfarin and a commercial ginseng product. Cardiology 2003; 99:111.

27. Srivastava KC. Aqueous extract of onion, garlic and ginger inhibit platelet aggregation and alter arachidonic acid metabolism. Biomed Biochim Acta 1984; 43:335–346.

28. Srivastava KC. Isolation and effects of some ginger components of platelet aggregation and eicosanoid biosynthesis. Prostaglandins Leukot Med 1986; 25:187–198.

29. Kruth P, Brosi E, Fux R, Morike K, Gleiter C. Ginger-associated overanticoagulation by phenprocoumon. Ann Pharmacother 2004; 38:257–260.

30. Ho M, Korzekwa KR, Jones JP, Rettie AE, Trager WF. Structural forms of phenprocoumon and warfarin that are metabolized by the active site of CYP2C9. Arch Biochem Biophys 1999; 372:16–28.

31. Kirchheiner J, Ufer M, Walter E, et al. Effects of CYP2C9 polymorphisms on the pharmacokinetics of R- and S-phenprocoumon in healthy volunteers. Pharmacogenetics 2004; 14:19–26.

32. Hogan RP. Hemorrhagic diathesis caused by drinking an herbal tea. JAMA 1983; 249:2679–2680.

33. Dorso CR, Levin RI, Eldor A, Jaffe EA, Weksler BB. Chinese food and platelet. N Engl J Med 1980; 303:756–757.

34. Srivastava KC. Effect of onion and ginger consumption on platelet thromboxane production in humans. Prostaglandins Leukot Essent Fatty Acids 1989; 35:183–185.

35. Lumb AB. Effect of dried ginger on human platelet function. Thromb Haemost 1994; 71:110–111.

36. Janssen PL. Consumption of ginger (*Zingiber officinale* roscoe) does not affect ex vivo platelet thromboxane production in humans. Eur J Clin Nutr 1996; 50:772–774.

37. Hodges PJ, Kam PCA. The perioperative implications of herbal medicines. Anaesthesia 2002; 57:889–899.

38. Yin ZZ. The effect of dong quai (*Angelica sinensis*) and its ingredient ferulic acid on rat platelet aggregation and release of 5-HT. Acta Pharmaceut Sinica 1980; 15:321–330.

39. Ko FN, Wu TS, Lious MJ, Huang TF, Teng CM. Inhibition of platelet thromboxane formation and phosphoinositides breakdown by osthole from *Angelica pubescens*. Thromb Haemost 1989; 62:996–999.

40. Chang Q, Zuo Z, Harrison F, Chow MS. Hawthorn. J Clin Pharmacol 2002; 42:605–612.

41. Degenring FH, Suter A, Weber M, Saller R. A randomized double blind placebo controlled clinical trial of a standardized extract of fresh Crataegus

berries (Crataegisan) in the treatment of patients with congestive heart failure NYHA II. Phytomedicine 2003; 10:363–369.

42. Pittler MH, Schmidt K, Ernst E. Hawthorn extract for treating chronic heart failure: meta-analysis of randomized trial. Am J Med 2003; 114:665–674.

43. Abstract of Herbal Literature 1979:72, published in Chinese.

44. Tankanow R, Tamer HR, Streetman DS, et al. Interaction study between digoxin and a preparation of hawthorn (*Crataegus oxyacantha*). J Clin Pharmacol 2003; 43:637–642.

45. Dasgupta A, Szele-Stevens KA. Neutralization of free digoxin-like immunoreactive components of oriental medicines Dan Shen and Lu-Shen-Wan by the Fab fragment of antidigoxin antibody (Digibind). Am J Clin Pathol 2004; 121:276–281.

46. Wahed A, Dasgupta A. Positive and negative in vitro interferences of Chinese medicine dan shen in serum digoxin measurement. Elimination of interference by monitoring free digoxin concentration. Am J Clin Pathol 2001; 116:403–408.

47. Panesar NS. Bufalin and unidentified substance(s) in traditional Chinese medicine cross-react in commercial digoxin assay. Clin Chem 1992; 38:2155–2156.

48. Riedlinger JE, Tan PW, Lu W. Ping wei san, a Chinese medicine for gastrointestinal disorders. Ann Pharmacother 2001; 35:228–235.

49. Takahashi K, Uejima E, Morisaki T, Takahashi K, Kurokawa N, Azuma J. In vitro inhibitory effects of Kampo medicines on metabolic reactions catalyzed by human liver microsomes. J Clin Pharm Ther 2003; 28:319–327.

50. Guo LQ, Taniguchi M, Chen QY, Baba K, Yamazoe Y. Inhibitory potential of herbal medicines on human cytochrome P450-mediated oxidation; properties of umbelliferous or citrus crude drugs and their relative prescriptions. Jpn J Pharmacol 2001; 85:399–408.

51. Homma M, Oka K, Ikeshima K, et al. Different effects of traditional Chinese medicines containing similar herbal constituents on prednisolone pharmacokinetics. J Pharm Pharmacol 1995; 47:687–692.

52. Chen MF, Shimada F, Kato H, Yano S, Kanaoka M. Effect of oral administration of glycyrrhizin on the pharmacokinetics of prednisolone. Endocrinol Jpn 1991; 38:167–174.

53. Hasegawa T, Yamaki K, Nadai M, et al. Lack of effect of Chinese medicines on bioavailability of ofloxacin in healthy volunteers. Int J Clin Pharmacol Ther 1994; 32:57–61.

7

Drug Interactions of Grapefruit and Other Citrus—What Have We Learned?

**S. U. Mertens-Talcott, I. Zadezensky, W. V. De Castro,
Veronika Butterweck, and Hartmut Derendorf**

*Department of Pharmaceutics, Center for Food Drug Interaction Research and
Education, University of Florida, Gainesville, Florida, U.S.A.*

INTRODUCTION

The first report of grapefruit juice (GFJ) interacting with a drug, altering its bioavailability, was published in 1991. This accidental discovery was made in a study on ethanol–drug interactions—the bioavailability of felodipine was increased when subjects were consuming GFJ concomitantly with felodipine, associated with a lower dehydrofelodipine/felodipine area under the curve (AUC) ratio, decreased diastolic blood pressure, and an increased heart rate (1). Subsequent research in the area of fruit–drug interactions focused on grapefruit and grapefruit compounds of which several were found to affect the absorption or metabolism of certain drugs. GFJ was shown to alter the pharmacokinetics of several drugs such as statins, calcium channel blockers, antibiotics, and others (1–8). Other fruits, vegetables, and dietary supplements also have the potential to cause an adverse interaction with conventional drugs (9). Over 16% of all prescription drug users reported that they concurrently use at least one plant-based dietary supplement, including grapefruit and citrus products (10).

Many consumers have become more aware of the health benefits of antioxidants, phytochemical-rich fruits and vegetables, and products that contain these. In 1997, GFJ was purchased by 21% of all households as a popular antioxidant breakfast juice (11), predominantly preferred by the elderly. By-products from the citrus-processing industry, such as grapefruit seed extract, flavonoids, essential oils from the peel, and pectins may be added to other food products to improve taste, consistency, or overall quality. These by-products also may be used in the production of dietary supplements. Consequently, citrus compounds that have a potential for an interaction with drugs may find their way into other food products.

Hence, increased availability and consumption of drugs, dietary supplements, and phytochemical-containing antioxidant foods may increase the likelihood of an adverse interaction between foods and certain drugs. Absorption and metabolism of a drug may be adversely affected, shifting the administered dose outside of the therapeutic range, which may lead to a lower effectiveness of the drug or to an overdose associated with undesired or even dangerous side effects.

Based on our current knowledge, grapefruit compounds interact with drugs that are metabolized by cytochrome P450 3A4 (CYP3A4) and also have a low or variable oral bioavailability. The major mechanism leading to a grapefruit–drug interaction appears to be the reduction of the "pre-systemic" metabolism through the inhibition of intestinal CYP3A4 (12). Some hydroxymethylglutaryl-coenzyme A (HMG-CoA) reductase inhibitors and calcium channel antagonists are among the affected drugs (13).

Other mechanisms of interaction have also been reported, such as altered activity of other enzymes within the CYP450 family (14–17). Moreover, GFJ may also inhibit the intestinal P-glycoprotein (P-gp)-mediated efflux transport of drugs such as cyclosporine to increase its oral bioavailability (18–21). GFJ and other fruit juices have recently been shown to be potent in vitro inhibitors of a number of organic anion-transporting polypeptides (OATPs) (22,23).

Grapefruits and GFJ have a potential to interact with several oral medications when consumed in moderate amounts, such as one or two servings of GFJ (24). The concern that the concomitant administration of grapefruit products with certain drugs may lessen the effect of a drug or cause a toxic effect based on the increases in oral drug bioavailability has lead to the recommendation to avoid the consumption of grapefruit products in combination with these drugs of concern. The Food and Drug Administration (FDA) requires some drugs such as cyclosporine, sirolimus, simvastatin, lovastatin, and felodipine to carry a warning label regarding the possibility of an interaction. For example, Neoral[R], an immunosuppressant drug, carries a label stating " . . . Grapefruit and GFJ affect metabolism, increasing blood concentrations of cyclosporine, thus should be avoided" (25). Procardia[®] is labeled " . . . Co-administration of nifedipine with GFJ resulted in approximately a 2-fold increase in nifedipine AUC and C_{max} with no change in half-life. The increased plasma concentrations are most likely due to inhibition of CYP3A4 related first-pass metabolism. Co-administration of nifedipine with GFJ is to be avoided" (26).

In addition to GFJ, interactions with certain medications also have been shown for Seville orange juice, although Seville oranges are usually not processed to juice (27,28).

For most drugs in question, definitive recommendations regarding their concomitant administration with GFJ are not available, because conclusions regarding the clinical significance of the observed or predicted grapefruit–drug interactions are still limited and most of the data available are derived from in vitro experiments. Furthermore, the determination of the clinical relevance of observed interactions in human intervention trials is complicated by interindividual variability. Whereas the attention of patients and health care professionals is currently focused mainly on interactions of drugs with grapefruit products, other fruits and vegetables and dietary supplements, such as St. John's wort, green tea, and ginseng are an additional potential source for drug interactions (29). On the other hand, it should be noted that almost all drugs that show an interaction with grapefruit can be replaced by another drug within the same drug class that is without a known potential for an interaction.

PHENOLIC COMPOUNDS IN GRAPEFRUIT AND CITRUS WITH POTENTIAL DRUG INTERACTIONS

A major group of citrus compounds interacting with drugs are phenolics, which include hydroxycinnamic acids, flavonoids such as flavanones, flavones, and flavonols, and anthocyanins, as well as coumarins (Table 1, Fig. 1) (30). Many of these phenolic compounds have been shown to have antioxidant and anticancer properties that may play an important role in cancer prevention, but also in prevention of other chronic diseases such as coronary heart disease, gout, and arthritis (58–60).

Interactions with numerous drugs have been demonstrated for furanocoumarins, especially for bergamottin (BG) and 6′7′-dihydroxybergamottin (DHBG). Overall, furanocoumarins appear to interact with susceptible drugs through CYP3A4 and P-gp, but also were shown to influence OATP. In vitro studies, BG and DHBG have been demonstrated to inhibit the activity of CYP3A4 by reversible and irreversible mechanism-based inhibition (41,53,56). Several studies report an inhibitory effect of BG on the activity of CYP3A4, which leads to an increased C_{max} and AUC of diazepam in dogs, of nifedipine in rats, and of felodipine in humans (50–52). BG and DHBG inhibited CYP3A4 in human liver microsomes in vitro, leading to a decreased metabolism of saquinavir, whereas naringin and DHBG decreased the ratio of basolateral-to-apical to apical-to-basolateral (BA/AB) transport of saquinavir (41). BG, DHBG, bergaptol, and bergapten increased the steady-state uptake of [^{3}H]-vinblastine sulfate by Caco-2 cells (54), and BG and DHBG decreased the OATP-B–mediated uptake of estrone-3-sulfate into human embryonic kidney cells (23).

Table 1 Examples of Phenolic Compounds in Selected Citrus Varieties with Drug Interactions

Phenolic compound[a]	Citrus variety	Drug-interaction
Hydroxycinnamic acids		
Sinapic acid	*C. sinensis*	
p-Coumaric acid		
Ferulic acid		
Caffeic acid		
Flavonoids		
Flavanones		
Narirutin	*C. paradisi, C. aurantium, C. sinensis, C. clementina, C. tangerina*	
Hesperidin	*C. paradisi, C. aurantium, C. sinensis, C. clementina, C. tangerine, C. limon*	
Neohesperidin	*C. paradisi, C. aurantium, C. limon*	
Naringin, Naringenin	*C. paradisi, C. aurantium, C. limon*	vt (41–43), an (44)
Neoponcirin	*C. paradisi, C. aurantium, C. sinensis, C. clementina, C. tangerina*	
Flavones		
Luteolin	*C. sinensis, C. tangerine, C. limon*	
Rutin	*C. paradisi, C. aurantium, C. sinensis, C. clementina, C. tangerine, C. limon*	vt (45)
Tangeretin	*Citrus sinensis, Citrus aurantium,*	vt (23,46)
Nobiletin	*C. limon*	
Sinensetin	*Citrus sinensis*	
Flavonols		
Quercetin	*C. sinensis, C. clementina, C. tangerina*	vt (47–49)
Taxifolin		
Coumarins		
Bergamottin	*C. paradisi, C. aurantium, C. sinensis,*	hm (50), an (51,52), vt (38,41), (53–55)
Dihydroxybergamottin	*C. paradisi, C. aurantium, C. sinensis,*	vt (38,41,54,56)
Bergaptol	*C. paradisi*	vt (54)
Bergapten	*C. paradisi*	vt (43,54)
Coumarin dimers and trimers	*C. paradisi, C. aurantium*	vt (56,57)

[a]Names of phenolics include their conjugated forms which occur in citrus.
Abbreviations: an, animal study; C, citrus; hm, human trial; vt, in vitro study.
Source: From Refs. 30–40.

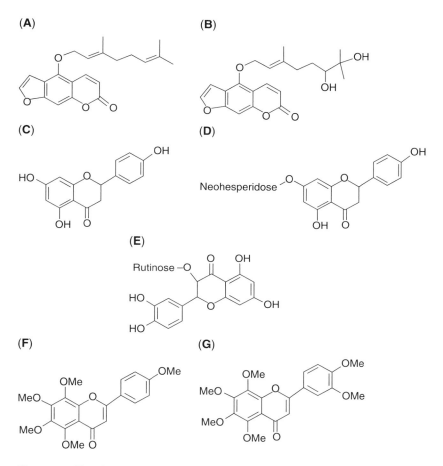

Figure 1 Chemical structure of polyphenolics in citrus. (**A**) Bergamottin, (**B**) 6'7' dihydroxybergamottin, (**C**) Naringenin, (**D**) Naringin, (**E**) Rutin, (**F**) Tangeretin, and (**G**) Nobiletin.

Several human intervention studies confirm the contribution of BG and DHBG to drug interactions with GFJ (14,61,62). After previous reports had been inconsistent regarding the potency of BG and DHBG, Paine et al. investigated the kinetics of reversible and mechanism-based inhibition of CYP3A4 by BG and DHBG, using midazolam and testosterone as probes in human intestinal microsomes (63). In this study, it was found that the inhibition caused by DHBG was substrate-independent, reversible, and mechanism-based. BG was found to be a substrate-dependent reversible inhibitor, with an eightfold higher inhibition for midazolam than for testosterone.

Interactions with drugs have also been demonstrated for flavonoids from citrus. Naringin and naringenin were shown to interact with simvastatin and saquinavir in in vitro experiments (41,42) and caused alterations in the pharmacokinetics of quinine in rats (44). Moreover, naringenin and naringin were found to inhibit the OATP-B–mediated uptake of estrone-3-sulfate into human embryonic kidney cells (23).

Quercetin has been found to inhibit P-gp–mediated efflux of ritonavir in Caco-2 cells (47), to reduce the oxidation of acetaminophen in rat liver microsomes and HepG2 cells (48), and to inhibit the metabolism of midazolam and quinidine in human liver microsomes (49). It did not have an effect on CYP3A4-mediated metabolism and P-gp–mediated transport of saquinavir (41). Rutin was demonstrated to moderately increase the uptake of idarubicin in an isolated perfused rat lung model, and also the outflow recovery of the major metabolite idarubicinol, possibly by affecting P-gp (45). Nobelitin and tangeretin were shown to inhibit OATP-B–mediated uptake of estrone-3-sulfate into human embryonic kidney cells (23).

For several phenolics from citrus, such as eriocitrin, poncirin, and sinapic acid and anthocyanins, which occur in red grapefruit varieties and blood oranges, no specific drug interactions and also no interactions with CYP3A4 and P-gp are reported.

The clinical relevance of data obtained from studies with single compounds is questionable, because most studies were performed in in vitro systems, limiting the predictability of the effects of the examined compounds in vivo. Moreover, some polyphenolics, such as quercetin, were shown to interact with the absorption or metabolism of drugs only at very high concentrations (50–100 µmol/L), which are likely to exceed the expected in vivo concentration after the consumption of a moderate amount of a grapefruit/citrus product. Also, flavonoids have been demonstrated to potentially induce apoptosis in cell lines at concentrations comparable to those used for some in vitro drug interaction studies (64–66). This potentially could have impaired the investigation of enzyme and transporter activities.

In summary, studies with single compounds demonstrate that furanocoumarins and their dimers are primarily responsible for the interactions of GFJ and drugs.

In conclusion, grapefruit, sour orange (Seville), and also limes, which contain BG (61) seem to have the highest potential among the citrus species for interacting with drugs, whereas other citrus varieties such as sweet orange seem to have an overall low potential for interfering with medications. However, in studies using juices rather than single compounds, orange juice has also been shown to interact with drugs in some studies. A more recent study in rats demonstrated that orange juice (and apple juice) decreased the oral exposure of fexofenadine, possibly through an inhibition of the influx transporter OATP (67). The interaction of orange juice and fexofenadine has also been demonstrated in HeLa cells, where orange juice at 5% strength inhibited the uptake of fexofenadine in a concentration-dependent manner by an array of human and rat OATPs (22). Also, orange juice inhibited the uptake of estrone-3-sulfate into human embryonic kidney 293 cells, probably mediated through OATP-B (23).

Overall it can be concluded that orange juice has a minor potential for drug interactions.

POSSIBLE MECHANISMS OF INTERACTION

A food–drug interaction can be defined as the alteration of absorption, metabolism, or effects of a drug by food. The underlying mechanisms can be classified into two broad categories. The first category is pharmacokinetics, which includes alterations in absorption, distribution, metabolism, and excretion. The second category is pharmacodynamics, which describes alterations in the drug concentration–effect relationship (68). Changes in the pharmacokinetics of drugs are the more common consequences of citrus–drug interactions, which may shift the effect of the drug outside of its therapeutic window, possibly leading either to loss of effect or undesired side effects, or even toxicity (24). Originally, the liver was expected to be the major site of grapefruit–drug interactions. However, for felodipine, it was shown that the interaction only occurred when drugs are administered orally, but not intravenously, which indicated that the interaction may take place during the gastrointestinal absorption phase (69,70). For several other drugs such as cyclosporine, midazolam, and nifedipine, the gastrointestinal mucosa has been demonstrated to be a major metabolic organ, where an inhibition of CYP3A4 caused an increase in oral bioavailability (71). Because most drugs exhibiting an interaction with GFJ are metabolized primarily by CYP3A4, it has been suggested that the effect of GFJ may be due to the inhibition of CYP3A4 activity. This effect may be particularly important for orally administered drugs, because CYP3A4 is located not only in the hepatocytes, but also in the epithelial cells of the intestine, where major interactions occur (24).

In addition to CYP3A4, enterocyte efflux transport proteins such as P-gp, and enterocyte uptake proteins, such as OATPs also appear to be involved in grapefruit–drug interactions (24,72). The activity of P-gp has been reported to be altered by GFJ and orange juice in in vitro experiments (73,74), whereas the clinical relevance currently seems unclear, as demonstrated by inconsistent results from human clinical trials (22,75–77).

Regarding interactions between citrus and OATP, data from in vitro, animal and also human clinical studies are available. These studies demonstrated the inhibition of OATP-A in HeLa cells and of OATP-B–mediated uptake of estrone-3-sulfate in human embryonic kidney cells and also in the oral intake of fexofenadine in rats by fruit juices, including GFJ and orange juice. Human clinical trials suggest a potential role of OATP in grapefruit-drug interactions using fexofenadine as substrate (22,23,67,78,79).

Cytochrome P450 Family

The cytochrome P450 (CYP) enzyme family is the major catalyst of phase I drug biotransformation reactions. CYP enzymes are bound to membranes of the endoplasmatic reticulum and are predominantly expressed in the liver, although they are also present in extrahepatic tissues such as the gut mucosa. In humans, 16 gene families and 29 subfamilies have been identified to date. CYP3A4 is the most abundantly expressed isoform and represents approximately 30% to 40% of the total CYP protein in human adult liver (80). CYP3A4 is located mainly in the liver and in apical enterocytes of the small intestine. The high expression levels in the intestinal mucosa and the broad substrate specificity may contribute to the high susceptibility of CYP3A4 for citrus–drug interactions (81). Many drugs for which interactions with citrus have been demonstrated are metabolized by CYP3A4. Grapefruit inhibits the activity of intestinal CYP3A4, which can lead to an interaction with drugs during their first passage from the intestinal lumen into the systemic circulation (82). The alteration of intestinal CYP3A4 by GFJ includes reversible and mechanism-based inhibition and also destruction of the CYP3A4 protein (57,83), whereas mRNA levels remain unaltered, indicating an accelerated degradation after mechanism-based inhibition (82). A moderate consumption does not appear to lead to an inhibition of hepatic CYP3A4 activity (63). Several drug classes such as dihydropyridine calcium antagonists and HMG-CoA-reductase inhibitors are affected by grapefruit-induced inhibition of CYP3A4. GFJ increased the AUC and maximal plasma concentration (C_{max}) for these calcium antagonists within an approximated range of 1.5- to 2.5-fold on average in a single-dose study design [reviewed in (81)]. For the HMG-CoA reductase inhibitor atorvastatin, double-strength GFJ increased the AUC 2.5-fold but not the C_{max}, when the GFJ was administered over three days and the drug was given on day three (84). In a very similar study design performed by the same group with simvastatin, double-strength GFJ increased the AUC 16-fold and C_{max} ninefold (85). The same group demonstrated that one glass of GFJ caused an increase of plasma triazolam concentrations, and the repeated consumption of GFJ induced a higher increase in triazolam concentrations and a prolonged half-life of triazolam. The repeated consumption may cause an inhibition of hepatic CYP3A4 (86). In a three day study, GFJ increased the AUC of simvastatin 3.6-fold and that of simvastatin acid 3.3-fold. C_{max} of simvastatin and simvastatin acid were increased 3.9-fold and 4.3-fold, respectively, when the GFJ was administered for three days and simvastatin on day three (87). In an in vitro study performed with several grapefruit compounds, it was shown that BG, DHBG, and the furanocoumarin dimers GF-I-1 and GF-I-4 inhibited CYP3A4-catalyzed nifedipine oxidation in a concentration-and time-dependent manner, which is consistent with the mechanism-based inhibition. DHBG was more potent than BG, while the dimers were more potent than the monomers. Not only CYP3A4 but also CYP2C9, CYP2C19, and CYP2D6 seem to be affected by citrus compounds. In the same study, the inhibitory effect of BG was stronger on CYP1A2, CYP2C9, CYP2C19, and CYP2D6 than on CYP3A4 (38). In an intervention trial with healthy volunteers, GFJ (twice daily) decreased the activity of CYP1A2, as determined with caffeine as a probe (88). In another human study, GFJ and naringenin caused a minor reduction of the activity of CYP1A2 (89). Overall, the inhibition of CYP enzymes other than CYP3A4 does not appear to be of great magnitude and may clinically be relevant only for drugs with a narrow therapeutic range (81).

Not much information is available regarding the reversible and mechanism-based inhibition kinetics for grapefruit compounds. In a study conducted with human intestinal microsomes by Paine and coworkers, DHB induced a substrate-independent reversible and mechanism-based inhibition on CYP3A4. In contrast, BG, being more lipophilic, was a substrate-dependent reversible inhibitor and a substrate-independent mechanism-based inhibitor. Similar trends resulted with cDNA-expressed CYP3A4. For BG, the inhibition for testosterone was more potent than for midazolam, possibly due to the higher affinity of BG for the testosterone-binding site than for the midazolam-binding site. As mechanism-based inhibitors, BG and DHBG are substrates for CYP3A4, but the binding sites are not known. The authors conclude that both furanocoumarins inactivate CYP3A4 by the binding of the furanoepoxide to the apoprotein, presumably at or near their respective substrate domains (63). The same group determined the onset time of inhibition by both compounds (90). It was found that DHBG inhibited 85% of CYP3A4 activity independent of substrate within 30 minutes, whereas the onset for BG-induced inhibition was much later—a 70% inhibition was reached after three hours. The substrate-dependent inhibition caused by BG was more than 50% after 0.5 to 3 hours for testosterone 6-hydroxylation, while midazolam 1'-hydroxylation was unaffected, or activated, within one hour. Both furanocoumarins caused 40% to 50% reduction of CYP3A4 protein, probably due to intracellular degradation of the enzyme caused by mechanism-based inactivation. These data imply that, after the consumption of GFJ, DHBG causes the enzyme inhibition earlier than BG. Greenblatt et al. determined, in a human intervention trial, the time of recovery of intestinal CYP3A4 after the consumption of 300 mL of regular-strength GFJ and a single dose of midazolam at 2, 26, 50, or 74 hours after administering the juice. After two hours, the AUC was 1.65-fold increased and after 26, 50, and 74 hours, the AUC was 1.29-, 1.21-, and 1.06-fold increased, respectively, in comparison to the control. The recovery half-life was estimated at 23 hours. These results indicate that a single dose of GFJ was able to impair the intestinal presystemic metabolism of midazolam when administered orally, which appeared to recover after 74 hours, consistent with a mechanism-based inhibition (15).

In summary, the presented in vitro studies confirm the inhibitory effects of grapefruit compounds on CYP-enzymes, with major effects on CYP3A4 with both, mechanism-based and reversible inhibition. Overall, DHBG appears to be more potent than BG; however, coumarin dimers seem to be more effective than monomers in the inhibition of CYP3A4. The human intervention trials examining the pharmacokinetic interaction of GFJ revealed a great interindividual variability, where subjects with the highest content of CYP3A4 showed the largest reduction of this enzyme after the consumption of grapefruit. Overall, GFJ seems to interact with orally administered drugs, not with intravenously administered drugs.

P-Glycoprotein

The interest in transporters as mediators of interactions between grapefruit and drugs is increasing. One of the most studied drug transporters is P-gp. P-gp is a 170 kDa plasma glycoprotein, which is encoded by the multidrug resistance (MDR) 1 gene and belongs to the family of ATP-binding cassette transporters (91,92). P-gp was first characterized in tumor cells, where it contributes to the MDR (91). P-gp is expressed constitutively at high levels on the apical surface of the small intestines, liver, pancreas, kidney, colon, and adrenal glands, but also can be found at the blood–brain barrier and blood–cerebrospinal fluid barriers (92–94). Striking overlaps of substrates and inhibitors between CYP3A4 and P-gp were reported by Wacher et al. (95). Consequently, the inhibition of P-gp function may also play a role in the effects of GFJ.

Earlier studies demonstrated that GFJ did not influence the activity of P-gp; Lown and coworkers found that 8 oz of GFJ (three times per day for six days) did not alter P-gp concentrations in healthy volunteers (82). Eagling et al. confirmed these findings in their in vitro study in Caco-2 cells, where compounds from grapefruit were not found to modulate P-gp (41). In 1999, it was reported that GFJ increased P-gp–mediated transport in Madin-Darby canine kidney epithelial cells (MDCK)–MDR1 cells (96). However, this finding is controversial to the later findings and was attributed to an equipment-generated artifact by the authors (40). Takanaga et al. were the first group to demonstrate the inhibition of P-gp by GFJ in Caco-2 cells with vinblastine as probe (97). Vinblastine also is a substrate of CYP3A4, which limits the conclusions regarding the inhibition of P-gp. Therefore, the same group showed that GFJ and phenolic compounds from orange, such as tangeretin, nobiletin, and heptamethoxyflavone, which have been demonstrated not to alter CYP3A4 activity, increased the net influx of vincristine into adriamycin-resistant human myelogenous leukemia cells conclusively, through the inhibition of P-gp (46).

Clinical studies that compare the effects of orange juice with GFJ on drug bioavailability confirm the involvement of P-gp in grapefruit-induced alterations in drug absorption. A clinical intervention study conducted by Edwards et al. in the same year indicated that GFJ may interact with P-gp activity. In this study, AUC and peak concentrations of cyclosporine, a P-gp substrate, were increased by GFJ, whereas Seville orange juice did not have an influence on cyclosporine, while it reduced enterocyte concentrations of CYP3A4. DHBG did not inhibit P-gp in vitro. These data imply that the inhibition of P-gp activity by other compounds in GFJ may be responsible for the increased bioavailability of cyclosporine (98). These results were confirmed by Malhotra et al. (40) in a randomized three-way crossover intervention study in healthy volunteers who received felodipine with Seville orange juice, dilute GFJ (normalized to equivalent total concentration of BG and DHBG), and sweet orange juice. Seville orange juice and GFJ increase the AUC of felodipine. While Seville orange juice and GFJ probably interact with felodipine through inactivation of intestinal CYP3A4, the lack of interaction between Seville orange juice and cyclosporine indicates that grapefruit may cause interactions also through the inhibition of intestinal P-gp.

Several in vitro studies with different probes (talinolol, digoxin, and vinblastine) also confirm the findings that GFJ inhibits the efflux of P-gp substrates (20,54,73).

In addition to GFJ, orange juice and pomelo juice also have been shown to inhibit the activity of P-gp in vitro (73). Flavones from orange juice have been shown to be more potent than compounds from grapefruit in the inhibition of P-gp (97).

The pharmacokinetics of several drugs that are known P-gp substrates were not altered by GFJ in several clinical studies that investigated the effect of GFJ on the bioavailability of digoxin, amlodipine, and indinavir (27,75,99). Possible other unknown mechanisms and factors such as strength of the administered juices and length of consumption are relevant for the interactions of citrus with drugs (100).

Overall, it can be stated that grapefruit and other citrus may interact with several drugs through the combined inhibition of CYP3A4 and P-gp. The magnitude of interactions may strongly depend on variations in the polyphenolic profile of the GFJs and study design (101,102). The clinical significance of P-gp–related interactions between drugs and GFJ needs to be clarified in further clinical studies.

Organic Anion Transporting Polypeptides

The family of OATPs consists of membrane carriers that mediate the transport of anionic molecules, although not exclusively, and more recently, transport of nonanionic molecules has been observed. OATPs are located in the small intestines on luminal membranes of enterocytes, where they mediate the uptake of drugs. In the liver, OATPs facilitate the uptake of drugs into the hepatocytes (103,104). Whereas OATP-A is predominantly located in the brain, OATP-B has been found to be expressed on the membranes of intestinal epithelial cells (105,106). The inhibition of drug uptake mediated by OATP may alter the plasma concentration of OATP substrates.

In a more recent work, GFJ and orange juice have been reported to reduce the availability of fexofenadine and celiprolol (22,76,107). Both drugs are substrates for P-gp and OATP, but not CYP3A4 (108,109). If P-gp had played a major role in the observed interactions, the bioavailability would have been increased instead of decreased. This led to the conclusion that a mechanism other than P-gp was involved. In theory, the inhibition of OATP could lead to a decreased absorption of OATP substrates into intestinal enterocytes. This hypothesis was tested by several in vitro studies.

Dresser et al. determined that GFJ and orange juice decreased OATP-A–mediated fexofenadine uptake into HeLa cells, and that this inhibition of OATP was more potent than the inhibition of P-gp. In a corresponding human trial, the same authors found that GFJ and orange juice decreased the bioavailability of fexofenadine in healthy volunteers (22). These results imply that citrus juices may be able to inhibit both forms of OATP, namely OATP-A, which occurs in the brain and was used in the in vitro experiments, and OATP-B, which occurs in the intestine and may be responsible for the reduction of the availability of fexofenadine in the human trial. The authors also considered that the apparent decreased bioavailability of fexofenadine in human subjects may have been caused indirectly by an increased drug intake when the drug was administered with water, due to the lower osmolarity of water. Therefore a nonpolar fraction of GFJ was tested in a clinical trial. This nonpolar fraction also significantly reduced the bioavailability of fexofenadine. In a study with human embryonic kidney 293 cells expressing OATP-B, different citrus juices were tested in their effect on the uptake of estrone-3-sulfate. GFJ, orange juice, BG, DHBG, quercetin, naringin, and naringenin significantly inhibited OATP-B–mediated uptake of estrone-3-sulfate. The citrus compounds DHBG and tangeretin significantly inhibited OATP-B–mediated influx of the probe ibenclamide (23). The effects of fruit juices on the oral availability of fexofenadine also have been tested in rats. In this study, orange juice decreased the oral bioavailability of the drug to a lesser extent than that observed in humans (67). The clinical relevance of this study for the situation in humans is not clear, because fexofenadine mainly is substrate for OATP-A, which in humans predominantly occurs in the brain, whereas OATP-B occurs in the intestines. Overall, it has to be considered that genetic differences in the OATPs between humans and other species may contribute to differences in the susceptibility to grapefruit-induced inhibition, which also is true for other transporters and enzymes.

Two reports of human clinical trials discuss the potential role of OATP in grapefruit-drug interactions using fexofenadine as substrate. These studies in human healthy volunteers revealed that consumption of GFJ reduced the rate and extent of absorption of fexofenadine, an OATP substrate. The C_{max} and AUC was decreased by a range of 30% to 60% compared to when the drug was taken with water. Both studies suggested an inhibition of the influx mediated drug transporter OATP by GFJ (78,79). A recent report evaluates the effect of GFJ on disposition of talinolol in healthy human volunteers. A single glass of GFJ decreased the talinolol area under the serum concentration-time curve (AUC), peak serum drug concentration (C_{max}) and urinary excretion values to around 55%, compared with water. In addition repeated ingestion of GFJ had a similar effect. Because both single and repeated ingestion of GFJ lowered rather than increased talinolol AUC, the findings suggest that constituents present in GFJ preferentially inhibit an intestinal uptake process such as OATP rather than P-glycoprotein (110).

In summary, OATPs appear to play an important role in the influx of a number of drugs into enterocytes and hepatocytes. The inhibition of OATP activity has been demonstrated for orange and GFJ in in vitro experiments. The clinical relevance of this mechanism remains to be investigated in further human intervention trials.

CLASSES OF DRUGS INTERACTING WITH GFJ

The major drug classes for which grapefruit or other citrus interactions have been reported are described below and the interactions are summarized. Predicting the clinical significance of pharmacokinetic drug interactions is sometimes difficult especially for drugs where there are no robust methods to quantify effects or side effects. There has been recent effort in the United States by the FDA and the Pharmaceutical Research and Manufacturers of America (PhRMA) to establish some general guidelines to help drug companies, prescribers, and patients interpret the clinical significance of drug interactions (111). These are based on the clinical experience gained from some well-known drug interactions, such as the inhibition of CYP3A4. For this interaction, it could be shown that the benzodiazepine midazolam is a reproducible probe that allows quantitative determination of the interaction potential of an enzyme inhibitor. The degree of interaction can be measured in the form of an increase in the AUC of the midazolam serum concentrations. It was recently proposed to classify changes of midazolam AUC being less than twofold as "weak," which is the case observed on midazolam coadministration with ranitidine, relatively small volumes of GFJ, roxithromycin, fentanyl, or azithromycin (111). AUC changes that range from two- to fivefold, which occur on midazolam coadministration with erythromycin, diltiazem, fluconazole, verapamil, relatively large volumes of GFJ, and cimetidine are classified as "moderate." Changes that exceed a fivefold increase in midazolam AUC are labeled as "strong." Examples of drugs demonstrating strong midazolam interactions include: ketoconazole, itraconazole, mibefradil, clarithromycin, and nefazodone. Strong drug interactions are considered clinically significant and result in contraindications or strong warnings on the product label. The clinical significance of moderate inhibitors may include decisions about dose adjustments that should be based on the concentration–effect relationship.

Where applicable, the clinical relevance of GFJ interactions in the present paper was assessed according to the PhRMA classification (111). If not otherwise stated studies are performed with human subjects. An overview is given in Table 2.

Antiallergics

Interaction studies were performed for the antiallergic drugs desloratadine (78), fexofenadine (78), and terfenadine (7,112–114). When taken with GFJ, the mean exposure for desloratadine was not altered, whereas for fexofenadine it was decreased. In one of the terfenadine interaction studies, the concentrations of the control group could not be quantified (7). Three other studies demonstrated a significant increase in exposure to terfenadine (112–114). The maximum difference in exposure to terfenadine of 2.4-fold was shown by Clifford et al. No significant changes were observed in electrocardiogram (ECG) parameters for desloratadine and fexofenadine. A statistically significant increase in rate-corrected QT (QTc) intervals was reported for terfenadine when administered with GFJ and this drug was taken off the market. The mean effect of GFJ on desloratadine pharmacokinetics seems to be unlikely to be clinically relevant.

Antibiotics

The effects of GFJ were studied for clarithromycin (115) and erythromycin (116). A decrease in the time to reach the maximal plasma concentration (T_{max}) was found for clarithromycin. The exposure of erythromycin was mildly increased when administered concomitantly with GFJ. It seems unlikely that the reported interactions with the above drugs would be relevant in a clinical setting.

Anticoagulants

Data derived from studies performed with coumarin are inconsistent. In one study, the percentage of 7-hydroxycoumarin excreted in urine was decreased (117); in a second study the appearance of the metabolite was delayed when 300 mL GFJ were given concomitantly, but the recovery in urine was unchanged (118), whereas four times 250 mL juice in 30-minute intervals increased the recovery by 100%. The delay in appearance of the metabolite could also be confirmed in a third study (119). A study performed with

Table 2 Drugs for Which Grapefruit–Drug Interactions Have Been Investigated

Drug	GFJ parameters	Pharmacokinetics	Pharmacodynamics	References
Antiallergics				
Desloratadine	240 mL DS GFJ t.i.d.	AUC $\leftrightarrow$, $C_{max} \leftrightarrow$, $T_{max} \leftrightarrow$, $t_{1/2} \leftrightarrow$	NS changes in ECG parameters were observed	(78)
Fexofenadine	240 mL DS GFJ t.i.d.	AUC $\downarrow$, $C_{max} \downarrow$, $T_{max} \leftrightarrow$, $t_{1/2} \uparrow$	NS changes in ECG parameters were observed	(78)
Terfenadine	240 mL DS GFJ with terfenadine intake or 2 hr after	Concentrations were not quantifiable in control group	SS increase in QTc interval in GFJ group	(7)
	250 mL RS or DS GFJ	(RS and DS) AUC $\uparrow$, $C_{max} T_{max} \uparrow$, $t_{1/2} \leftrightarrow$ (terfenadine carboxylate)	QTc interval $\leftrightarrow$	(112)
	240 mL DS GFJ b.i.d.	AUC $\uparrow$, $C_{max} \uparrow$ (NS), $T_{max} \uparrow$, ke $\leftrightarrow$	QTc interval $\uparrow$, ECG $\leftrightarrow$	(113)
	300 mL freshly squeezed GFJ 30 min before drug administration	AUC $\uparrow$, $C_{max} \uparrow$, $T_{max} \uparrow$ (NS), $t_{1/2} \leftrightarrow$ (terfenadine acid)	QTc interval $\leftrightarrow$	(114)
Antibiotics				
Clarithromycin	240 mL freshly squeezed GFJ at time 0 and 2 hr	AUC $\leftrightarrow$, $C_{max} \leftrightarrow$, $T_{max} \uparrow$, $t_{1/2} \leftrightarrow$	N/A	(115)
Erythromycin	300 mL DS GFJ 30 min before drug administration	AUC $\uparrow$, $C_{max} \uparrow$, $T_{max} \leftrightarrow$, $t_{1/2} \leftrightarrow$	N/A	(116)
Anticoagulants				
Coumarin	300 mL GFJ 30 min before or with drug administration	Percentage of excreted 7-hydroxycoumarin in urine $\downarrow$	N/A	(117)

(Continued)

Table 2 Drugs for Which Grapefruit–Drug Interactions Have Been Investigated (*Continued*)

Drug	GFJ parameters	Pharmacokinetics	Pharmacodynamics	References
	(i) 300 mL GFJ with drug administration or (ii) 4 × 250 mL GFJ in 30 min intervals	(i) Retarded appearance of fluorescent metabolite, recovery in urine unchanged, (ii) retarded appearance of metabolite and increased the recovery in urine to 100%	N/A	(118)
Warfarin	300 mL GFJ or 1 L juice + various combinations of GFJ and Naringenin ($n = 1$)	Increasing amounts of GFJ delay the excretion of 7-hydroxycoumarin by 2 hr	N/A	(119)
	8 oz of freshly prepared GFJ from concentrate t.i.d. for 1 wk	N/A	Prothrombin time $\leftrightarrow$, international normalized ratio $\leftrightarrow$	(120)
Antimalaria drugs				
Artemether	350 mL DS GFJ with drug administration	AUC $\uparrow$, C_{max} $\uparrow$, T_{max} $\downarrow$, $t_{1/2}$ $\downarrow$	No sign of bradycardia, QTc interval $\leftrightarrow$	(121)
	350 mL DS GFJ with drug administration	AUC $\uparrow$, C_{max} $\uparrow$, T_{max} $\leftrightarrow$, $t_{1/2}$ $\leftrightarrow$	N/A	(122)
Chloroquine	4 mL/kg freshly squeezed GFJ (study performed in chicken)	Cloroquine concentration $\uparrow$ (7–37%)	No overt signs of toxicity were observed	(123)
	4 mL/kg freshly squeezed GFJ (study performed in mice)	AUC $\uparrow$, C_{max} $\uparrow$, median T_{max} $\uparrow$	N/A	(124)
Halofantrine	250 mL RS GFJ at 8:00 A.M. and 72, 48, 24, 12 before the study	AUC $\uparrow$, C_{max} $\uparrow$, T_{max} $\leftrightarrow$, $t_{1/2}$ $\leftrightarrow$	QTc prolongation $\uparrow$	(125)
Quinidine	250 mL RS GFJ b.i.d.	median C_{max} $\leftrightarrow$, median T_{max} $\leftrightarrow$, median Clren $\leftrightarrow$, median $t_{1/2}$ $\uparrow$	N/A	(88)

Drug	Dose	Pharmacokinetics	Pharmacodynamics	Ref.
	8 oz GFJ at 8:00 A.M.	AUC ↔, C_{max} ↔, T_{max} ↑, $t_{1/2}$ ↔	SS change in QTc interval prolongation only at 1 hr after drug administration	(126)
Quinine	200 mL RS or HS GFJ for 5 days b.i.d.	AUC ↔, C_{max} ↔, T_{max} ↔, $t_{1/2}$ ↔	N/A	(127)
Antiparasitic drugs				
Albendazole	250 mL DS GFJ	AUC ↑, C_{max} ↑, T_{max} ↑, $t_{1/2}$ ↓	N/A	(195)
Praziquantel	250 mL commercially squeezed GFJ	AUC ↑, C_{max} ↑, T_{max} ↔, $t_{1/2}$ ↔	N/A	(129)
Anxiolytics				
Alprazolam	(i) 200 mL RS GFJ t.i.d. for 8 days before and 2 days after treatment (ii) predosing with alprazolam existed for 2 to 10 weeks, 200 mL RS GFJ were administered t.i.d. for 7 days	(i) AUC ↔, C_{max} ↔, $t_{1/2}$ ↔, (ii) nonsmoker: AUC ↔, smokers: AUC ↑	(i) Psychomotor function ↔, thinking speed ↓ GFJ treatment at time points 1 and 2 hr (ii) Psychomotor function ↔	(130)
Buspirone	200 mL DS GFJ b.i.d. for 2 days and 1/2 and 1½ hr after drug administration	AUC ↑, C_{max} ↑, T_{max} ↑, $t_{1/2}$ ↑	Subjective overall effect ↑, psychomotor function ↔	(131)
Diazepam	250 mL RS GFJ	AUC ↑, C_{max} ↑, T_{max} ↑	N/A	(132)
Midazolam	(i) 300 mL GFJ (ii) 300 mL GFJ + 750 mg erythromycin	(i) N/A (ii) mean plasma conc. ↑	(i) Digit substitution test ↓, flicker fusion test ↓ (ii) N/A	(133)
	200 mL RS GFJ 60 and 15 min before drug (p.o. or i.v.) administration	p.o. AUC ↑, F (%) ↑ i.v. AUC ↔ F(%) ↔	Psychomotor function ↓	(6)

(Continued)

Table 2   Drugs for Which Grapefruit–Drug Interactions Have Been Investigated (*Continued*)

Drug	GFJ parameters	Pharmacokinetics	Pharmacodynamics	References
	200 mL RS GFJ 60 and 15 min before drug administration	AUC↑, C_{max}↑ (NS), T_{max}↑ (NS), $t_{1/2}$ ↔	N/A	(134)
	10 oz RS GFJ	AUC↑, C_{max}↑, $t_{1/2}$ ↔, CL↓ Recovery close to complete after 3 days	N/A	(15)
Triazolam	200 mL (1) RS, (2) DS or (3) multiple dose (t.i.d.) DS GFJ	(i) AUC↑, C_{max}↑, T_{max} ↔, $t_{1/2}$ ↔ (ii) AUC↑, C_{max}↑, T_{max} ↔, $t_{1/2}$ ↔ (iii) AUC↑, C_{max}↑, T_{max} ↔, $t_{1/2}$ ↑	(i) and (ii) psychomotor function ↔, subjective overall effect ↔ (iii) psychomotor function ↓, drowsiness ↑	(86)
	300 mL	N/A	Slight but SS psychomotor function →	(133)
	250 mL RS GFJ	AUC↑, C_{max}↑, T_{max}↑, $t_{1/2}$ ↔	Drowsiness ↑, psychomotor function ↔	(3)
Calcium channel blocker				
Amlodipine	250 mL fresh GFJ	AUC↑, C_{max}↑, T_{max} ↔, $t_{1/2}$ ↔	Blood pressure ↔, heart rate ↔	(99)
	240 mL GFJ with drug administration 200 mL GFJ for 8 days after drug administration	AUC↔, C_{max}↔, T_{max} ↔, $t_{1/2}$ ↔	Blood pressure ↔, heart rate ↔	(135)
Diltiazem	250 mL GFJ	AUC↑, C_{max}↑ (NS), T_{max} ↔, $t_{1/2}$ ↔	Blood pressure ↔, heart rate ↔	(77)

	Treatment	Pharmacokinetic effect	Pharmacodynamic effect	Ref.
Felodipine	200 mL fresh prepared GFJ at 0, 2, 4, 8, and 12 hr after drug administration	$AUC \leftrightarrow$, $C_{max} \leftrightarrow$, $T_{max} \leftrightarrow$, $t_{1/2} \uparrow$	Arterial blood pressure $\leftrightarrow$, heart rate $\leftrightarrow$, PR interval $\uparrow$ (NSR)	(136)
	(i) 250 mL GFJ or (ii) 2, (iii) 6, or (iv) 12 mg bergamottin	(i) $AUC \uparrow$, $C_{max} \uparrow$, $T_{max} \leftrightarrow$, $t_{1/2} \leftrightarrow$ (ii) $C_{max} \uparrow$ (iii) $C_{max} \uparrow$ (iv) $AUC \uparrow$, $C_{max} \uparrow$	N/A	(50)
	200 mL GFJ	$AUC \uparrow$, $C_{max} \uparrow$, $T_{max} \leftrightarrow$, $t_{1/2} \leftrightarrow$	Heart rate $\uparrow$, blood pressure $\uparrow$	(69)
	250 mL RS GFJ	$AUC \uparrow$, $C_{max} \uparrow$, $t_{1/2} \leftrightarrow$	N/A	(137)
	8 oz RS GFJ t.i.d.	$AUC \uparrow$, $C_{max} \uparrow$	N/A	(82)
	200 mL fresh frozen GFJ	$AUC \uparrow$, $C_{max} \uparrow$, $T_{max} \leftrightarrow$, $t_{1/2} \leftrightarrow$	N/A	(138)
	250 mL RS GFJ	$AUC \uparrow$, $C_{max} \uparrow$, $T_{max} \leftrightarrow$, $t_{1/2} \leftrightarrow$	Single dose: heart rate $\uparrow$, blood pressure $\downarrow$ steady state: heart rate $\uparrow$, blood pressure $\leftrightarrow$	(139)
	240 mL supernatant fraction, particulate fraction 9 g, 250 mL whole GFJ	(GFJ) $AUC \uparrow$, $C_{max} \uparrow$, $T_{max} \downarrow$, $t_{1/2} \leftrightarrow$	N/A	(62)
	240 mL diluted GFJ 1.3:1	$AUC \uparrow$, $C_{max} \uparrow$, $T_{max} \leftrightarrow$, $t_{1/2} \leftrightarrow$	N/A	(40)
	200 mL GFJ 14-day period	(day 1) $AUC \uparrow$, $C_{max} \uparrow$, $T_{max} \leftrightarrow$, $t_{1/2} \leftrightarrow$ (day 14) $AUC \uparrow$, $C_{max} \uparrow$, $T_{max} \leftrightarrow$	Heart rate $\uparrow$	(140)
	240 mL GFJ	$AUC \uparrow$, $C_{max} \uparrow$ (compared to OJ)	N/A	(14)
	200 mL GFJ	$AUC \uparrow$, $C_{max} \uparrow$, $T_{max} \uparrow$ (NS), $t_{1/2} \leftrightarrow$	Supine heart rate $\uparrow$, diastolic blood pressure $\downarrow$	(141)

(Continued)

Table 2 Drugs for Which Grapefruit–Drug Interactions Have Been Investigated (*Continued*)

Drug	GFJ parameters	Pharmacokinetics	Pharmacodynamics	References
	250 mL DS GFJ	AUC ↑, C_{max} ↑, T_{max} ↑	Blood pressure ↓, heart rate ↑	(1)
Nicardipine	250 mL RS GFJ	AUC ↑, C_{max} ↑, T_{max} ↔, $t_{1/2}$ ↔	N/A	(142)
	300 mL concentrated GFJ	AUC ↑, CL_{oral} ↓	Arterial blood pressure ↔, heart rate ↑ (1 and 2 hr) ECG ↔	(143)
Nifedipine	200 mL GFJ at 0, 2, 4, 8, and 12 hr after drug administration	AUC ↑, C_{max} ↑, T_{max} ↑, $t_{1/2}$ ↔	N/A	(144)
	200 mL DS GFJ	AUC ↑, C_{max} ↔, T_{max} ↔, $t_{1/2}$ ↔	N/A	(16)
	250 mL DS GFJ	AUC ↑, C_{max} ↔, T_{max} ↑, $t_{1/2}$ ↓	N/A	(1)
Nimodipine	250 mL GFJ	AUC ↑, C_{max} ↑, $t_{1/2}$ ↔	Maximum heart rates ↔, blood pressure ↔	(145)
Nisoldipine	250 mL GFJ	AUC ↑, C_{max} ↑, T_{max} ↓	N/A	(4)
	200 mL GFJ t.i.d. for 7 days (drug intake 0, 14, 38, 72, and 96 hr after last GFJ dose)	AUC ↑ (at 0, 14, 38, and 72 hr) C_{max} ↑ (0, 14hr) T_{max} ↔, $t_{1/2}$ ↔	Blood pressure ↓	(146)
Nitrendipine	150 mL reconstituted frozen GFJ	AUC ↑, C_{max} ↑, T_{max} ↔, $t_{1/2}$ ↔	Heart rate ↔, blood pressure ↔	(2)
Pranidipine	250 mL GFJ	AUC ↑, C_{max} ↑, T_{max} ↔, $t_{1/2}$ ↔	Blood pressure ↔, heart rate ↑	(147)
Verapamil	Four times 250 mL (at time 0, 3, 8, 12h)	AUCss ↑, C_{max}, ss ↑, peak to trough fluctuation ↑ (NSR)	PR interval ↑	(148)
	200 mL GFJ b.i.d. 5 days pretreatment	AUC ↑, $t_{1/2}$ ↔	Blood pressure ↔, heart rate ↔, PR interval ↔	(149)

Drug	GFJ dose	Effect	Comments	Ref.
	200 mL RS GFJ	AUC ↔, C_{max} ↔, T_{max} ↔	N/A	(150)
HIV protease inhibitors				
Amprenavir	200 mL GFJ	AUC ↔ ($P < 0.15$), C_{max} ↓ ($P < 0.09$), T_{max} ↑ ($P < 0.13$)	No adverse events reported	(151)
Indinavir	8 oz RS GFJ	AUC ↔, C_{max} ↔, T_{max} ↔, $t_{1/2}$ ↔	N/A	(27)
Saquinavir	180 mL DS GFJ	AUC ↔, C_{max} ↔, T_{max} ↑	N/A	(152)
	200 mL RS GFJ 45 and 15 min before drug administration	AUC ↑, C_{max} ↔, T_{max} ↔, $t_{1/2}$ ↔, F(%) ↑	N/A	(8)
	250 mL RS GFJ ($n = 1$)	AUC ↑ (NSR)	N/A	(153)
HMG CoA reductase inhibitors				
Atorvastatin	250 mL RS GFJ t.i.d. for 2 days	AUC ↑, C_{max} ↔, T_{max} ↔, $t_{1/2}$ ↔	N/A	(154)
	200 mL DS GFJ t.i.d. for 2 days	AUC ↑, C_{max} ↔, median T_{max} ↑, median $t_{1/2}$ ↑	Active inhibitors: AUC ↑, C_{max} ↔, median T_{max} ↑, $t_{1/2}$ ↔, total inhibitors: AUC ↑, C_{max} ↔ median T_{max} ↑, $t_{1/2}$ ↑	(82)
Lovastatin	200 mL DS GFJ t.i.d. for 2 days	AUC ↑, C_{max} ↑, T_{max} ↔, $t_{1/2}$ ↔	N/A	(155)
	200 mL RS GFJ for 3 days	AUC ↑, C_{max} ↑, T_{max} ↔, $t_{1/2}$ ↔	Active inhibitors: AUC ↑, C_{max} ↑, T_{max} ↔ Total inhibitors: AUC ↑, C_{max} ↑, T_{max} ↔	(156)
Pravastatin	250 mL RS GFJ t.i.d. for 2 days	AUC ↔, C_{max} ↔, T_{max} ↔, $t_{1/2}$ ↔	N/A	(154)

(Continued)

Table 2 Drugs for Which Grapefruit–Drug Interactions Have Been Investigated (*Continued*)

Drug	GFJ parameters	Pharmacokinetics	Pharmacodynamics	References
	200 mL DS GFJ t.i.d. for 2 days	AUC ↔, C_{max} ↔, T_{max} ↔, $t_{1/2}$ ↔	Active inhibitors: AUC ↔, C_{max} ↔, median T_{max} ↑ Total inhibitors: AUC ↔, C_{max} ↔, T_{max} ↔, $t_{1/2}$ ↔	(84)
Simvastatin	200 mL DS GFJ (drug administration at time 1, 3, 7, days after last GFJ intake)	(0 and 24hr) AUC ↑, C_{max} ↑, T_{max} (0) ↑, T_{max} (24) ↔, $t_{1/2}$ ↔, (3 days) AUC ↔, C_{max} ↔, T_{max} ↔, $t_{1/2}$ ↔ (7 days) AUC ↔, C_{max} ↔, T_{max} ↔, $t_{1/2}$ ↓	N/A	(157)
	200 mL RS GFJ for 2 days	AUC ↑, C_{max} ↑, T_{max} ↔, $t_{1/2}$ ↔	N/A	(87)
	200 mL DS GFJ t.i.d. for 2 days	AUC ↑, C_{max} ↑, T_{max} ↔, $t_{1/2}$ ↔	Active inhibitors: AUC ↑, C_{max} ↔, median T_{max} ↑, $t_{1/2}$ ↔ Total inhibitors: AUC ↑, C_{max} ↑, T_{max} ↑, $t_{1/2}$ ↔	(85)
Hormones				
17-Beta estradiol	200 mL GFJ	AUC ↔, C_{max} ↔, T_{max} ↔	No adverse events reported	(158)
Ethinyl-estradiol	2 times 100 mL GFJ	AUC ↑, C_{max} ↑	N/A	(159)
Prednisone	150 mL GFJ q.3.h. over 30 hr	AUC ↔, C_{max} ↔, T_{max} ↔	N/A	(160)
Methyl-prednisolone	200 mL DS GFJ t.i.d. for 2 days	AUC ↑, C_{max} ↑, T_{max} ↑, $t_{1/2}$ ↑	Morning plasma cortisol concentrations ↓ ($p < 0.09$)	(161)

Immunosuppressants

Drug	Dose	Effect	Notes	Ref.
Cyclosporine	8 oz GFJ at time −30 min, $3_{1/2}$ h, $7_{1/2}$ h, $11_{1/2}$ h	AUC ↑, C_{max} ↑, T_{max} ↔	N/A	(98)
	250 mL GFJ	AUC ↑, C_{max} ↑, T_{max} ↑, $t_{1/2}$ ↔	N/A	(70)
	150 mL GFJ b.i.d.	AUC ↑, C_{max} ↔	1 patient showed neurological side effects	(162)
	250 mL GFJ	AUC ↑, C_{max} ↔, T_{max} ↔	N/A	(163)
	240 mL RS GFJ	AUC ↔, C_{max} ↔, T_{max} ↔ λz (cyclosporine solution) ↑	N/A	(164)
	8 oz GFJ	AUC ↑, C_{max} ↔, C_{min} ↑, T_{max} ↑	N/A	(165)
	6 oz GFJ (0, 30, 90 min after drug administration)	AUC ↑, C_{max} ↑, T_{max} ↑ (NS), $t_{1/2}$ ↔	N/A	(166)
	250 mL GFJ	AUC ↑, C_{max} ↔, T_{max} ↔, $t_{1/2}$ ↔	N/A	(167)
	240 mL RS GFJ with each daily dose for 3 days	AUC ↑, C_{max} ↔, T_{max} ↔, C_{min} ↑	N/A	(168)
	150 mL GFJ q.3.h. for 30 hr	AUC ↑ ($P < 0.252$), C_{max} ↑, T_{max} ↔, $t_{1/2}$ ↑, C_{min} ↔	No clinical symptoms	(160)
	6 oz RS GFJ at time 0, 30 min and 90 min after drug administration	AUC ↑, C_{max} ↑, T_{max} ↔, $t_{1/2}$ ↔	N/A	(169)
	8 oz GFJ	C_{min} ↑	N/A	(5)
	250 mL GFJ 15 min before and 250 mL with drug intake	Median AUC ↑, C_{max} ↔, T_{max} ↔, $t_{1/2}$ ↔	N/A	(170)

Antitumor drugs

Drug	Dose	Effect	Notes	Ref.
Etoposide	100 mL GFJ	Mean AUC ↓ (no statistics provided)	N/A	(171)
Vinblastine (in vitro)	Ethyl acetate extract from GFJ	uptake of [³H]-vinblastine ↑	N/A	(172)

(Continued)

Table 2 Drugs for Which Grapefruit–Drug Interactions Have Been Investigated (*Continued*)

Drug	GFJ parameters	Pharmacokinetics	Pharmacodynamics	References
Vinblastine (in vitro)	Ethyl acetate extract from GFJ or 20 μmol/L DHB	LLC-PK1: uptake ↓ LLC-GA5-COL300 cells: uptake ↑	N/A	(172)
Vinblastine (in vitro)	Ethyl acetate extract of 10 mL GFJ	Uptake ↑	N/A	(97)
OTC drugs				
Caffeine	200 mL GFJ	AUC ↔, ke ↔	Blood pressure ↔, heart rate ↔	(173)
	300 mL GFJ with drug administration and q.6.h. for the sampling period	AUC ↑, cloral ↓, $t_{1/2}$ ↑	N/A	(89)
Dextromethorphan	200 mL GFJ from concentrate (1:3 dilution with water)	F↑, percent excreted ↑	N/A	(28)
Beta-blocker				
Celiprolol	200 mL RS GFJ t.i.d. for 2 days	AUC ↓, C_{max} ↓, Cl renal ↔	Blood pressure ↔, heart rate ↔	(76)
Talinolol (in rats)	GFJ	AUC ↑, C_{max} ↑, T_{max} ↔, $t_{1/2}$ ↔		(174)
Other drugs				
Carbamazepine	300 mL fresh GFJ	AUCss ↑, C_{max} ss↑, T_{max} ↔, C_{min}ss ↑		(175)
Cisapride	250 mL GFJ	AUC ↑, C_{max} ↑, T_{max} ↑, $t_{1/2}$ ↔	Heart rate ↔, blood pressure ↔, QTc interval ↔	(176)
	250 mL GFJ	AUC ↑, C_{max} ↑, T_{max} ↔, $t_{1/2}$ ↔	QTc interval ↔	(177)
	200 mL DS GFJ t.i.d. for 2 days	AUC ↑, C_{max} ↑, T_{max} ↑, $t_{1/2}$ ↑	QTc interval ↔	(178)
	200 mL DS GFJ t.i.d. for 2 days	AUC ↑, C_{max} ↑, T_{max} ↑, $t_{1/2}$ ↑ for (−) Cisapride	QTc interval ↔	(179)

Drug	Intervention	Pharmacokinetic effect	Clinical/other effect	Reference
Clozapine	250 mL yellow GFJ	No significant difference in mean plasma levels		(180)
	250 mL RS GFJ b.i.d. for 2 wk	No significant difference in mean plasma levels	Clinical Global Impressions Scale scores ↔, Calgary Depression Scale scores ↔, side effects profiles ↔	(181)
Diclofenac (in rats)	DS GFJ 10 mL/kg	N/A	SS increase in effect in the 2.5 mg/kg and 5 mg/kg diclofenac group, no significant increase in the 1 mg/kg group	(182)
Digoxin	220 mL RS GFJ at time −30 min and 1.5, 7.5, 11.5 hr	AUC ↑ (NS), C_{max} ↑ (NS)	PR prolongation in $n=2$	(183)
	240 mL RS GFJ t.i.d. for 5 days	Ka ↓, T_{lag}↑, AUC ↔, $t_{1/2}$ ↔, Clrenal ↔	N/A	(75)
Fluvoxamine	250 mL RS GFJ t.i.d. for 5 days	AUC ↑, C_{max} ↑, T_{max} ↔, $t_{1/2}$ ↔	N/A	(184)
Itraconazole	350 mL RS GFJ	AUC ↔, C_{max} ↔, T_{max} ↔, $t_{1/2}$ ↔	N/A	(185)
	240 mL DS GFJ	AUC ↑, C_{max} ↓ (NS), T_{max} ↑	N/A	(186)
	240 mL RS GFJ t.i.d. for 2 days	AUC ↑, C_{max} ↔, T_{max} ↔	N/A	(187)
Losartan	200 mL GFJ	AUC ↑ (NS), T_{lag} ↑, C_{max} ↔, T_{max} ↔, $t_{1/2}$ ↔	Blood pressure ↔, pulse ↔	(188)
Methadone	200 mL GFJ 30 min before drug intake	AUC ↑, C_{max} ↑, T_{max} ↔, $t_{1/2}$ ↔	Side effects ↓, withdrawal symptoms ↔	(189)
Omeprazole	300 mL GFJ	AUC ↔, C_{max} ↔, T_{max} ↔, $t_{1/2}$ ↔	N/A	(190)

(Continued)

Table 2 Drugs for Which Grapefruit–Drug Interactions Have Been Investigated (*Continued*)

Drug	GFJ parameters	Pharmacokinetics	Pharmacodynamics	References
Scopolamine	150 mL fresh squeezed GFJ	AUC ↑, C_{max} ↔, T_{max} ↑, $t_{1/2}$ ↔	Alertness ↓, contentment ↔, calmness ↔	(191)
Sertraline	240 mL GFJ	Mean serum trough levels ↑	Side effects ↔	(192)
Sildenafil	GFJ (1 subject)	AUC ↔, C_{max} ↑, T_{max} ↔, $t_{1/2}$ ↔ (NSR)	Blood pressure ↔, ECG ↔	(193)
Theophylline	250 mL GFJ	AUC ↑, C_{max} ↔, $t_{1/2}$ ↔		(194)
	100 mL GFJ	AUC ↔, C_{max} ↔, T_{max}↔, $t_{1/2}$ ↔ (NSR)	Blood pressure ↔, ECG ↔	(195)
Haloperidol	200 mL RS GFJ t.i.d. for 7 days	Mean plasma concentrations ↔	BPRS ↔	(196)

Abbreviations: λz, terminal elimination rate constant; AUC, area under the curve; AUCss, area under the curve at steady state; b.i.d., two times per day; Cl, clearance; Cloral, oral clearance; Clren, renal clearance; DS, double strength; ECG, electrocardiogram; F, bioavailability; GFJ, grapefruit juice; HS, half strength; i.v., intravenous; ke, eliminariont rate constant; N/A, not available; NS, not significant; NSR, no statistics reported; OJ, orange juice; p.o., per os: q.3.h., every 3 hr; RS, regular strength; SS, statistically significant; $t_{1/2}$, half-life; t.i.d., three times per day; T_{lag}, lag time; T_{max}, time to reach peak concentration; BPRS, Brief Psychiatric Rating Scale; QTc, rate-corrected QT interval; ↑, increase; ↔, no change; ↓, decrease; *n*, number of volunteers.

warfarin did not assess any pharmacokinetic parameters. However, when patients were pretreated with 8 oz GFJ three times a day for one week, no change in prothrombin time or International Normalized Ratio could be observed (120). More conclusive clinical studies are necessary to assess the overall effect of GFJ on these anticoagulants.

Antimalaria Drugs

GFJ increases the exposure of artemether (121,122), chloroquine in chicken and mice (123,124), and halofantrine (125). No signs of bradycardia or changes in the QTc interval were observed when artemether was adminis-tered with GFJ. No overt signs of toxicity of chloroquine were observed in the chicken study. Furthermore, it was reported that GFJ increased the QTc interval when administered concomitantly with halofantrine. No changes in pharmacokinetic parameters were observed when quinidine (88,126) or quinine (127) was coadministered with GFJ. However, one study assessing the interaction with quinidine reported a significant change in QTc interval prolongation, although this change was only seen at one hour after drug administration. According to the classification of Bjornsson et al. (111) the interactions of quinidine and quinine would be considered weak and unlikely to be clinically relevant. However, a further evaluation of the phar-macodynamic parameters would be desirable. Artemether showed a moder-ate interaction and halofantrine exhibited a strong interaction. GFJ should be avoided with halofantrine and should be consumed only after a cautious risk and benefit assessment with artemether.

Antiparasitic Drugs

The interactions of GFJ with albendazole (128) and praziquantel (129) can be considered moderate and weak, respectively. GFJ increases the AUC of albendazole 3.1-fold and the C_{max} 3.2-fold. A concomitant consumption should only be considered after a cautious risk and benefit assessment. Regarding the pharmacokinetic parameters, an interaction of GFJ with pra-ziquantel seems unlikely to be clinically relevant (AUC increases 1.62-fold and C_{max} increases 1.9-fold).

Anxiolytics

Alprazolam did not exhibit any changes in pharmacokinetic parameters when administered concomitantly with GFJ (130) in a single dose experi-ment. When predosing existed, GFJ increased the exposure of alprazolam only in smokers. However, this interaction seems unlikely to be clinically rele-vant. In both parts of this study psychomotor function remained unchanged; however, there was a small decrease in cognitive speed in the single dose part at one and two hours after dosing. Midazolam (6,15,133,134) and triazolam

(3,86,133) exposure increased when administered concomitantly with GFJ, but these increases fall into the category of weak interactions. However, changes in psychomotor function have been reported. On the other hand, one study showed a 2.06-fold increase in exposure in patients with liver cirrhosis. These results would be considered a moderate interaction and cannot easily be extrapolated to healthy patients. Diazepam plasma concentrations in dogs were increased by GFJ (52). Buspirone plasma concentrations also were increased, as was the overall subjective effect (197). No changes in psychomotor function were observed. Patients should not consume buspirone concomitantly with GFJ, because they may exhibit a strong pharmacokinetic interaction. More human intervention trials will have to be conducted to confirm results from previous studies.

Calcium Channel Blockers

Amlodipine (99,135), diltiazem (77,136), nimodipine (145), nifedipine (1,16,144), pranidipine (147), and verapamil (148–150) exhibit a weak interaction with GFJ with regard to their mean exposure. However, only for amlodipine, diltiazem, nimodipine, and verapamil, no changes in the pharmacodynamic parameters heart rate and blood pressure were reported. Blood pressure was increased after verapamil and GFJ administration only at eight hours after drug administration. No pharmacodynamic parameters were recorded in the studies performed with nifedipine and GFJ. Heart rate was increased after pranidipine administration with GFJ, however the blood pressure remained constant. Felodipine (14,40,50,62,69,82,99,137–142), nicardipine (143), nisoldipine (4,146), and nitrendipine (2) exhibit a moderate interaction with GFJ. However, blood pressure decreased in one study with nisoldipine and no change in pharmacodynamic parameters were observed in the study examining nitrendipine. The heart rates after concomitant nicardipine and GFJ administration changed only at two hours. Changes in pharmacodynamic parameters were reported after GFJ was administered with felodipine. Felodipine-, nicardipine-, nisoldipine-, and nitrendipine-containing products should only be consumed with GFJ after a cautious risk and benefit assessment.

HIV Protease Inhibitors

Amprenavir (151) and indinavir (27,152) showed no changes in pharmacokinetic parameters when administered concomitantly with GFJ. Even 180 mL double-strength GFJ had no effect on indinavir pharmacokinetics. The AUC of saquinavir was increased after predosing with GFJ. The mean increase was 1.5-fold (8). In a study performed with one subject, a 5-fold (153) increase was reported. The reported interactions can be considered weak and are unlikely to be clinically relevant.

HMG-CoA Reductase Inhibitors

Increases in exposure were reported for atorvastatin (84,154), lovastatin (155,156), and simvastatin (85,87,157). GFJ was shown not to have an effect on the pharmacokinetics of pravastatin (84,154). Atorvastatin exhibited a moderate interaction with GFJ regarding the overall exposure. Lovastatin and simvastatin exhibited a strong interaction. Pravastatin could be chosen as an alternative drug if patients want to ensure a lack of interaction.

Hormones

No effect of GFJ was observed on 17-beta estradiol (158) or prednisone (160) pharmacokinetics. AUCs were increased for ethinyl-estradiol (159) and methylprednisolone (161). The increases in exposure can be considered weak and seem to be unlikely to be clinically relevant. It has to be mentioned that a decrease in morning cortisol plasma concentrations has been observed after administration of methylprednisolone with GFJ.

Immunosupressants

An increase in cyclosporine exposure was reported by 11 out of a total of 13 studies (5,70,98,162,163,165–170). Two studies reported no change in AUC induced by GFJ (160,164). Even administration of a large amount of GFJ was shown to increase the AUC only by 7% (160). Regarding the exposure to cyclosporine, the reported interactions seem unlikely to be clinically relevant.

Antitumor Drugs

GFJ was demonstrated to decrease the mean AUC of etoposide when administered concomitantly (171). However, there was no indication of whether the results were statistically significant. Furthermore, an increased uptake has been shown for vinblastine in Caco-2 cells (22,97). These results can only serve as an estimate. Further research will have to be conducted to develop recommendations for this drug class.

Over-the-Counter Drugs

Contradicting results were reported for GFJ when administered with caffeine. One study reported no changes in AUC, blood pressure, and heart rate (173). A second study reported increases in AUC and half-life. However, no assessment of pharmacodynamic parameters was performed (89). Furthermore, GFJ increased the fraction absorbed and the percentage of excreted dextromethorphan (28). The above-mentioned interactions can be considered weak regarding the overall exposure. Furthermore, dextromethorphan has a broad therapeutic window. The interactions of GFJ with caffeine and dextromethorphan do not seem to be of clinical relevance.

Hence, no clinically significant interactions of an over-the-counter drug with GFJ have been reported.

Beta-Blockers

When celiprolol was administered concomitantly with GFJ, AUC and C_{max} of celiprolol decreased by 95% (76); however, heart rate and blood pressure remained the same. The authors of this study conclude the observed interactions to be clinically relevant. In an animal study, talinolol exposure has been reported to increase after GFJ administration (174). Further human studies will have to be conducted to derive reliable conclusions.

Other Drugs

GFJ has been shown to increase the exposure of carbamazepine (175), cisapride (176–179), fluvoxamine (184), losartan (188), methadone (189), scopolamine (191), and sertraline (192). However, only the interaction of GFJ with carbamazepine and cisapride seems to be clinically relevant. No alteration in exposure was observed for clozapine (180,181), heophylline (195), haloperidol (196), and omeprazole (190). Reports of increased pharmacokinetic parameters of clozapine, theophylline, and haloperidol suggest that an interaction is unlikely to be clinically relevant. Contradicting results were reported for itraconazole (185–187), digoxin (75,183), and sildenafil (193,194). An increased effect on concomitant use of diclofenac and GFJ was observed in rats (182). Overall, the clinical relevance for this drug class appears to be low.

CONCLUSIONS

Citrus-based products, and grapefruit in particular, can interact with several orally administered medications. In most cases, the expected interactions will be minor and of little clinical relevance. However, the overall observation that a single serving of GFJ can induce a long-lasting increase in oral bioavailability of some drugs, which may lead to potential drug toxicity, does call for caution. In situations where toxicity can be expected, GFJ and other citrus products with a known interaction should be avoided during the whole period of drug treatment. For those patients who want to consume GFJ while they are being medicated, many of the drugs showing an interaction could be replaced by other drugs that have been shown to not interact with GFJ. It also should be considered that, for patients who regularly consumed GFJ before the dose of their medication was adjusted and continued with a constant consumption of GFJ during their medication, a potential toxicity appears relatively unlikely, because the dose for these patients would be lower than for those not consuming GFJ (12).

There are a few situations in which toxicity could potentially occur: (i) in patients taking unusually high doses of a susceptible drug, who then consume GFJ for the first time, where the GFJ may lead to a sudden decrease of intestinal CYP3A4 activity, (ii) in patients with severe liver disease, the exposure to the drug would be expected to be higher with the intestines being the major site of metabolism. Also in these patients a sudden decrease in CYP activity in the intestines may lead to an increase of drug concentration, and (iii) patients susceptible to toxic effects from drugs are likely to exhibit drug toxicity when the bioavailability is increased (12).

Additionally, it has to be considered that patients consuming GFJ are also prone to consume other fruits and vegetables and dietary supplements, which may cause an interaction. Sales of dietary supplements containing phytochemicals have been expanding, in part driven by increased health awareness. In particular, patients with chronic diseases have a high propensity to consume prescription drugs and concomitant dietary supplements. Between 1990 and 1995, the use of alternative medicines, including dietary supplements, increased from 34% to 42%, leading to an expenditure of $27 billion for patients. Worldwide, up to 75% of cancer patients use alternative medicine (198). In a survey conducted in 2002, 54.9% of all users of alternative medicines, including dietary supplements, thought that the natural remedy would help when consumed in combination with the conventional drug (199). Although GFJ can cause a drug interaction by itself, it should not be taken out of the context of the complete diet, which may also contribute to drug interactions.

The extent of the grapefruit–drug interaction in the case of CYP3A4 appears to be dependent on the patient intestinal enzyme activity. Subjects with a high activity of CYP3A4 appear to show a higher inhibition by GFJ, whereas the inhibition of CYP was lower for subjects with a low initial CYP activity. Theoretically, the concomitant administration of GFJ with a susceptible drug would cause the highest increase in AUC in subjects with a high intestinal CYP3A4 activity; however unexpectedly, these subjects tend to have a low AUC after intake of a standard dose of drugs without the administration of GFJ (82,176). More studies will have to be performed, especially in the area of P-gp and OATP-mediated drug interactions, before sound recommendations for the concomitant intake of citrus with certain drugs can be given.

FUTURE DIRECTIVES

According to the current, still limited knowledge, responsible recommendations should be communicated effectively to health care personnel and patients. Here care must be taken to avoid careless prescription of susceptible drugs without unnecessary overreaction leading to complete avoidance of citrus products, because these contain significant amounts of antioxidant phytochemicals with significant health benefits.

It also appears possible to develop grapefruit furanocoumarins as additives to certain drugs in order to improve their oral bioavailability and reduce the variability. On the other hand, citrus juice manufacturers could develop GFJs without furanocoumarins, which would reduce the potential for a drug interaction (12). Citrus fruits, other than grapefruit, and other food products, in general, will have to be investigated further in their potential to induce a drug interaction.

Further clinical research will have to be conducted to conclusively determine the mechanisms and clinical relevance of these interactions.

REFERENCES

1. Bailey DG, Spence JD, Munoz C, Arnold JM. Interaction of citrus juices with felodipine and nifedipine. Lancet 1991; 337(8736):268–269.
2. Soons PA, Vogels BA, Roosemalen MC, et al. Grapefruit juice and cimetidine inhibit stereoselective metabolism of nitrendipine in humans. Clin Pharmacol Ther 1991; 50(4):394–403.
3. Hukkinen SK, Varhe A, Olkkola KT, Neuvonen PJ. Plasma concentrations of triazolam are increased by concomitant ingestion of grapefruit juice. Clin Pharmacol Ther 1995; 58(2):127–131.
4. Bailey DG, Arnold JM, Strong HA, Munoz C, Spence JD. Effect of grapefruit juice and naringin on nisoldipine pharmacokinetics. Clin Pharmacol Ther 1993; 54(6):589–594.
5. Ducharme MP, Provenzano R, Dehoorne-Smith M, Edwards DJ. Trough concentrations of cyclosporine in blood following administration with grapefruit juice. Br J Clin Pharmacol 1993; 36(5):457–459.
6. Kupferschmidt HH, Ha HR, Ziegler WH, Meier PJ, Krahenbuhl S. Interaction between grapefruit juice and midazolam in humans. Clin Pharmacol Ther 1995; 58(1):20–28.
7. Benton RE, Honig PK, Zamani K, Cantilena LR, Woosley RL. Grapefruit juice alters terfenadine pharmacokinetics, resulting in prolongation of repolarization on the electrocardiogram. Clin Pharmacol Ther 1996; 59(4):383–388.
8. Kupferschmidt HH, Fattinger KE, Ha HR, Follath F, Krahenbuhl S. Grapefruit juice enhances the bioavailability of the HIV protease inhibitor saquinavir in man. Br J Clin Pharmacol 1998; 45(4):355–359.
9. Butterweck V, Derendorf H, Gaus W, Nahrstedt A, Schulz V, Unger M. Pharmacokinetic herb-drug interactions: are preventive screenings necessary and appropriate? Planta Med 2004; 70(9):784–791.
10. Kaufman DW, Kelly JP, Rosenberg L, Anderson TE, Mitchell AA. Recent patterns of medication use in the ambulatory adult population of the United States: the Slone survey. JAMA 2002; 287(3):337–344.
11. Lesser PF. Florida grapefruit juice developments. Second International Fruit-Juice Conference, Amsterdam, The Netherlands, 1997.
12. Huang SM, Hall SD, Watkins P, et al. Drug interactions with herbal products and grapefruit juice: a conference report. Clin Pharmacol Ther 2004; 75(1): 1–12.

13. Dahan A, Altman H. Food-drug interaction: grapefruit juice augments drug bioavailability—mechanism, extent and relevance. Eur J Clin Nutr 2004; 58(1):1–9.

14. Kakar SM, Paine MF, Stewart PW, Watkins PB. 6'7'-Dihydroxybergamottin contributes to the grapefruit juice effect. Clin Pharmacol Ther 2004; 75(6): 569–579.

15. Greenblatt DJ, von Moltke LL, Harmatz JS, et al. Time course of recovery of cytochrome p450 3A function after single doses of grapefruit juice. Clin Pharmacol Ther 2003; 74(2):121–129.

16. Rashid TJ, Martin U, Clarke H, Waller DG, Renwick AG, George CF. Factors affecting the absolute bioavailability of nifedipine. Br J Clin Pharmacol 1995; 40(1):51–58.

17. Veronese ML, Gillen LP, Burke JP, et al. Exposure-dependent inhibition of intestinal and hepatic CYP3A4 in vivo by grapefruit juice. J Clin Pharmacol 2003; 43(8):831–839.

18. Mitsunaga Y, Takanaga H, Matsuo H, et al. Effect of bioflavonoids on vincristine transport across blood-brain barrier. Eur J Pharmacol 2000; 395(3): 193–201.

19. Takanaga H, Ohnishi A, Yamada S, et al. Polymethoxylated flavones in orange juice are inhibitors of P-glycoprotein but not cytochrome P450 3A4. J Pharmacol Exp Ther 2000; 293(1):230–236.

20. Spahn-Langguth H, Langguth P. Grapefruit juice enhances intestinal absorption of the P-glycoprotein substrate talinolol. 2001; 12(4):361–367.

21. Tian R, Koyabu N, Takanaga H, Matsuo H, Ohtani H, Sawada Y. Effects of grapefruit juice and orange juice on the intestinal efflux of P-glycoprotein substrates. Pharm Res 2002; 19(6):802–809.

22. Dresser GK, Bailey DG, Leake BF, et al. Fruit juices inhibit organic anion transporting polypeptide-mediated drug uptake to decrease the oral availability of fexofenadine. Clin Pharmacol Ther 2002; 71(1):11–20.

23. Satoh H, Yamashita F, Tsujimoto M, et al. Citrus juices inhibit the function of human organic anion transporting polypeptide OATP-B. Drug Metab Dispos 2005; 33(4):518–253.

24. Bailey DG, Dresser GK. Interactions between grapefruit juice and cardiovascular drugs. Am J Cardiovasc Drugs 2004; 4(5):281–297.

25. FDA/CDER. CDER New and Generic Drug Approvals: 1998–2004. In: FDA CDER; 2004, http://www.fda.gov/cder/approval/index.htm (accessed in 1/2005).

26. Pfizer. Procardia (nifedipine) CAPSULES For Oral Use. New York, NY: Pfizer Labs, Division of Pfizer Inc., http://www.pfizer.com/download/uspi_procardia.pdf, 2000 (accessed in 1/2005).

27. Penzak SR, Acosta EP, Turner M, et al. Effect of Seville orange juice and grapefruit juice on indinavir pharmacokinetics. J Clin Pharmacol 2002; 42(10):1165–1170.

28. Di Marco MP, Edwards DJ, Wainer IW, Ducharme MP. The effect of grapefruit juice and seville orange juice on the pharmacokinetics of dextromethorphan: the role of gut CYP3A and P-glycoprotein. Life Sci 2002; 71(10):1149–1160.

29. Izzo AA, Di Carlo G, Borrelli F, Ernst E. Cardiovascular pharmacotherapy and herbal medicines: the risk of drug interaction. Int J Cardiol 2005; 98(1):1–14.

30. Berhow MTB, Kanes K, Vandercook C. Survey of Phenolic Compounds Produced in Citrus. Technical Bulletin Number 1856. United States Department of Agriculture, 1998.

31. Kawaii S, Tomono Y, Katase E, Ogawa K, Yano M. Quantitation of flavonoid constituents in citrus fruits. J Agric Food Chem 1999; 47(9):3565–3571.

32. Gil-Izquierdo A, Gil MI, Ferreres F, Tomas-Barberan FA. In vitro availability of flavonoids and other phenolics in orange juice. J Agric Food Chem 2001; 49(2):1035–1041.

33. Albach RF, Redman GH. Composition and inheritance of flavanones in citrus fruit. 1969; 8(1):127.

34. Fukuda K, Ohta T, Oshima Y, Ohashi N, Yoshikawa M, Yamazoe Y. Specific CYP3A4 inhibitors in grapefruit juice: furocoumarin dimers as components of drug interaction. Pharmacogenetics 1997; 7(5):391–396.

35. Rouseff RL, Dettweiler GR, Swaine RM, Naim M, Zehavi U. Solid-phase extraction and HPLC determination of 4-vinyl guaiacol and its precursor, ferulic acid, in orange juice. J Chromatogr Sci 1992; 30(10):383–387.

36. Hillebrand S, Schwarz M, Winterhalter P. Characterization of anthocyanins and pyranoanthocyanins from blood orange *Citrus sinensis* (L.) Osbeck juice. J Agric Food Chem 2004; 52(24):7331–7338.

37. Clifford MN. Chlorogenic acids and other cinnamates—nature, occurrence and dietary burden. J Sci Food Agric 1999; 79:362–372.

38. Tassaneeyakul W, Guo LQ, Fukuda K, Ohta T, Yamazoe Y. Inhibition selectivity of grapefruit juice components on human cytochromes P450. Arch Biochem Biophys 2000; 378(2):356–363.

39. Manners GD, Breksa AP III, Schoch TK, Hidalgo MB. Analysis of bitter limonoids in citrus juices by atmospheric pressure chemical ionization and electrospray ionization liquid chromatography-mass spectrometry. J Agric Food Chem 2003; 51(13):3709–3714.

40. Malhotra S, Bailey DG, Paine MF, Watkins PB. Seville orange juice-felodipine interaction: comparison with dilute grapefruit juice and involvement of furocoumarins. Clin Pharmacol Ther 2001; 69(1):14–23.

41. Eagling VA, Profit L, Back DJ. Inhibition of the CYP3A4-mediated metabolism and P-glycoprotein-mediated transport of the HIV-1 protease inhibitor saquinavir by grapefruit juice components. Br J Clin Pharmacol 1999; 48(4): 543–552.

42. Ubeaud G, Hagenbach J, Vandenschrieck S, Jung L, Koffel JC. In vitro inhibition of simvastatin metabolism in rat and human liver by naringenin. Life Sci 1999; 65(13):1403–1412.

43. Ho PC, Saville DJ, Wanwimolruk S. Inhibition of human CYP3A4 activity by grapefruit flavonoids, furanocoumarins and related compounds. J Pharm Pharm Sci 2001; 4(3):217–227.

44. Zhang H, Wong CW, Coville PF, Wanwimolruk S. Effect of the grapefruit flavonoid naringin on pharmacokinetics of quinine in rats. Drug Metabol Drug Interact 2000; 17(1–4):351–363.

45. Kuhlmann O, Hofmann HS, Muller SP, Weiss M. Pharmacokinetics of idarubicin in the isolated perfused rat lung: effect of cinchonine and rutin. Anticancer Drugs 2003; 14(6):411–416.

46. Ikegawa T, Ushigome F, Koyabu N, et al. Inhibition of P-glycoprotein by orange juice components, polymethoxyflavones in adriamycin-resistant human myelogenous leukemia (K562/ADM) cells. Cancer Lett 2000; 160(1):21–28.

47. Patel J, Buddha B, Dey S, Pal D, Mitra AK. In vitro interaction of the HIV protease inhibitor ritonavir with herbal constituents: changes in P-gp and CYP3A4 activity. Am J Ther 2004; 11(4):262–277.

48. Li Y, Wang E, Patten CJ, Chen L, Yang CS. Effects of flavonoids on cytochrome P450-dependent acetaminophen metabolism in rats and human liver microsomes. Drug Metab Dispos 1994; 22(4):566–571.

49. Ha HR, Chen J, Leuenberger PM, Freiburghaus AU, Follath F. In vitro inhibition of midazolam and quinidine metabolism by flavonoids. Eur J Clin Pharmacol 1995; 48(5):367–371.

50. Goosen TC, Cillie D, Bailey DG, et al. Bergamottin contribution to the grapefruit juice-felodipine interaction and disposition in humans. Clin Pharmacol Ther 2004; 76(6):607–617.

51. Mohri K, Uesawa Y. Effects of furanocoumarin derivatives in grapefruit juice on nifedipine pharmacokinetics in rats. Pharm Res 2001; 18(2):177–182.

52. Sahi J, Reyner EL, Bauman JN, Gueneva-Boucheva K, Burleigh JE, Thomas VH. The effect of bergamottin on diazepam plasma levels and P450 enzymes in beagle dogs. Drug Metab Dispos 2002; 30(2):135–140.

53. He K, Iyer KR, Hayes RN, Sinz MW, Woolf TF, Hollenberg PF. Inactivation of cytochrome P450 3A4 by bergamottin, a component of grapefruit juice. Chem Res Toxicol 1998; 11(4):252–259.

54. Ohnishi A, Matsuo H, Yamada S, et al. Effect of furanocoumarin derivatives in grapefruit juice on the uptake of vinblastine by Caco-2 cells and on the activity of cytochrome P450 3A4. Br J Pharmacol 2000; 130(6):1369–1377.

55. Le Goff-Klein N, Koffel JC, Jung L, Ubeaud G. In vitro inhibition of simvastatin metabolism, a HMG-CoA reductase inhibitor in human and rat liver by bergamottin, a component of grapefruit juice. Eur J Pharm Sci 2003; 18(1):31–35.

56. Schmiedlin-Ren P, Edwards DJ, Fitzsimmons ME, et al. Mechanisms of enhanced oral availability of CYP3A4 substrates by grapefruit constituents. Decreased enterocyte CYP3A4 concentration and mechanism-based inactivation by furanocoumarins. Drug Metab Dispos 1997; 25(11):1228–1233.

57. Guo LQ, Fukuda K, Ohta T, Yamazoe Y. Role of furanocoumarin derivatives on grapefruit juice-mediated inhibition of human CYP3A activity. Drug Metab Dispos 2000; 28(7):766–771.

58. Sun J, Chu YF, Wu X, Liu RH. Antioxidant and antiproliferative activities of common fruits. J Agric Food Chem 2002; 50(25):7449–7454.

59. Kim HY, Kim OH, Sung MK. Effects of phenol-depleted and phenol-rich diets on blood markers of oxidative stress, and urinary excretion of quercetin and kaempferol in healthy volunteers. J Am Coll Nutr 2003; 22(3):217–223.

60. Vinson JA, Liang X, Proch J, Hontz BA, Dancel J, Sandone N. Polyphenol antioxidants in citrus juices: in vitro and in vivo studies relevant to heart disease. Adv Exp Med Biol 2002; 505:113–122.

61. Bailey DG, Dresser GK, Bend JR. Bergamottin, lime juice, and red wine as inhibitors of cytochrome P450 3A4 activity: comparison with grapefruit juice. 2003; 73(6):529–537.

62. Bailey DG, Dresser GK, Kreeft JH, Munoz C, Freeman DJ, Bend JR. Grapefruit-felodipine interaction: effect of unprocessed fruit and probable active ingredients. Clin Pharmacol Ther 2000; 68(5):468–477.

63. Paine MF, Criss AB, Watkins PB. Two major grapefruit juice components differ in intestinal CYP3A4 inhibition kinetic and binding properties. Drug Metab Dispos 2004; 32(10):1146–1153.

64. Mertens-Talcott SU, Percival SS. Ellagic acid and quercetin interact synergistically with resveratrol in the induction of apoptosis and cause transient cell cycle arrest in human leukemia cells. Cancer Lett 2005; 218(2):141–151.

65. Chen YC, Shen SC, Chow JM, Ko CH, Tseng SW. Flavone inhibition of tumor growth via apoptosis in vitro and in vivo. Int J Oncol 2004; 25(3):661–670.

66. Iwashita K, Kobori M, Yamaki K, Tsushida T. Flavonoids inhibit cell growth and induce apoptosis in B16 melanoma 4A5 cells. 2000; 64(9):1813–1820.

67. Kamath AV, Yao M, Zhang Y, Chong S. Effect of fruit juices on the oral bioavailability of fexofenadine in rats. J Pharm Sci 2005; 94(2):233–239.

68. Dresser GK, Spence JD, Bailey DG. Pharmacokinetic-pharmacodynamic consequences and clinical relevance of cytochrome P450 3A4 inhibition. 2000; 38(1):41–57.

69. Lundahl J, Regardh CG, Edgar B, Johnsson G. Effects of grapefruit juice ingestion—pharmacokinetics and haemodynamics of intravenously and orally administered felodipine in healthy men. Eur J Clin Pharmacol 1997; 52(2):139–145.

70. Ducharme MP, Warbasse LH, Edwards DJ. Disposition of intravenous and oral cyclosporine after administration with grapefruit juice. Clin Pharmacol Ther 1995; 57(5):485–491.

71. Doherty MM, Charman WN. The mucosa of the small intestine: how clinically relevant as an organ of drug metabolism? Clin Pharmacokinet 2002; 41(4): 235–253.

72. Dresser GK, Bailey DG. The effects of fruit juices on drug disposition: a new model for drug interactions. Eur J Clin Invest 2003; 33(suppl 2):10–16.

73. Xu J, Go ML, Lim LY. Modulation of digoxin transport across Caco-2 cell monolayers by citrus fruit juices: lime, lemon, grapefruit, and pummelo. Pharm Res 2003; 20(2):169–176.

74. Romiti N, Tramonti G, Donati A, Chieli E. Effects of grapefruit juice on the multidrug transporter P-glycoprotein in the human proximal tubular cell line HK-2. Life Sci 2004; 76(3):293–302.

75. Parker RB, Yates CR, Soberman JE, Laizure SC. Effects of grapefruit juice on intestinal P-glycoprotein: evaluation using digoxin in humans. Pharmacotherapy 2003; 23(8):979–987.

76. Lilja JJ, Backman JT, Laitila J, Luurila H, Neuvonen PJ. Itraconazole increases but grapefruit juice greatly decreases plasma concentrations of celiprolol. Clin Pharmacol Ther 2003; 73(3):192–198.

77. Christensen H, Asberg A, Holmboe AB, Berg KJ. Coadministration of grapefruit juice increases systemic exposure of diltiazem in healthy volunteers. Eur J Clin Pharmacol 2002; 58(8):515–520.

78. Banfield C, Gupta S, Marino M, Lim J, Affrime M. Grapefruit juice reduces the oral bioavailability of fexofenadine but not desloratadine. Clin Pharmacokinet 2002; 41(4):311–318.

79. Dresser GK, Kim RB, Bailey DG. Effect of grapefruit juice volume on the reduction of fexofenadine bioavailability: Possible role of organic anion transporting polypeptides, 170–177.
80. Donato MT, Castell JV. Strategies and molecular probes to investigate the role of cytochrome P450 in drug metabolism: focus on in vitro studies. Clin Pharmacokinet 2003; 42(2):153–178.
81. Harris RZ, Jang GR, Tsunoda S. Dietary effects on drug metabolism and transport. Clin Pharmacokinet 2003; 42(13):1071–1088.
82. Lown KS, Bailey DG, Fontana RJ, et al. Grapefruit juice increases felodipine oral availability in humans by decreasing intestinal CYP3A protein expression. J Clin Invest 1997; 99(10):2545–2553.
83. Bailey DG, Malcolm J, Arnold O, Spence JD. Grapefruit juice-drug interactions. Eur J Pharm Sci 1998; 46(2):101–110.
84. Lilja JJ, Kivisto KT, Neuvonen PJ. Grapefruit juice increases serum concentrations of atorvastatin and has no effect on pravastatin. Clin Pharmacol Ther 1999; 66(2):118–127.
85. Lilja JJ, Kivisto KT, Neuvonen PJ. Grapefruit juice-simvastatin interaction: effect on serum concentrations of simvastatin, simvastatin acid, and HMG-CoA reductase inhibitors. Clin Pharmacol Ther 1998; 64(5):477–483.
86. Lilja JJ, Kivisto KT, Backman JT, Neuvonen PJ. Effect of grapefruit juice dose on grapefruit juice-triazolam interaction: repeated consumption prolongs triazolam half-life. Eur J Clin Pharmacol 2000; 56(5):411–415.
87. Lilja JJ, Neuvonen M, Neuvonen PJ. Effects of regular consumption of grapefruit juice on the pharmacokinetics of simvastatin. Br J Clin Pharmacol 2004; 58(1):56–60.
88. Damkier P, Hansen LL, Brosen K. Effect of diclofenac, disulfiram, itraconazole, grapefruit juice and erythromycin on the pharmacokinetics of quinidine. Br J Clin Pharmacol 1999; 48(6):829–838.
89. Fuhr U, Klittich K, Staib AH. Inhibitory effect of grapefruit juice and its bitter principal, naringenin, on CYP1A2 dependent metabolism of caffeine in man. Br J Clin Pharmacol 1993; 35(4):431–436.
90. Paine MF, Criss AB, Watkins PB. Two major grapefruit juice components differ in time to onset of intestinal Cyp3a4 inhibition. J Pharmacol Exp Ther 2004; 33(4):518–523.
91. Ambudkar SV, Dey S, Hrycyna CA, Ramachandra M, Pastan I, Gottesman MM. Biochemical, cellular, and pharmacological aspects of the multidrug transporter. Annu Rev Pharmacol Toxicol 1999; 39:361–398.
92. Schinkel AH, Jonker JW. Mammalian drug efflux transporters of the ATP binding cassette (ABC) family: an overview. Adv Drug Deliv Rev 2003; 55(1):3–29.
93. Gottesman MM, Pastan I. Biochemistry of multidrug resistance mediated by the multidrug transporter. Annu Rev Biochem 1993; 62:385–427.
94. Schinkel AH. The roles of P-glycoprotein and MRP1 in the blood-brain and blood-cerebrospinal fluid barriers. Adv Exp Med Biol 2001; 500:365–372.
95. Wacher VJ, Wu CY, Benet LZ. Overlapping substrate specificities and tissue distribution of cytochrome P450 3A and P-glycoprotein: implications for drug delivery and activity in cancer chemotherapy. Mol Carcinog 1995; 13(3):129–134.

96. Soldner A, Christians U, Susanto M, Wacher VJ, Silverman JA, Benet LZ. Grapefruit juice activates P-glycoprotein-mediated drug transport. Pharm Res 1999; 16(4):478–485.

97. Takanaga H, Ohnishi A, Matsuo H, Sawada Y. Inhibition of vinblastine efflux mediated by P-glycoprotein by grapefruit juice components in caco-2 cells. Biol Pharm Bull 1998; 21(10):1062–1066.

98. Edwards DJ, Fitzsimmons ME, Schuetz EG, et al. 6′,7′-Dihydroxybergamottin in grapefruit juice and Seville orange juice: effects on cyclosporine disposition, enterocyte CYP3A4, and P-glycoprotein. Clin Pharmacol Ther 1999; 65(3):237–244.

99. Josefsson M, Zackrisson AL, Ahlner J. Effect of grapefruit juice on the pharmacokinetics of amlodipine in healthy volunteers. Eur J Clin Pharmacol 1996; 51(2):189–193.

100. Zhou S, Lim LY, Chowbay B. Herbal modulation of P-glycoprotein. Drug Metab Rev 2004; 36(1):57–104.

101. Zhang Y, Benet LZ. The gut as a barrier to drug absorption: combined role of cytochrome P450 3A and P-glycoprotein. Clin Pharmacokinet 2001; 40(3): 159–168.

102. Kane GC, Lipsky JJ. Drug-grapefruit juice interactions. 2000; 75(9):933–942.

103. Mikkaichi T, Suzuki T, Tanemoto M, Ito S, Abe T. The organic anion transporter (OATP) family. Drug Metab Pharmacokinet 2004; 19(3):171–179.

104. Kim RB. Organic anion-transporting polypeptide (OATP) transporter family and drug disposition. Eur J Clin Invest 2003; 33(suppl 2):1–5.

105. Kullak-Ublick GA, Stieger B, Meier PJ. Enterohepatic bile salt transporters in normal physiology and liver disease. Gastroenterology 2004; 126(1):322–342.

106. Kobayashi D, Nozawa T, Imai K, Nezu J, Tsuji A, Tamai I. Involvement of human organic anion transporting polypeptide OATP-B (SLC21A9) in pH-dependent transport across intestinal apical membrane. J Pharmacol Exp Ther 2003; 306(2):703–708.

107. Lilja JJ, Juntti-Patinen L, Neuvonen PJ. Orange juice substantially reduces the bioavailability of the beta-adrenergic-blocking agent celiprolol. Clin Pharmacol Ther 2004; 75(3):184–190.

108. Karlsson J, Kuo SM, Ziemniak J, Artursson P. Transport of celiprolol across human intestinal epithelial (Caco-2) cells: mediation of secretion by multiple transporters including P-glycoprotein. Br J Pharmacol 1993; 110(3):1009–1016.

109. Cvetkovic M, Leake B, Fromm MF, Wilkinson GR, Kim RB. OATP and P-glycoprotein transporters mediate the cellular uptake and excretion of fexofenadine. Drug Metab Dispos 1999; 27(8):866–871.

110. Schwarz UI, Seemann D, Oertel R, et al. Grapefruit juice ingestion significantly reduces talinolol bioavailability. Clin Pharmacol Ther 2005; 77(4):291–301.

111. Bjornsson TD, Callaghan JT, Einolf HJ, et al. The conduct of in vitro and in vivo drug-drug interaction studies: a PhRMA perspective. J Clin Pharmacol 2003; 43(5):443–469.

112. Rau SE, Bend JR, Arnold MO, Tran LT, Spence JD, Bailey DG. Grapefruit juice-terfenadine single-dose interaction: magnitude, mechanism, and relevance. Clin Pharmacol Ther 1997; 61(4):401–409.

113. Honig PK, Wortham DC, Lazarev A, Cantilena LR. Grapefruit juice alters the systemic bioavailability and cardiac repolarization of terfenadine in poor metabolizers of terfenadine. J Clin Pharmacol 1996; 36(4):345–351.
114. Clifford CP, Adams DA, Murray S, et al. The cardiac effects of terfenadine after inhibition of its metabolism by grapefruit juice. Eur J Clin Pharmacol 1997; 52(4):311–315.
115. Cheng KL, Nafziger AN, Peloquin CA, Amsden GW. Effect of grapefruit juice on clarithromycin pharmacokinetics. Antimicrob Agents Chemother 1998; 42(4):927–929.
116. Kanazawa S, Ohkubo T, Sugawara K. The effects of grapefruit juice on the pharmacokinetics of erythromycin. Eur J Clin Pharmacol 2001; 56(11): 799–803.
117. Merkel U, Sigusch H, Hoffmann A. Grapefruit juice inhibits 7-hydroxylation of coumarin in healthy volunteers. Eur J Clin Pharmacol 1994; 46(2):175–177.
118. Runkel M, Tegtmeier M, Legrum W. Metabolic and analytical interactions of grapefruit juice and 1,2-benzopyrone (coumarin) in man. Eur J Clin Pharmacol 1996; 50(3):225–230.
119. Runkel M, Bourian M, Tegtmeier M, Legrum W. The character of inhibition of the metabolism of 1,2-benzopyrone (coumarin) by grapefruit juice in human. Eur J Clin Pharmacol 1997; 53(3–4):265–269.
120. Sullivan DM, Ford MA, Boyden TW. Grapefruit juice and the response to warfarin. Am J Health Syst Pharm 1998; 55(15):1581–1583.
121. van Agtmael MA, Gupta V, van der Wosten TH, Rutten JP, van Boxtel CJ. Grapefruit juice increases the bioavailability of artemether. Eur J Clin Pharmacol 1999; 55(5):405–410.
122. van Agtmael MA, Gupta V, van der Graaf CA, van Boxtel CJ. The effect of grapefruit juice on the time-dependent decline of artemether plasma levels in healthy subjects. Clin Pharmacol Ther 1999; 66(4):408–414.
123. Ali BH, Al-Qarawi A, Mousa HM. Effect of grapefruit juice and cimetidine on the concentration of chloroquine in plasma of chicken. Indian J Pharmacol 2001; 33(4):289–290.
124. Ali BH, Al-Qarawi A, Mousa HM. Effect of grapefruit juice on plasma chloroquine kinetics in mice. Clin Exp Pharmacol Physiol 2002; 29(8):704–706.
125. Charbit B, Becquemont L, Lepere B, Peytavin G, Funck-Brentano C. Pharmacokinetic and pharmacodynamic interaction between grapefruit juice and halofantrine. Clin Pharmacol Ther 2002; 72(5):514–523.
126. Min DI, Ku YM, Geraets DR, Lee H. Effect of grapefruit juice on the pharmacokinetics and pharmacodynamics of quinidine in healthy volunteers. J Clin Pharmacol 1996; 36(5):469–476.
127. Ho PC, Chalcroft SC, Coville PF, Wanwimolruk S. Grapefruit juice has no effect on quinine pharmacokinetics. Eur J Clin Pharmacol 1999; 55(5):393–398.
128. Nagy J, Schipper HG, Koopmans RP, Butter JJ, Van Boxtel CJ, Kager PA. Effect of grapefruit juice or cimetidine coadministration on albendazole bioavailability. Am J Trop Med Hyg 2002; 66(3):260–263.
129. Castro N, Jung H, Medina R, Gonzalez-Esquivel D, Lopez M, Sotelo J. Interaction between grapefruit juice and praziquantel in humans. Antimicrob Agents Chemother 2002; 46(5):1614–1616.

130. Yasui N, Kondo T, Furukori H, et al. Effects of repeated ingestion of grape-fruit juice on the single and multiple oral-dose pharmacokinetics and pharma-codynamics of alprazolam. Psychopharmacology (Berl) 2000; 150(2):185–190.

131. Lilja JJ, et al. Grapefruit juice substantially increases plasma concentrations of buspirone. Clin Pharmacol Ther 1998; 64(6):655–660.

132. Ozdemir M, et al. Interaction between grapefruit juice and diazepam in humans. Eur J Drug Metab Pharmacokinet 1998; 23(1):55–59.

133. Vanakoski J, Mattila MJ, Seppala T. Grapefruit juice does not enhance the effects of midazolam and triazolam in man. Eur J Clin Pharmacol 1996; 50(6):501–508.

134. Andersen V, Pedersen N, Larsen NE, Sonne J, Larsen S. Intestinal first pass metabolism of midazolam in liver cirrhosis—effect of grapefruit juice. Br J Clin Pharmacol 2002; 54(2):120–124.

135. Vincent J, Harris SI, Foulds G, Dogolo LC, Willavize S, Friedman HL. Lack of effect of grapefruit juice on the pharmacokinetics and pharmacodynamics of amlodipine. Br J Clin Pharmacol 2000; 50(5):455–463.

136. Sigusch H, Henschel L, Kraul H, Merkel U, Hoffmann A. Lack of effect of grapefruit juice on diltiazem bioavailability in normal subjects. Pharmazie 1994; 49(9):675–679.

137. Bailey DG, Bend JR, Arnold JM, Tran LT, Spence JD. Erythromycin-felodipine interaction: magnitude, mechanism, and comparison with grape-fruit juice. Clin Pharmacol Ther 1996; 60(1):25–33.

138. Bailey DG, Arnold JM, Munoz C, Spence JD. Grapefruit juice—felodipine interaction: mechanism, predictability, and effect of naringin. Clin Pharmacol Ther 1993; 53(6):637–642.

139. Dresser GK, Bailey DG, Carruthers SG. Grapefruit juice—felodipine interac-tion in the elderly. Clin Pharmacol Ther 2000; 68(1):28–34.

140. Lundahl JU, Regardh CG, Edgar B, Johnsson G. The interaction effect of grapefruit juice is maximal after the first glass. Eur J Clin Pharmacol 1998; 54(1):75–81.

141. Edgar B, Bailey D, Bergstrand R, Johnsson G, Regardh CG. Acute effects of drinking grapefruit juice on the pharmacokinetics and dynamics of felodipine—and its potential clinical relevance. Eur J Clin Pharmacol 1992; 42(3):313–317.

142. Bailey DG, Arnold JM, Bend JR, Tran LT, Spence JD. Grapefruit juice-felodipine interaction: reproducibility and characterization with the extended release drug formulation. Br J Clin Pharmacol 1995; 40(2):135–140.

143. Uno T, Ohkubo T, Sugawara K, Higashiyama A, Motomura S, Ishizaki T. Effects of grapefruit juice on the stereoselective disposition of nicardipine in humans: evidence for dominant presystemic elimination at the gut site. Eur J Clin Pharmacol 2000; 56(9–10):643–649.

144. Sigusch H, Hippius M, Henschel L, Kaufmann K, Hoffmann A. Influence of grapefruit juice on the pharmacokinetics of a slow release nifedipine formula-tion. Pharmazie 1994; 49(7):522–524.

145. Fuhr U, Maier-Bruggemann A, Blume H, et al. Grapefruit juice increases oral nimodipine bioavailability. Int J Clin Pharmacol Ther 1998; 36(3):126–132.

146. Takanaga H, Ohnishi A, Murakami H, et al. Relationship between time after intake of grapefruit juice and the effect on pharmacokinetics and

pharmacodynamics of nisoldipine in healthy subjects. Clin Pharmacol Ther 2000; 67(3):201–214.

147. Hashimoto K, Shirafuji T, Sekino H, et al. Interaction of citrus juices with pranidipine, a new 1,4-dihydropyridine calcium antagonist, in healthy subjects. Eur J Clin Pharmacol 1998; 54(9–10):753–760.

148. Fuhr U, Muller-Peltzer H, Kern R, et al. Effects of grapefruit juice and smoking on verapamil concentrations in steady state. Eur J Clin Pharmacol 2002; 58(1):45–53.

149. Ho PC, Ghose K, Saville D, Wanwimolruk S. Effect of grapefruit juice on pharmacokinetics and pharmacodynamics of verapamil enantiomers in healthy volunteers. Eur J Clin Pharmacol 2000; 56(9–10):693–698.

150. Zaidenstein R, Dishi V, Gips M, et al. The effect of grapefruit juice on the pharmacokinetics of orally administered verapamil. Eur J Clin Pharmacol 1998; 54(4):337–340.

151. Demarles D, Gillotin C, Bonaventure-Paci S, Vincent I, Fosse S, Taburet AM. Single-dose pharmacokinetics of amprenavir coadministered with grapefruit juice. Antimicrob Agents Chemother 2002; 46(5):1589–1590.

152. Shelton MJ, Wynn HE, Hewitt RG, DiFrancesco R. Effects of grapefruit juice on pharmacokinetic exposure to indinavir in HIV-positive subjects. J Clin Pharmacol 2001; 41(4):435–442.

153. Hugen PW, Burger DM, Koopmans PP, et al. Saquinavir soft-gel capsules (Fortovase) give lower exposure than expected, even after a high-fat breakfast. Pharm World Sci 2002; 24(3):83–86.

154. Fukazawa I, Uchida N, Uchida E, Yasuhara H. Effects of grapefruit juice on pharmacokinetics of atorvastatin and pravastatin in Japanese. Br J Clin Pharmacol 2004; 57(4):448–455.

155. Kantola T, Kivisto KT, Neuvonen PJ. Grapefruit juice greatly increases serum concentrations of lovastatin and lovastatin acid. Clin Pharmacol Ther 1998; 63(4):397–402.

156. Rogers JD, Zhao J, Liu L, et al. Grapefruit juice has minimal effects on plasma concentrations of lovastatin-derived 3-hydroxy-3-methylglutaryl coenzyme A reductase inhibitors. Clin Pharmacol Ther 1999; 66(4):358–366.

157. Lilja JJ, Kivisto KT, Neuvonen PJ. Duration of effect of grapefruit juice on the pharmacokinetics of the CYP3A4 substrate simvastatin. Clin Pharmacol Ther 2000; 68(4):384–390.

158. Schubert W, Cullberg G, Edgar B, Hedner T. Inhibition of 17 beta-estradiol metabolism by grapefruit juice in ovariectomized women. Maturitas 1994; 20(2–3):155–163.

159. Weber A, Jager R, Borner A, et al. Can grapefruit juice influence ethinylestradiol bioavailability? Contraception 1996; 53(1):41–47.

160. Hollander AA, van Rooij J, Lentjes GW, et al. The effect of grapefruit juice on cyclosporine and prednisone metabolism in transplant patients. Clin Pharmacol Ther 1995; 57(3):318–324.

161. Varis T, Kivisto KT, Neuvonen PJ. Grapefruit juice can increase the plasma concentrations of oral methylprednisolone. Eur J Clin Pharmacol 2000; 56(6–7):489–493.

162. Ioannides-Demos LL, Christophidis N, Ryan P, Angelis P, Liolios L, McLean AJ. Dosing implications of a clinical interaction between grapefruit juice and cyclosporine and metabolite concentrations in patients with autoimmune diseases. J Rheumatol 1997; 24(1):49–54.

163. Yee GC, Stanley DL, Pessa LJ, et al. Effect of grapefruit juice on blood cyclosporin concentration. Lancet 1995; 345(8955):955–956.

164. Brunner LJ, Pai KS, Munar MY, Lande MB, Olyaei AJ, Mowry JA. Effect of grapefruit juice on cyclosporin A pharmacokinetics in pediatric renal transplant patients. Pediatr Transplant 2000; 4(4):313–321.

165. Min DI, Ku YM, Perry PJ, et al. Effect of grapefruit juice on cyclosporine pharmacokinetics in renal transplant patients. Transplantation 1996; 62(1): 123–125.

166. Ku YM, Min DI, Flanigan M. Effect of grapefruit juice on the pharmacokinetics of microemulsion cyclosporine and its metabolite in healthy volunteers: does the formulation difference matter? J Clin Pharmacol 1998; 38(10):959–965.

167. Hermann M, Asberg A, Reubsaet JL, Sather S, Berg KJ, Christensen H. Intake of grapefruit juice alters the metabolic pattern of cyclosporin A in renal transplant recipients. Int J Clin Pharmacol Ther 2002; 40(10):451–456.

168. Brunner LJ, Munar MY, Vallian J, et al. Interaction between cyclosporine and grapefruit juice requires long-term ingestion in stable renal transplant recipients. Pharmacotherapy 1998; 18(1):23–29.

169. Lee M, Min DI, Ku YM, Flanigan M. Effect of grapefruit juice on pharmacokinetics of microemulsion cyclosporine in African American subjects compared with Caucasian subjects: does ethnic difference matter? J Clin Pharmacol 2001; 41(3):317–323.

170. Bistrup C, Nielsen FT, Jeppesen UE, Dieperink H. Effect of grapefruit juice on Sandimmun Neoral absorption among stable renal allograft recipients. Nephrol Dial Transplant 2001; 16(2):373–377.

171. Reif S, Nicolson MC, Bisset D, et al. Effect of grapefruit juice intake on etoposide bioavailability. Eur J Clin Pharmacol 2002; 58(7):491–494.

172. Ohnishi A, Matsuo H, Yamada S, et al. Effect of furanocoumarin derivatives in grapefruit juice on the uptake of vinblastine by Caco-2 cells and on the activity of cytochrome P450 3A4. Br J Pharmacol 2000; 130(6):1369–1377.

173. Maish WA, Hampton EM, Whitsett TL, Shepard JD, Lovallo WR. Influence of grapefruit juice on caffeine pharmacokinetics and pharmacodynamics. Pharmacotherapy 1996; 16(6):1046–1052.

174. Spahn-Langguth H, Langguth P. Grapefruit juice enhances intestinal absorption of the P-glycoprotein substrate talinolol. Eur J Pharm Sci 2001; 12(4):361–367.

175. Garg SK, Kumar N, Bhargava VK, Prabhakar SK. Effect of grapefruit juice on carbamazepine bioavailability in patients with epilepsy. Clin Pharmacol Ther 1998; 64(3):286–288.

176. Gross AS, Goh YD, Addison RS, Shenfield GM. Influence of grapefruit juice on cisapride pharmacokinetics. Clin Pharmacol Ther 1999; 65(4):395–401.

177. Offman EM, Freeman DJ, Dresser GK, Munoz C, Bend JR, Bailey DG. Red wine-cisapride interaction: comparison with grapefruit juice. Clin Pharmacol Ther 2001; 70(1):17–23.

178. Kivisto KT, Lilja JJ, Backman JT, Neuvonen PJ. Repeated consumption of grapefruit juice considerably increases plasma concentrations of cisapride. Clin Pharmacol Ther 1999; 66(5):448–453.
179. Desta Z, Kivisto KT, Lilja JJ, et al. Stereoselective pharmacokinetics of cisapride in healthy volunteers and the effect of repeated administration of grapefruit juice. Br J Clin Pharmacol 2001; 52(4):399–407.
180. Vandel S, Netillard C, Perault MC, Bel AM. Plasma levels of clozapine and desmethylclozapine are unaffected by concomitant ingestion of grapefruit juice. Eur J Clin Pharmacol 2000; 56(4):347–348.
181. Lane HY, Jann MW, Chang YC, et al. Repeated ingestion of grapefruit juice does not alter clozapine's steady-state plasma levels, effectiveness, and tolerability. J Clin Psychiatry 2001; 62(10):812–817.
182. Mahgoub AA. Grapefruit juice potentiates the anti-inflammatory effects of diclofenac on the carrageenan-induced rat's paw oedema. Pharmacol Res 2002; 45(1):1–4.
183. Becquemont L, Verstuyft C, Kerb R, et al. Effect of grapefruit juice on digoxin pharmacokinetics in humans. Clin Pharmacol Ther 2001; 70(4):311–316.
184. Hori H, Yoshimura R, Ueda N, et al. Grapefruit juice-fluvoxamine interaction—is it risky or not? J Clin Psychopharmacol 2003; 23(4):422–424.
185. Kawakami M, Suzuki K, Ishizuka T, Hidaka T, Matsuki Y, Nakamura H. Effect of grapefruit juice on pharmacokinetics of itraconazole in healthy subjects. Int J Clin Pharmacol Ther 1998; 36(6):306–308.
186. Penzak SR, Gubbins PO, Gurley BJ, Wang PL, Saccente M. Grapefruit juice decreases the systemic availability of itraconazole capsules in healthy volunteers. Ther Drug Monit 1999; 21(3):304–309.
187. Gubbins PO, McConnell SA, Gurley BJ, et al. Influence of grapefruit juice on the systemic availability of itraconazole oral solution in healthy adult volunteers. Pharmacotherapy 2004; 24(4):460–467.
188. Zaidenstein R, Soback S, Gips M, et al. Effect of grapefruit juice on the pharmacokinetics of losartan and its active metabolite E3174 in healthy volunteers. Ther Drug Monit 2001; 23(4):369–373.
189. Benmebarek M, Devaud C, Gex-Fabry M, et al. Effects of grapefruit juice on the pharmacokinetics of the enantiomers of methadone. Clin Pharmacol Ther 2004; 76(1):55–63.
190. Tassaneeyakul W, Vannaprasaht S, Yamazoe Y. Formation of omeprazole sulphone but not 5-hydroxyomeprazole is inhibited by grapefruit juice. Br J Clin Pharmacol 2000; 49(2):139–144.
191. Ebert U, Oertel R, Kirch W. Influence of grapefruit juice on scopolamine pharmacokinetics and pharmacodynamics in healthy male and female subjects. Int J Clin Pharmacol Ther 2000; 38(11):523–531.
192. Lee AJ, Chan WK, Harralson AF, Buffum J, Bui BC. The effects of grapefruit juice on sertraline metabolism: an in vitro and in vivo study. Clin Ther 1999; 21(11):1890–1899.
193. Lee M, Min DI. Determination of sildenafil citrate in plasma by high-performance liquid chromatography and a case for the potential interaction of grapefruit juice with sildenafil citrate. Ther Drug Monit 2001; 23(1):21–26.

194. Jetter A, Kinzig-Schippers M, Walchner-Bonjean M, et al. Effects of grape-fruit juice on the pharmacokinetics of sildenafil. Clin Pharmacol Ther 2002; 71(1):21–29.

195. Fuhr U, Maier A, Keller A, Steinijans VW, Sauter R, Staib AH. Lacking effect of grapefruit juice on theophylline pharmacokinetics. Int J Clin Pharma-col Ther 1995; 33(6):311–314.

196. Yasui N, Kondo T, Suzuki A, et al. Lack of significant pharmacokinetic inter-action between haloperidol and grapefruit juice. Int Clin Psychopharmacol 1999; 14(2):113–118.

197. Lilja JJ, Kivisto KT, Backman JT, Lamberg TS, Neuvonen PJ. Grapefruit juice substantially increases plasma concentrations of buspirone. Clin Pharma-col Ther 1998; 64(6):655–660.

198. Richardson MA. Biopharmacologic and herbal therapies for cancer: research update from NCCAM. J Nutr 2001; 131(11 suppl):3037S–3040S.

199. Barnes PP-GE, McFann K, Nahin R. Complementary and Alternative Med-icine Use Among Adults: United States, 2002. National Center for Comple-mentary and Alternative Medicine, National Institutes of Health, 2004.

8

Quality Assurance and Standardization in Botanical Product–Drug Interaction: Evaluation and Documentation

Lucas R. Chadwick and Harry H. S. Fong

Program for Collaborative Research in the Pharmaceutical Sciences, WHO Collaborating Center for Traditional Medicine and UIC/NIH Center for Botanical Dietary Supplements Research, College of Pharmacy, University of Illinois, Chicago, Illinois, U.S.A.

INTRODUCTION

The popularity of botanical products in the United States is reflected in a survey on complementary and alternative medicine that showed that American consumers had spent an estimated $5.1 billion on botanical products in 1997 (1). In the same year, the global market for botanical medicinal products was estimated to be approximately $20 billion (2,3). It has been estimated that currently more than 1500 botanical products are available in the U.S. market alone (4). This popularity has been fueled, in part, by the perception that botanicals are naturally derived products, and hence are safe and devoid of adverse effects. This perception appeared to be justified by a paper summarizing the fatality of pharmaceutical drugs and botanical products in the 1981–1993 period, in which statistics compiled by the National Center for Health Statistics, the American Association of Poison Control Centers, Centers for Disease Control and Prevention, the *Journal of the American Medical Association*, and the U.S. Consumer Product Safety Commission showed an annual mortality rate of 100,000 deaths for pharmaceuticals and none for botanical products (5). However, because the information covered was only to the end of 1993, this report did not take into consideration the subsequent fatalities attributed to *Ephedra* and ephedrine products. With the increase in the number of incidents of adverse reactions being reported, a database on adverse reactions of botanical products has been created as part of the World Health Organization (WHO) International Drug Monitoring System (6).

In recent years, it has become increasingly apparent that even therapeutically safe botanical products can manifest toxic effects as a result of botanical product–drug interaction, when administered concomitantly with synthetic pharmaceutical agents. The best-documented examples have been cases involving grapefruit juice and St. John's wort with a variety of drugs. Grapefruit (*Citrus × paradisi* Macfad.) juice has been documented to interact with calcium channel blockers as well as to increase the level of cyclosporin in the blood of transplant patients (7,8). St. John's wort (*Hypericum perforatum* L.), a botanical used in the management of mild to moderate depression, has been found to increase the effects of monoamine oxidase inhibitors or serotonin reuptake inhibitors; reduce the blood levels, and hence the pharmacological effects of anticonvulsants (carbamazepine and phenobarbitone), anticoagulants (warfarin and phenprocoumon), oral contraceptives, theophylline, digoxin, cyclosporin, HIV reverse transcriptase inhibitors (nevirapine and efavirenz), and protease inhibitors (indinavir); increase photosensitivity with other such drugs; prolong narcotic-induced sleeping time; and decrease the level of cyclosporin in organ transplant patients (9–18). The adverse effects recorded for these and some other botanical products are due to true pharmacological interactions. There are, however, botanical product–drug interactions reported for botanical products that may not be true pharmacological/physiological events, and that can be avoided if in-process quality control (QC) is in place during the manufacturing process. Botanical products adulterated with synthetic drugs such as phenylbutazone, indomethacin, corticoid steroids, caffeine, acetaminophen, indomethacin, hydrochlorothiazide, ethoxybenzamide, theophylline, diazepam, chlorpheniramine maleate, ibuprofen, phenobarbital, mefenamic acid, prioxicam, salicylamide, diethylstilbestrol, and warfarin (19–21) have led to botanical product–drug interactions. Multicomponent Chinese or Ayurvedic botanical remedies, known to contain heavy metals such as lead and mercury as active ingredients (19,22,23), can likewise lead to adverse events and/or botanical product–drug interactions.

On the other hand, a number of adverse event reports recorded in the literature are themselves erroneous in nature due to the quality of the assessment and reporting, with Siegel's report of the so-called "ginseng-abuse-syndrome" (GAS) being a prime example (24). In this report, the author simply recorded adverse reactions in patients who had ingested "ginseng" without reference to which of a number of plants having the same common name (25) were actually ingested. Further, the author did not take into account the concomitant pharmaceutical drugs and drugs of abuse used by the patients being reported to have adverse drug reactions to "ginseng."

In monitoring botanical product–drug interactions, the quality of the data obtained may be influenced by a number of factors. Among the important issues to be addressed include raw material source and sourcing practices; intrinsic and extrinsic factors affecting the occurrence and concentration of active or marker chemical constituents in both the starting and finished products; the meaning of the word "standardization"; the methods of chemical and biological analyses employed; the manufacturing practices employed; substitution; adulteration of botanical products with pharmaceutical drugs or contamination with foreign toxic substances; formulation of the dosage form; regulatory requirements; and clinical experimental design and data interpretation. In this chapter, the influence of these quality assurance (QA)/QC and standardization issues on botanical product safety will be examined.

MATERIAL QUALITY AND QUALITY CONTROL ISSUES

The quality of presently available botanical products varies from very high to very low. Our study on selected commercial ginseng products prepared from *Panax ginseng* C.A. Meyer, *P. quinquefolius* L., and *Eleutherococcus senticosus* Max. (Araliaceae)[a] and marketed as botanical supplements in North America in the 1995–1998 period showed that 74% of these products met label claims, with the ginsenoside contents of the *P. ginseng* and *P. quinquefolius* products analyzed ranging from 0.00% to 13.54% and 0.009% to 8.00%, respectively (26). The eleutherosides B and E content of *E. senticosus* root powder and other formulated products also showed similarly large variations (26). Studies on the quality of St. John's wort products showed that hypericin content ranged from 22% to 165% and that silymarin content in milk thistle [*Silybum marianum* (L.) Gaertn.] products ranged from 58% to 116% of the labeled claims (27). These content variations not only will influence the efficacy, but also could affect the safety of botanical products, because chemically induced drug interactions may be active compound–concentration dependent. Why are there such wide variations in the content of active/marker compounds in these products? Are such variations intrinsic to botanical products or are they due to external factors, or both?

---

[a] In botanical nomenclature, the name of a plant consists of its genus name (first letter in upper case) and specific name (all lower case letters), both italicized; the author citation (abbreviation of the name of the botanist who first described the plant); and within parentheses, the name of the family to which it belongs.

INTRINSIC AND EXTRINSIC FACTORS

It is well established that intrinsic and extrinsic factors including plant species differences, organ specificity, diurnal and seasonal variation, environment, field collection and cultivation methods, contamination, substitution, adulteration, processing, and manufacturing practices greatly affect botanical quality (28–32). Intrinsically, plants are dynamic living organisms, each of which is capable of being genetically influenced to be slightly different in its physical and chemical characters. For example, a study on the accumulation of hypericin in *H. perforatum* showed that narrow-leafed populations have greater concentrations than the broader-leafed variety (33,34); variations of phytochemicals are greater in wild than in domesticated populations of the same species, as exemplified by the results of studies on the content of artemisinin, an antimalarial agent, in *Artemisia annua* L. (32); on michellamine B, a compound with in vitro anti-HIV activity, in *Ancistrocladus korupensis* D.W. Thomas & R.E. Gereau (32); and on the essential oil composition of *Ocimum basilicum* L. (32). Also, the secondary chemical constituents of medicinal plants differ qualitatively as well as quantitatively from species to species as demonstrated by the presence of structurally different alkylamides in the roots of *Echinacea angustifolia* D.C. and *E. purpurea* (L.) Moench, and by their total absence in *E. pallida* (Nutt.) Nutt. (35,36). Organ specificity is yet another intrinsic factor influencing chemical variation because the site of biosynthesis and the site of accumulation and storage are normally different. Chemical biosynthesis usually takes place in the leaves, and then the product synthesized is transported through the stems to the roots for storage, with the chemical profiles in these organs being different from each other. Accumulation and storage can also take place in the leaves, but to a much lower extent, and very infrequently in the stems. An example of site-specific accumulation, as well as species specificity, is that of the compounds considered responsible for the immunostimulant effect of *Echinacea* species. These compounds encompass five groups of chemicals: caffeic acid derivatives, alkylamides, polyacetylenes (ketodialkenes and ketodialkynes), glycoproteins, and polysaccharides. As indicated above, alkylamides are found in the roots of *E. angustifolia* and *E. purpurea*, but they are structurally different, and are totally absent in *E. pallida* roots. Polyacetylenes, on the other hand, are present abundantly in the roots of *E. pallida*, but are absent in *E. angustifolia* and *E. purpurea* roots. Whereas the glycoproteins and polysaccharides are present in the aerial parts of all three species, they occur only in minute quantities in the roots (35,36).

Diurnal variation and seasonal variation are other intrinsic factors affecting chemical accumulation in both wild and cultivated plants. Depending on the plant, the accumulation of chemical constituents can occur at any time during the various stages of growth. In a majority of cases, maximum chemical accumulation occurs at the time of flowering, followed by a decline beginning at the fruiting stage. The time of harvest or field collection can thus influence the quality, efficacy, and safety of the final botanical product (37,38).

With respect to extrinsic factors, there are many that can affect the quality of medicinal plants. It has been well established that environmental factors such as soil, light, water, temperature, and nutrients can affect phytochemical accumulation in plants. For example, alkaloid concentrations in *Atropa belladonna* L. have been found to vary from 0.3% to 1.3%, when grown in different areas of the world (30). Also, the silymarin content in milk thistle was found to be highest in the fruits of plants grown under 60% water/field capacity (1.39%) and nitrogen level of 100 (1.46%) per acre (39). The methods employed in field collection from the wild, as well as in commercial cultivation, harvest, postharvest processing, shipping, and storage can also influence the physical appearance and chemical quality of the botanical source materials. Contaminations by microbial and chemical agents (pesticides, herbicides and heavy metals) as well as by insects, animals, animal parts, and animal excreta during any of the stages of source plant material production and collection can lead to lower quality and/or unsafe source materials (28,30,32). Heavy-metal contamination can occur at the cultivation, postharvest treatment, or product-manufacturing stages. Lead and thallium contaminations have been reported in multicomponent botanical mixtures, and cases of lead, thallium, mercury, arsenic, gold, and cadmium poisoning from the consumption of such products have been documented (19,40).

Botanical source materials collected in the wild often include nontargeted species either by accidental substitution or by intentional adulteration. However, substitution and adulteration of cultivated botanicals can also occur. Substitution of *Periploca sepium* Bunge for *E. senticosus* (eleuthero) has been widely documented and is regarded as being responsible for the "hairy baby" case involving maternal/neonatal androgenization (41). Adverse reactions due to plantain (*Plantago ovata* Forskal) being contaminated by *Digitalis lanata* Ehr. during harvest is another example of accidental adulteration by human error (42).

Adulteration of botanical products with synthetic drugs represents another problem in product quality and botanical product–drug interactions. Foremost among the documented cases are multicomponent Chinese or Ayurvedic botanical remedies. Chemical analyses of some arthritis remedies have led to the finding that synthetic anti-inflammatory drugs such as phenylbutazone, indomethacin, and/or corticoid steroids have been added (19). In a classic study of chemical adulteration of traditional medicine in Taiwan, 23.7% (618 of 2609) of botanical remedy samples collected by eight major hospitals were found to contain one or more synthetic therapeutic agents, including caffeine, acetaminophen, indomethacin, hydrochlorothiazide, prednisolone, ethoxybenzamide, phenylbutazone, betamethasone, theophylline, dexamethasone, diazepam, bucetin, chlorpheniramine maleate, prednisone, oxyphenbutazone, diclofenac sodium, ibuprofen, cortisone, ketoprofen, phenobarbital, hydrocortisone acetate, niflumic acid, triamcinolone, diethylpropion, mefenamic acid, prioxicam, and salicylamide (20). The most frequent adulterants were caffeine, acetaminophen, indomethacin, hydrochlorothiazide, prednisone, and chloroxazone. Obviously, such adulterated botanical products are prime candidates for botanical product–drug interactions.

Besides the unintentional in-process adulteration of heavy metals, it is well established that Ayurvedic medicine and traditional Chinese medicine sometimes employ complex mixtures of plant, animal, and mineral substances, and it is not uncommon to find appreciable quantities of heavy metals such as lead, mercury, cadmium, arsenic, and gold in certain formulations (19,22,23).

With respect to the words/claims, "active compound," "marker compounds," "standardization," and "standardized products," the clinician should be vigilant about their meaning when monitoring botanical safety. In the case of prescription and over-the-counter (OTC) drugs, each product has a single, defined "active" chemical constituent, which is used to measure or standardize product quality and determine shelf life. The active principle(s) of botanical products/dietary supplements, on the other hand, are largely unknown. For example, there is no evidence that the marker compounds eleutherosides B and E are the active principles in eleuthero (*E. senticosus*). Presently, there is also considerable disagreement as to whether hypericin or hyperforin is the active antidepressant principle in St. John's wort, with the latter being the current leading candidate. Further, even when the active principles of a medicinal plant have been identified, the compound may not be commercially available for use as a reference standard. Hence, major constituent(s) of the source plant, whether biologically active or not, are currently employed as marker compounds for the standardization of most of the botanical products marketed (43), so that one manufacturer may not use the same reference standard as another (44). Compounding the issue of standardizing is the meaning of a "standardized extract," which may refer to (i) an extract made to a consistent standard such as a ratio of the starting plant material to that of the dried extract, (ii) an extract manufactured to contain a specific concentration of a marker compound(s), or (iii) any one of a number of botanical, agricultural, and/or manufacturing process control measures in the production of a material of reasonable consistency (45). With these inconsistencies in the meaning of standardization and standardized products, variations in efficacy and adverse events/drug interactions can, and will, occur.

REGULATORY INFLUENCE

Botanical product quality and safety can also be influenced by regulatory status, which varies from country to country (46). In some countries, botanical products are regulated as medicine and are subject to mandated standards of quality, whereas in the United States a majority of botanicals are marketed as dietary supplements. Good manufacturing practices (GMPs) are required in the production of prescription and OTC drugs, but the regulatory provisions under the Dietary Supplement Health and Education Act (DSHEA) of 1994 provide little assurance of identity, quality, or purity for botanical dietary supplements (43). Thus, botanical dietary supplement products have not been subjected to mandated QA/QC standards as in the case of prescription and OTC drugs. Although the Food and Drug Administration advanced a notice of proposed rulemaking on current good manufacturing practice in the labeling and manufacturing standards on dietary supplements in March 2003 (47), such standards have not yet been implemented. Elsewhere in the world, e.g., in the European Union and in most of Asia and Southeast Asia, national policies exist, but in some countries, these products are totally unregulated. Consequently, product quality, efficacy, and safety differ internationally, nationally, and from product brand to product brand, and even from lot to lot within the same brand.

QUALITY ASSURANCE AND QUALITY CONTROL

For effective monitoring of botanical product–drug interaction in clinical studies or application, the clinician must be aware that standards of quality for botanical products do not exist in many countries, including the United States. Therefore, the products being evaluated must be accurately defined as to the quality of botanicals employed, and information on the QC measures employed to ensure their quality must be taken into consideration. If such QC/QA information, including standardization and what is meant by the term, is lacking, it is not possible to attribute the drug interactions observed to the botanical product in the clinical study/use, and the data being published will be invalid and/or misleading.

Information on QC of the botanical product under investigation or in clinical use must be derived from measures taken, from the procurement of source material to the production of the final formulation. Whether by field collection from the wild or by cultivation, good agricultural and/or collection practices must be adhered to during the procurement process (48), because the quality of the finished botanical products is obviously directly related to the quality and safety of the raw materials. Hence, whether field-collected or produced by cultivation, the identification and authentication of plant species by a taxonomic botanist is critical to ensuring that the correct source material is acquired. It is essential that the plant materials are identified by their scientific names (Latin binomial), and a description of the macroscopic, microscopic, and organoleptic (sensory) characters be provided along with herbarium specimens, drawings, or photographs (31,49–52). In the field collection of medicinal plants, care must be exercised to avoid the acquisition of nontargeted species and to free the targeted source material of undesirable plant parts, soil, rock, insects, animals, animal excreta, and other contaminants. Postcollection treatments should mirror those accorded cultivated plant materials. Due to their genetic and chemical content variations, the site and date should be recorded for each collection. The production of raw materials by cultivation should normally lead to more uniform botanical products due to greater genetic uniformity. The production of quality raw materials can only be assured by employing good agricultural practices such as those described in the recently published WHO Guidelines on Good Agriculture and Collection Practices (48). The harvested source materials must be processed to produce the finished products under GMPs (53). GMP procedures employed for the manufacture of botanical products involving, at the raw material production end, botanical taxonomic identification to assure species identification must be implemented. Otherwise the efficacy, safety, and botanical product–drug interaction reported for one medicinal plant may in fact be those caused by another botanical product. It should be noted that although common names are most frequently used by the source material producers/collectors, a common name may apply to more than one plant. For example, "ginseng" may refer to American ginseng [*P. quinquefolius* L. (Araliaceae)], Asian/ Korean ginseng [*P. ginseng* C.A. Meyer (Araliaceae)], Russian/Siberian ginseng [*E. senticosus* (Rupr. & Maxim.) Maxim. (Araliaceae)], Blue ginseng [*Caulophyllum thalictroides* L. Michx. (Berberidaceae)], Brazilian ginseng [*Pfaffia paniculata* Kuntz (Amaranthaceae)], Indian ginseng [*Withania somnifera* L. Dunal (Solanaceae)], or Wild Red American ginseng [*Rumex hymenosepalus* (Polygonaceae)] (25). Thus, the identification of the source material from which the botanical product is being monitored must be by its Latin binomial.

At the processing and manufacturing stage, macroscopic, microscopic, and organoleptic analyses and analytical procedures similar to those employed for the manufacture of conventional drugs to assure quality and purity by appropriate protocols (31,51,52,54) must be used. Otherwise, the quality of the finished product under clinical investigation/use may be compromised, and this can lead to adverse events and/or botanical product–drug interactions. Microscopic and organoleptic examinations will help assure botanical identity and purity because each plant species possesses characteristic microscopic cellular features, and may have distinct sensory properties. Macroscopic examination will reveal the presence of deterioration and signs of contamination by molds, insects, rodents, and other animals, as well as by other plants.

As with pharmaceutical drugs, botanical products should be thoroughly evaluated biologically, employing not only in vitro methods, but also the more relevant in vivo animal studies, particularly with respect to acute and chronic toxicity.

Procedures for the QC analysis of active and/or marker chemical compounds in botanical products during the manufacturing and post-marketing surveillance processes can be accomplished by colorimetric, spectroscopic, and/or chromatographic methods. Colorimetric and direct spectroscopic methods are older analytical procedures that quantify the absorption of structurally related compounds at a specific wavelength of light, expressed as a concentration of a reference standard (marker), which is normally the active or major chemical constituent in that plant material. Because other plant constituents possessing the same absorbance are included in the measurement, a higher concentration is usually ascribed to the test material. The use of these procedures has recently been on the decline. Modern methods for the chemical analysis of secondary chemical constituent markers in botanical products involve some form of chromatography. Thin-layer chromatographic procedures have the advantages of being simple and rapid, and they can provide useful characteristic profile patterns and are inexpensive to use. However, their resolving power is limited and quantitative data for minor constituents is difficult to obtain. Gas chromatography can provide a high resolution of the more volatile complex mixtures, but is of limited value in the case of nonvolatile polar compounds, especially the polar polyhydroxylated and glycosidic compounds. High-performance liquid chromatography (HPLC) is capable of resolving complex mixtures of polar and nonpolar compounds, and has become the chromatographic method of choice for the qualitative and quantitative analysis of botanical extracts and products. HPLC can be coupled with a range of analytical techniques including ultraviolet (UV) spectroscopy, mass spectrometry, nuclear magnetic resonance (NMR), and evaporative light-scattering detection (ELSD). Combined with HPLC, any of these techniques is capable of producing a "fingerprint" of the botanical product. However, some of these detection methods may be inappropriate for the quantitative determination of a specific active or marker compound. The literature is replete with HPLC methods for the analysis of specific compounds in more than 95% of the botanical extracts or products in the market. Detection by UV is readily available in most labs, and is carried out either with a single- or dual-wavelength, or a full spectrum (e.g., photo-diode array) detector, and is the most appropriate technique for the routine analysis of compounds that contain a UV-active chromophore. Combined HPLC–mass spectrometry (LC–MS) and liquid chromatography–tandem mass spectrometry (LC–MS^n) is being used increasingly. The advantage of these methods is that as each compound is being eluted, it is captured by the mass spectrometer and provides a molecular ion and/or major mass fragment, which can provide a specific identification of the eluting "peak." However, ionization techniques compatible with HPLC, such as electrospray ionization, show a broad range of sensitivity to various compound classes. This technique is excellent for compounds such as alkaloids, phenols, and organic acids, but can be highly insensitive to others such as aliphatic hydrocarbons, sterols, and polysaccharides. All compounds containing protons, including virtually all medicinally significant phytochemicals, can be detected by NMR. This technique generally provides more structural information than any other single technique. However, LC–NMR is available in only a few labs worldwide, requires the use of deuterated solvents for chromatography, and will remain inaccessible and prohibitively expensive for routine use for some time. A vast majority of all plant secondary metabolites are detectable by ELSD, but this method provides no structural information.

There can exist no standardization regime that would be universally applicable to all medicinal botanical products. Ideally, the formulated product should be chemically assayed for an active constituent, using an analytical method appropriate for the given compound class, and also biologically assayed for in vitro and/or in vivo activity, using assay(s) relevant to the intended use of the product.

CLINICAL EXPERIMENTAL DESIGN AND DATA INTERPRETATION

For effective botanical product–drug interaction monitoring, there is a most critical need for a well-designed clinical experiment that not only takes into account the aforementioned QC issues, but also includes a safety monitoring component that will enable the clinician to delineate between adverse reactions caused by botanical product–drug interactions and those by drug–drug interactions due to concomitant ingestions of multiple pharmaceutical drugs by the patient, or adverse events owing to idiosyncratic causes. A system designed for careful and rational interpretation of study data should be devised so as to avoid erroneous conclusions such as those reported on the so-called GAS (24).

CONCLUSION

In monitoring botanical product–drug interactions, the quality of the data obtained may be influenced by a number of factors. Among the contributing factors are: raw material source and sourcing practices; intrinsic and extrinsic factors affecting the occurrence and concentration of active or marker chemical constituents in both the starting and the finished products; standardization and standardized products; the methods of chemical and biological analyses; manufacturing practices; substitution; adulteration of botanical products with pharmaceutical drugs or contamination with foreign toxic substances; regulatory requirements; and the quality of the clinical experimental design and data interpretation.

REFERENCES

1. Eisenberg DM, Davis RB, Ettner SL, et al. Trends in alternative medicine use in the United States, 1990–1997: results of a follow-up national survey. JAMA 1998; 280:1569–1575.
2. Dev S. Ethnotherapeutics and modern drug development: the potential of Ayurveda. Curr Sci 1997; 73:909–928.
3. Dev S. Ancient-modern concordance in Ayurvedic plants: some examples. Environ Health Perspect 1999; 107:783–789.
4. Anon. Medicinal herbs: NTP extracts the facts. Environmental Health Perspectives (NIEHS News) 1999; 107:A604–605 (accessed online at http://ehp.niehs.nih.gov/docs/1999/107–12/niehsnews.html via http://ehp.niehs.nih.gov/docs/montharch.html, 24 March, 2004).
5. Murray F. Vitamins-1. Drugs-100,000. Let's Live. 1996; September:12.
6. Fucik H, Backlund A, Farah M. Building a computerized herbal substance register for implementation and use in the World Health Organization International Drug Monitoring Programme. Drug Information J 2002; 36:839–854.
7. Ho PC, Ghose K, Saville D, Wanwimolruk S. Effect of grapefruit juice on pharmacokinetics and pharmacodynamics of verapamil enantiomers in healthy volunteers. Eur J Clin Pharmacol 2000; 56:693–698.
8. Takanaga H, Ohnishi A, Matsuo H, et al. Pharmacokinetic analysis of felodipine-grapefruit juice interaction based on an irreversible enzyme inhibition model. Br J Clin Pharmacol 2000; 49:49–58.
9. Barone GW, Gurley BJ, Kotel BL, Abul-Ezz SR. Herbal supplements: a potential for drug interactions in transplant recipients. Transplantation 2001; 71: 239–241.
10. Broughton A, Denahm A. Hypericum and drug interactions. Eur J Herbal Med 2001; 5:19–25.
11. de Maat MM, Hoetelmans RM, Math RA, et al. Drug interaction between St. John's wort and nevirapine. AIDS 2001; 15:420–421.
12. Ernst E. Second thoughts about safety of St. John's wort. Lancet 1999; 354: 2014–2016.
13. Izzo AA, Ernst E. Interactions between herbal medicines and prescribed drugs: a systematic review. Drugs 2001; 61:2163–2175.
14. Johne A, Brockmoller J, Bauer S, Maurer A, Langheinrich M, Roots I. Pharmacokinetic interaction of digoxin with an herbal extract from St. John's wort (*Hypericum perforatum*). Clin Pharmacol Ther 1999; 66:338–345.
15. Karliova M, Treichel U, Malago M, Frilling A, Gerken G, Broelsch CE. Interaction of Hypericum perforatum (St. John's wort) with cyclosporin A metabolism in a patient after liver transplantation. J Hepatol 2000; 33:853–855.
16. Pennachio DL. Drug-herb interactions: How vigilant should you be? Patient Care 2000; 19:41–68.
17. Piscitelli SC, Burstein AH, Chaitt D, Alfaro RM, Falloon J. Indinavir concentrations and St. John's wort. Lancet 2000; 355:547–548.
18. Ruschitzka F, Meier PJ, Turina M, Luscher TF, Noll G. Acute heart transplant rejection due to St. John's wort. Lancet 2000; 355:548–549.
19. Farnsworth NR. Relative safety of herbal medicines. HerbalGram 1993; 29: 36A–36H.

20. Huang WF, Wen KC, Hsiao ML. Adulteration by synthetic therapeutic substances of traditional Chinese medicines in Taiwan. J Clin Pharmacol 1997; 37:344–350.

21. Blumenthal M. The rise and fall of PC-SPES: new generation of herbal supplement, adulterated product, or new drug? Integrative Cancer Therapies 2002; 1:266–270.

22. Bhattacharyya PC. Herbal drugs. Curr Sci 1996; 71:341–349.

23. Ernst E, Thompson Coon J. Heavy metals in traditional Chinese medicines: a systematic review. Clin Pharmacol Therapeut 2001; 70:497–504.

24. Siegel RK. Ginseng abuse syndrome. Problems with the panacea. JAMA 1979; 241:1614–1615.

25. Awang DVC. Siberian ginseng toxicity may be case of mistaken identity. CMAJ 1996; 155:1237.

26. Fitzloff J, Yat P, Lu ZZ, et al. Perspectives on the quality assurance of ginseng products in North America. In: Huh H, Choi KJ, Kim YC, eds. Advances in Ginseng Research. 7th International Symposium on Ginseng. Seoul, Korea: The Korean Society of Ginseng, 1998:138–145.

27. Schulz V, Hubner WD, Ploch M. Clinical trials with phytopharmacological agents. Phytomedicine 1997; 4:379–387.

28. Busse W. The processing of botanicals. In: Eskinazi D, Blumenthal M, Farnsworth NR, Riggins CW, eds. Botanical Medicine – Efficacy, Quality Assurance and Regulation. Larchmont, NY: Mary Ann Liebert Inc., 1999:143–145.

29. Flaster T. Shipping, handling, receipt, and short-term storage of raw plant materials. In: Eskinazi D, Blumenthal M, Farnsworth NR, Riggins CW, eds. Botanical Medicine – Efficacy, Quality Assurance and Regulation. Larchmont, NY: Mary Ann Liebert Inc., 1999:139–142.

30. McChesney JD. Environmental issues and methodology for detecting environmental contaminants. In: Eskinazi D, Blumenthal M, Farnsworth NR, Riggins CW, eds. Botanical Medicine – Efficacy, Quality Assurance and Regulation. Larchmont, NY: Mary Ann Liebert Inc., 1999:127–131.

31. Reichling J, Saller R. Quality control in the manufacturing of modern herbal remedies. Quarterly Review of Natural Medicine 1998; Spring:21–28.

32. Simon JE. Domestication and production considerations in quality control of botanicals. In: Eskinazi D, Blumenthal M, Farnsworth NR, Riggins CW, eds. Botanical Medicine – Efficacy, Quality Assurance and Regulation. Larchmont, NY: Mary Ann Liebert Inc., 1999:133–137.

33. Southwell IA, Campbell MH. Hypericin content variation in *Hypericum perforatum* in Australia. Phytochemistry 1991; 30:475–478.

34. Campbell MH, May CE, Southwell IA, Tomlinson JD, Michael PW. Variation in *Hypericum perforatum* L. (St. John's wort) in New South Wales. Plant Protection Quart 1997; 12:64–66.

35. Bauer R. Echinacea: biological effects and active principles. In: Lawson LD, Bauer R, eds. Phytomedicines of Europe. Chemistry and Biological Activity. Washington, D.C.: American Chemical Society, 1988:140–157.

36. Bauer R, Wagner H. *Echinacea* species as potential immunostimulatory drugs. In: Wagner H, Farnsworth NR, eds. Economic and Medicinal Plant Research. Vol. 5. New York: Academic Press, 1991:253–321.

37. James WO. Alkaloids in the plants. In: Manske RHF, Holmes HL, eds. The Alkaloids. Vol. 1. New York: Academic Press, 1950:16–86.
38. Manske RHF. Sources of alkaloids and their isolation. In: Manske RHF, Holmes HL, eds. The Alkaloids. Vol. 1. New York: Academic Press, 1950:1–11.
39. Hammouda FM, Ismail SI, Hassan NM, Zaki AK, Kamel A. Evaluation of the silymarin content in *Silybum marianum* (L.) Gaertn. cultivated under different agricultural conditions. Phytother Res 1993; 7:90–91.
40. Espinosa EO, Mann MJ, Bleadsdell B. Toxic metals in selected traditional Chinese medicinals. J Forensic Sci 1996; 41:453–456.
41. Awang DVC. Quality control and good manufacturing practices: safety and efficacy of commercial herbs. Food Drug Law J 1997; 52:341–344.
42. Slifman NR, Obermeyer WR, Aloi BK, et al. Contamination of botanical dietary supplements by *Digitalis lanata*. N Engl J Med 1998; 339:806–811.
43. Mahady GB, Fong HHS, Farnsworth NR. Botanical Dietary Supplements: Quality, Safety and Efficacy. Lisse, Netherlands: Swets & Zeitlinger, 2001.
44. Miller MJS. Herbal medicine standardization. Problems and possibilities. J Am Nutraceut Assoc 2001; 3:1–2.
45. Bone K. Standardized extracts: Neither poison nor panacea. HerbalGram 2001; 53:50–55.
46. Anon. Regulatory Situation of Herbal Medicines: A Worldwide Review. Geneva, Switzerland: World Health Organization, 1998.
47. Anon. Federal Register March 28, 2003 (Volume 68, Number 60). Accessed online 24 March, 2004 at http://www.cfsan.fda.gov/~lrd/fr030328.html.
48. Anon. WHO Guidelines on Good Agricultural and Collection Practices (GACP) for Medicinal Plants. Geneva, Switzerland: World Health Organization, 2003.
49. Anon. Research Guidelines for Evaluating the Safety and Efficacy of Herbal Medicines. Manila, Philippines: World Health Organization, Regional Office for the Western Pacific, 1993.
50. Anon. Guidelines for the assessment of herbal medicines. WHO Technical Report Series No. 863. Geneva, Switzerland: World Health Organization, 1996: 178–184.
51. Anon. Quality Control Methods for Medicinal Plant Materials. Geneva, Switzerland: World Health Organization, 1998.
52. Houghton PJ. Establishing identification criteria for botanicals. Drug Inform J 1998; 32:461–469.
53. Anon. Good Manufacturing Practices: Supplementary Guidelines for the Manufacture of Herbal Medicinal Products. WHO Technical Report Series No. 863. Geneva, Switzerland: World Health Organization, 1996:109–113.
54. Nortier JL, Martinez MC, Schmeiser HH, et al. Urothelial carcinoma associated with the use of a Chinese herb (*Aristolochia fangchi*). N Engl J Med 2000; 342:1686–1692.

9

Pharmacokinetics of Botanical Products

Veronika Butterweck and Hartmut Derendorf

Department of Pharmaceutics, Center for Food Drug Interaction Research and Education, University of Florida, Gainesville, Florida, U.S.A.

INTRODUCTION

A general disillusionment with conventional medicines, coupled with the desire for a "natural" lifestyle has resulted in an increasing utilization of herbal medicinal products (HMPs) across the developed world. Sales of botanical products in the United States have increased sharply in recent years, according to industry reports. An estimated $4 billion was spent in health food stores in 2000 for botanical products in bulk, as well as capsules, tablets, extracts, and teas (1–4). A similar trend is noted for European countries (5).

Many consumers use HMPs in a holistic manner and mainly on the basis of their empirical and traditional applications. The use of HMPs in an evidence-based approach is known as "rational phytotherapy," which is in contrast to traditional medical herbalism. To obtain "rationality," HMPs must meet acceptable standards of quality, safety, and efficacy. Besides quality and safety issues, establishing the pharmacological basis for efficacy of HMPs is a constant challenge for researchers worldwide. In general, pharmacology can be defined as the study of the interaction of biologically active agents with living systems. The study of pharmacology can be further divided into two main areas: pharmacodynamics and pharmacokinetics. Whereas in recent years the number of studies investigating the pharmacodynamic effects of HMPs has increased rapidly, there is still limited information available regarding herbal pharmacokinetics. This might be due to the following reasons. The study of herbal pharmacokinetics is extraordinarily complex because HMPs are multicomponent mixtures, which contain several chemical constituents. Therefore, concentrations of single compounds in the final product are in the lower milligram range per dose. The resulting plasma concentrations are often in the microgram per liter to picogram per liter range. As a consequence, analytical methods determining bioavailability and pharmacokinetics of HMPs have to be sufficiently sensitive. Advanced techniques such as gas chromatography–mass spectrometry (GC–MS)/MS or high-performance liquid chromatography–MS/MS can be used nowadays to accomplish these goals (6).

For the majority of these multicomponent mixtures, the active constituents are often unknown. In other words, a substance that is detectable in body fluids is not necessarily the active compound of an extract. Further, the different compounds will have a different bioavailability, thereby complicating the design of pharmacokinetic studies with HMPs. Natural compounds are often prodrugs that are metabolized in the digestive tract. Moreover, HMPs can contain large polar molecules that might be expected to have poor and unpredictable bioavailability (7).

Bioavailability is defined as the rate and extent of active substances in the blood stream after oral doses. The bioavailability of a substance depends on several factors: the pharmaceutical preparation, the size of the molecule, the fat/water solubility of the compound, factors within the gut, first-pass effects, interaction with food, and individual factors in the patient, such as the influence of pathological factors (8). Bioavailability of compounds in the plant extract might also be influenced by other components in the mixture, which are not active themselves but can act to improve the stability, solubility, or the half-life time of the active compounds. Some authors divide their components into active and accompanying substances (so-called coeffectors) (9,10). Coeffectors have an influence on the physicochemical properties of active compounds of an extract and, as a consequence, on their biopharmaceutical parameters. There are several examples in the literature showing that such coeffectors improve not only the solubility but also the bioavailability of single compounds (11). Saponines were shown to significantly increase the absorption of corticosteroids, some antibiotics, flavones (12), phytosterols, and silicic acid (13). The concentration of kavain and yangonin in mouse brain samples is higher after administration of a *Piper methysticum* extract than after administration of the purified single compounds in the same amount (14). Similarly, the oral bioavailability of kavain from an extract of *P. methysticum* is 10 times higher than that of pure kavain (15). The improved bioavailability of ascorbic acid from a *Citrus* extract compared to pure ascorbic acid is explained by an increased absorption and an improved stability of vitamin C in presence of several flavonoids contained in the *Citrus* extract (16). List et al. (17) showed that the transport of L-hyoscyamin from the mucosal to the serosal side of the rat's isolated ileum is increased when a native extract prepared from the leaves of *Hyoscyamus niger* is used instead of pure hyoscyamin; they suggest unidentified flavonoid glycosides as the responsible compounds. Unfortunately, most investigations on this topic give few or no information about the mechanism of interaction and, in particular, about the compounds involved. One approach to identify the chemical structure of a coeffector was recently performed by Butterweck et al. [for study details see section "St. John's wort" (SJW) (18,19)].

Taken together, although the study of herbal pharmacokinetics appears to be difficult, the information derived from such investigations will become an important issue to link data from pharmacological assays and clinical effects. In particular, a better understanding of the pharmacokinetics and bioavailability of natural compounds can help in designing rational dosage regimen; and it can help to predict potential botanical product–drug interactions. In addition, those studies would provide supporting evidence for the synergistic nature of herbal medicines and would further help in optimizing the bioavailability and, hence, the efficacy of HMPs. In the following chapter, pharmacokinetic studies that have been conducted for some of the top-selling HMPs worldwide are listed, including SJW, ginkgo, garlic, willow bark, milk thistle, and horse chestnut.

GINKGO BILOBA

G. biloba L. is a member of the Ginkgoaceae family, a gymnosperm that has survived unchanged from the Triassic period. In traditional Chinese medicine, the seeds (nuts) of *G. biloba* were used as an antitussive, expectorant, and antiasthmatic, and in bladder infection (20). In China, the leaves of *G. biloba* were also used for the treatment of asthma and cardiovascular disorders (21). Today, standardized concentrated extracts prepared from the leaves of *G. biloba* are used for the treatment of peripheral circulatory insufficiency, cerebrovascular disorders, geriatric complaints, and for Alzheimer dementia. For a more extensive treatment, readers are referred to the many authoritative reviews available, e.g., Refs. (22–27).

Interestingly, no preclinical or clinical work has been done investigating the pharmacology, therapeutic efficacy, or safety of crude ginkgo leaf preparations. Almost all of the existing data focus on dry extracts characterized by 22% to 27% flavonol glycosides, 5% to 7% terpene trilactones, and less than 5 ppm ginkgolic acids (EGb 761) (Fig. 1). Other chemicals present in the extracts are hydroxykynurenic acid, shikimic acid, protocatechuic acid, vanillic acid, and *p*-hydroxybenzoic acid. The monograph published by the Commission E of the German Health Authorities states that acceptable extracts should have an herb-to-extract ratio in the average range of 50:1 (28). Extracts should be prepared with an acetone–water mixture and then be purified further. This standardization process eliminates unwanted

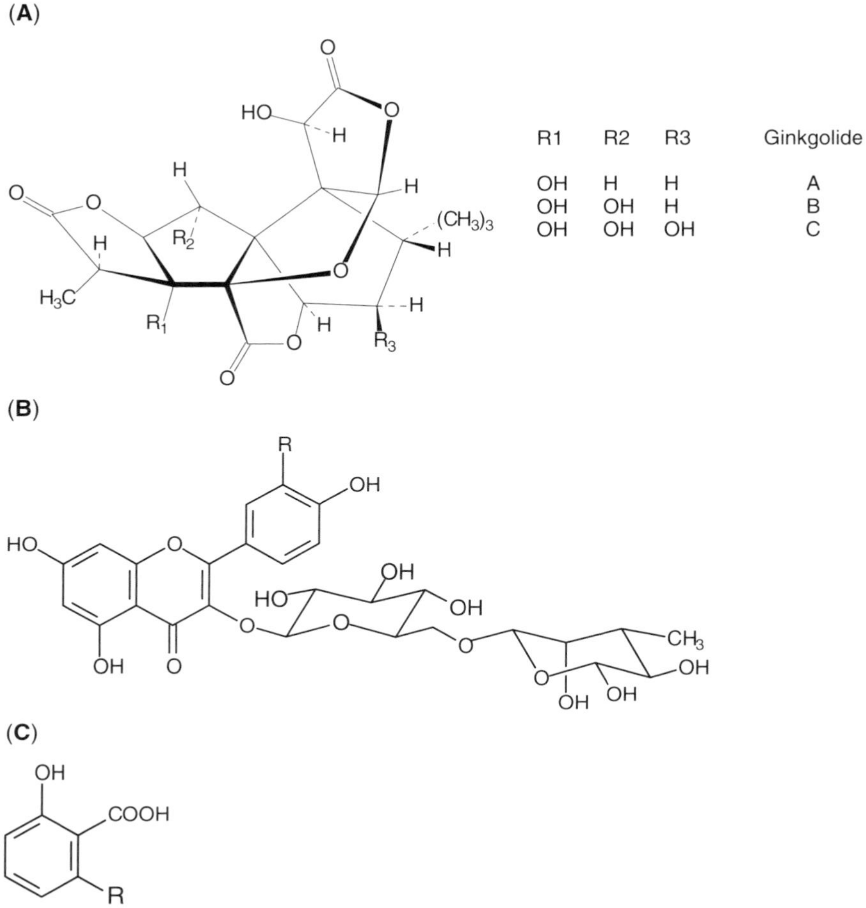

(A)

R1	R2	R3	Ginkgolide
OH	H	H	A
OH	OH	H	B
OH	OH	OH	C

(B)

(C)

Figure 1 Structures of (**A**) ginkgolide A, ginkgolide B, bilobalide, (**B**) flavonolglycosides (R=H: kaempferol-3-*O*-rutinoside; R=OH: quercetin-3-*O*-rutinoside; R=OCH$_3$: isorhamnetin-3-*O*-rutinoside) and (**C**) ginkgolic acids (R=C$_{13}$H$_{27}$, C$_{15}$H$_{31}$, C$_{15}$H$_{29}$, C$_{15}$H$_{33}$).

components that might have toxic effects. In particular, it has been shown that adverse effects such as allergies were related to ginkgolic acids (29–31). Therefore, extracts that are used in drug manufacture are free of ginkgolic acids (less than 5 ppm). The question of whether ginkgolic acids possess allergenic potential or not is still discussed controversially, especially because it has been shown that leaf extracts, if taken orally, showed adverse effects even if they contained ginkgolic acids in a concentration of 1000 ppm, whereas a pure ginkgolic acid extract showed allergic effects (32).

Pharmacokinetics

Both human and animal pharmacokinetic studies have been done on ginkgo flavonol aglycones (quercetin, kaempferol, and isorhamnetin) and terpene trilactones (ginkgolide A and B and bilobalide).

Flavonol Glycosides

Human clinical studies: In general, pharmacokinetic studies on flavonol glycosides are difficult to conduct because flavonoids are commonly present in the diet and their metabolites are numerous. An accurate pharmacokinetic assessment requires subjects to be maintained on a flavonoid-free diet for a period of time prior to dosing as has been done in the study by Pietta et al. (33). Six volunteers received the relatively high single oral dose of 4 g (equivalent to 1 g flavonol glycosides) of ginkgo leaf extract (EGb 761) following seven days of a flavonoid-free diet. The following flavonol metabolites were found in the urine over three days: 4-hydroxybenzoic acid conjugate, 4-hydroxyhippuric acid, 3-methoxy-4-hydroxyhippuric acid, 3,4-dihydroxybenzoic acid, 4-hydroxybenzoic acid, hippuric acid, and 3-methoxy-4-hydroxybenzoic acid, which represented less than 30% of the flavonols administered. The authors noted that the very high dose of extract administered to the subjects made it difficult to extrapolate the results to normal clinical dosages (40–240 mg extract daily).

The oral pharmacokinetics of the flavonol aglycones quercetin, kaempferol, and isorhamnetin in two healthy volunteers were studied by Nieder (34). Subjects were given 50, 100, and 300 mg of ginkgo leaf extract–coated tablets (LI 1370). Peak plasma concentrations (C_{max}) of 25 to 30, 65, and 130 ng/mL, respectively, were achieved within two to three hours with half-lives ($t_{1/2}$) of two to four hours. Values returned to baseline 24 hours after intake. There was a linear relationship between the dose administered and the peak plasma level. In the study by Wocjcicki et al. (35), the bioavailabilities of the same aglycones were determined using three different single oral dosage forms (capsule, liquid, and tablet). Results were similar to those of Nieder (34). However, the t_{max} was longer with the capsules. Values were back to baseline 24 hours after intake. The area under the curve (AUC) for the evaluated flavonoids did not differ significantly among formulations. The researchers concluded that the three formulations could be modeled by a one-compartment model with zero-order absorption without lag time, indicating that the aglycones were rapidly absorbed, and that the preparations had similar bioavailability (35). That the dosage form might have an influence on the bioavailability of ginkgolides and bilobalide was studied by Kressmann et al. (36,37) (see section "Triterpene lactones").

Increasing doses of a commercial special extract of *G. biloba* (LI 1370) were administered to two healthy volunteers (50, 100, and 300 mg) (38). The amounts of kaempferol and quercetin were significantly higher compared to baseline. The flavonoids were metabolized and excreted primarily as glucuronic acid conjugates in urine.

Animal studies: In the study by Pietta et al. (39), a single dose of ginkgo leaf extract (EGb 761) was administered orally to rats. Metabolites found in the urine represented less than 40% of the flavonoids administered. The presence of phenylalkyl acids in the rat urine but not in the human urine (33,39) indicates that the flavonols were more extensively metabolized in humans than in rats. In the study by Watanabe et al. (40), mice received a diet containing ginkgo leaf extract (EGb761; 36 mg/kg daily) or a standard diet without the extract for four weeks. Afterwards, plasma levels of quercetin (12.0 ng/mL vs. 4.8 ng/mL), kaempferol (7.0 ng/mL vs. 3.2 ng/mL), and isorhamnetin (49.6 ng/mL vs. 0 ng/mL) in both treatment groups were determined. The study indicates that these compounds can be absorbed intact into the blood stream.

Triterpene Lactones

Human clinical studies: Mauri et al. (41) investigated the pharmacokinetics of ginkgolides A, B, and bilobalide, after administration of ginkgo leaf extract (160 mg oral single dose) to 15 healthy subjects (Table 1). The product given contained either a phospholipid complex (Ginkgoselect Phytosome®) or not (Ginkgoselect®) (both products contained 24% flavonol glycosides and 6% terpene trilactones; Indena SpA). Administration with the phospholipids enhanced maximum absorption (C_{max}) of total ginkgolides and bilobalide two- to threefold (from 85.0 to 181.8 µg/mL), but delayed t_{max}1.5- to 2-fold. The AUC increased two- to threefold when the phospholipid complex was administered. In this single-compartment model, the mean elimination half-life ($t_{1/2}$) was approximately 120 to 180 minutes for all of the terpene trilactones, regardless of the product administered. Fourtillan et al. (42) studied the pharmacokinetics of terpene trilactones in 12 healthy volunteers after single-dose intravenous (i.v.) or oral administration of ginkgo leaf extract (EGb 761), given with or without a meal (Table 1). The authors could show that the consumption of a standard meal along with the oral dose of EGb 761 did not affect pharmacokinetic parameters. In a recent study, Drago et al. (43) focused on the pharmacokinetics of two different dosage regimens for orally administered ginkgo leaf extract (Egb 761) in healthy volunteers. The subjects received either 40 mg twice daily or 80 mg once daily, with an interval of 21 days between cycles. It could be shown that a dosage of 40 mg twice daily resulted in a significantly longer $t_{1/2}$ (11.6 ± 5.2 vs. 4.3 ± 0.5) and mean residence time (MRT) (13.1 ± 0.3 vs. 7.3 ± 0.6) than a single 80 mg dose (Fig. 2). t_{max} was reached two to three hours after administration with both dosages. The authors conclude that the twice-daily dosage regimen with the lower dose is superior to that of a higher single daily dose.

Table 1 Data of *Ginkgo biloba* Extracts in Humans

Compound(s)	Ginkgolide A	Ginkgolide B	Bilobalide	Ginkgolide A	Ginkgolide B	Bilobalide	Ginkgolide A	Ginkgolide B	Bilobalide
Subject	Humans	Humans	Humans	Humans	Humans	Humans	Humans	Humans	Humans
N	10–12	10–12	10–12	15	15	15	15	15	15
Application	i.v./oral[a]	i.v./oral[a]	i.v./oral[a]	Oral[b]	Oral[b]	Oral[b]	Oral[c]	Oral[c]	Oral[c]
Dose (mg)	40–120	40–120	40–120	160	160	160	160	160	160
C_{max} (ng/mL)	15 (80 mg)	4 (80 mg)	12 (80 mg)	41.8 ± 14	5.6±2.2	37.6 ± 14.2	108 ± 8	13.4 ± 2.2	60.3 ± 13
t_{max} (hr)	1–2	1–2	1–2	2	2	2	4	3	3
$t_{1/2 (\beta)}$ (hr)	4–6	5–11	~3	2.63 ± 0.45	2.34 ± 0.38	2.30 ± 0.24	1.88 ± 0.13	1.69 ± 0.30	3.16 ± 0.35
CL/F (mL/min)	130–200	140–250	600	—	—	—	—	—	—
V/F (L)	40–60	60–100	170	—	—	—	—	—	—
Oral bioavailability	80–98%	80–90%	70–80%	—	—	—	—	—	—
References	Fourtillan et al. (42), Kleijnen 1992			Mauri et al. (41)			Mauri et al. (41)		

[a]After administration of EGb 761 extract (24% ginkgo-flavone glycosides and 6% terpenoids).
[b]After administration of milligram Ginkgoselect[B] formulation (24% ginkgo-flavone glycosides and 6% terpenoids in free form).
[c]After administration of milligram Ginkgoselect Phytosome[B] formulation (24% ginkgo-flavone glycosides and 6% terpenoids in phospholipid complex, 1:2).
Abbreviations: N, number of subjects; i.v., intravenous; C_{max}, maximum plasma concentration; t_{max}, time at C_{max}; $t_{1/2(\beta)}$, elimination half-life; CL/F, clearance with regard to bioavailability; V/F, volume of distribution with regard to bioavailability.
Source: From Refs. 41, 42.

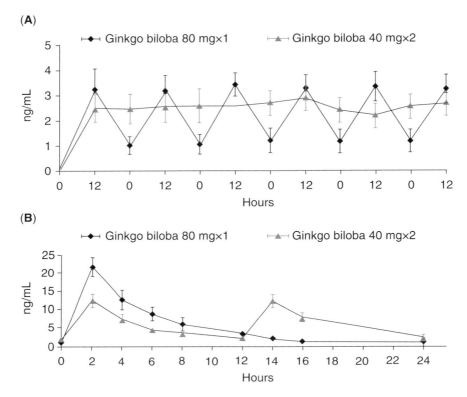

Figure 2 Plasma concentrations of (ng/mL) of ginkgolide B (**A**) from day 1 to day 6 and (**B**) on day 7 after oral administration of 40 and 80 mg tablets of *Ginkgo biloba* extract. *Source*: From Ref. 43.

The influence of the type of extract, the formulation, and dosage form on the bioavailability and pharmacokinetics of ginkolide A and B and bilobalide was recently investigated by Kressmann et al. (36,37). Twelve healthy volunteers received either Ginkgol® (containing Egb 761 = reference) or *G. biloba* capsules (= test compound) containing another commercial dry extract in an open, single-dose crossover design study. All subjects received an oral dose of 120 mg extract under fasting conditions. Pronounced differences could be detected between the test and reference formulations regarding the bioavailability of the investigated constituents, ginkgolide A, ginkgolide B, and bilobalide. The authors clearly could show that the type of extract, the formulation, and dosage form influence the pharmacokinetics and bioavailability of potential active *Ginkgo* ingredients.

Animal studies: The bioavailability of ginkgolides A and B and bilobalide was studied in rats after a single oral administration of 30, 55, and

100 mg/kg *Ginkgo* leaf extract (EGb 761) (44). The pharmacokinetics of these compounds was found to be dose-linear. Maximum plasma levels of ginkgolides A and B and bilobalide were reached in 30 to 60 minutes, with $t_{1/2}$ of ginkgolides A and B and bilobalide equaling 1.7, 2.0, and 2.2 hours, respectively, at the 30-mg dose and 1.8, 2.0, and 3.0 hours, respectively, at the 100-mg dose. Li and Wong (45) examined the pharmacokinetics of two *Ginkgo* leaf extracts in rabbits: one standardized to 27% flavonoids and 6% terpenoids and specially prepared to yield at least 80% higher levels of ginkgolide B compared to other standardized extracts (BioGinkgo®; Pharmanex), the other containing EGb 761 and standardized to 24% flavonoids and 6% terpenoids (Ginkoba®, Pharmaton). Plasma concentrations of ginkgolides from the BioGinkgo extract exhibited peaks at two and five hours post-treatment with the 40 mg/kg dose and at one and five hours with the 60 mg/kg dose. Mean C_{max} for the 40 and 60 mg/kg doses of the BioGinkgo extract were 18.8 ± 1.97 and $25.1 \pm 3.39\,\mu g/mL$, respectively, demonstrating dose dependency. With the Ginkoba preparation (40 mg/kg), a single peak in plasma concentration was observed at three hours with mean C_{max} of $17.8 \pm 0.59\,\mu g/mL$, similar to that of the former extract at the same dose. Twelve hours after the 40 mg/kg treatment, plasma ginkgolide levels were 2.6 times greater for BioGinkgo than for Ginkoba. The prolonged residence time and greater bioavailability was attributed to two factors: the slightly higher terpenoid content of the BioGinkgo preparation and, more importantly, the fact that the extract was enriched with ginkgolide B, which has a longer half-life than ginkgolide A.

ST. JOHN'S WORT

Hypericum perforatum (Clusiaceae), commonly known as SJW, is used in many countries for the treatment of mild-to-moderate forms of depression. Several clinical studies provide evidence that SJW is as effective as conventional synthetic antidepressants (46–51). From a phytochemical point of view, *H. perforatum* belongs to one of the best-investigated medicinal plants. A series of bioactive compounds have been detected in the crude material, namely phenylpropanes, flavonol derivatives, biflavones, proanthocyanidins, xanthones, phloroglucinols, some amino acids, naphthodianthrones, and essential oil constituents (Fig. 3) (52–54).

The pharmacological activity of SJW extracts has recently been reviewed (55–58). Recent reports have shown that the antidepressant activity of *Hypericum* extracts can be attributed to the phloroglucinol derivative hyperforin (59–62), to the naphthodianthrones hypericin and pseudohypericin (18,63–65), and to several flavonoids (66–69). The role and the mechanisms of action of these different compounds are still a matter of debate. But, taking these previous findings together, it is likely that several constituents are responsible for the clinically observed antidepressant efficacy of SJW.

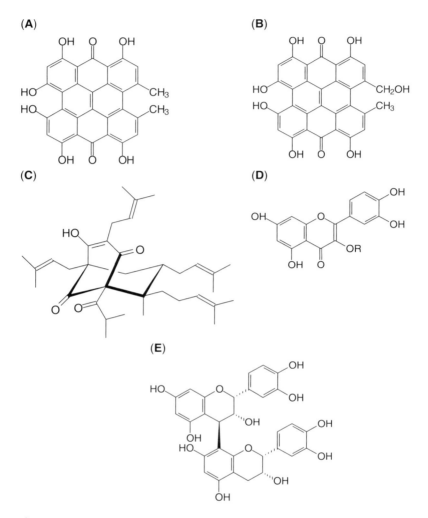

Figure 3 Structures of (**A**) hypericin (**B**) pseudohypericin (**C**) hyperforin (**D**) flavo-noids (R=H: quercetin; R=α-L-rhamnosyl: quercitrine; R=β-D-glucosyl: isoquerci-trine; R=β-D-galactosyl: hyperoside; R=β-D-rutinosyl: rutin; R=β-D-glucuronide: miquelianin) and (**E**) procyandin B2.

Pharmacokinetics

Single- and multiple-dose pharmacokinetic studies with extracts of SJW were performed in rats and humans, which focused on the determination of plasma levels of the naphthodianthrones hypericin and pseudohypericin and the phloroglucinol derivative hyperforin. Results from pharmacokinetic studies investigating plasma levels of different flavonoids after intake of SJW preparations are presently not available.

Naphthodianthrones

Human clinical studies: Detailed pharmacokinetic studies have been carried out with the hypericin-standardized SJW extract LI 160 (Jarsin® 300, Lichtwer GmbH, Berlin, Germany) (Table 2) (73–76). The preparation is reported to contain 300 mg of the dried extract of SJW, yielding 0.24% to 0.32% total hypericin. Administration of single oral doses of LI 160 (300, 900, and 1800 mg) to healthy male volunteers resulted in peak plasma hypericin concentrations of 1.5, 7.5, and 14.2 ng/mL for the three doses, respectively. Peak plasma concentrations were seen with hypericin between 2.0 and 2.6 hours and with pseudohypericin after 0.4 to 0.6 hours. The elimination half-life of hypericin was between 24.8 and 26.5 hours, and varied for pseudohypericin from 16.3 to 36.0 hours (76). The AUC showed a nonlinear increase on raising the dose—this effect was statistically significant for hypericin. Repeated doses of LI 160 (300 mg) three times daily resulted in steady-state concentrations after four days. Mean maximal plasma level during the steady-state treatment was 8.5 ng/mL for hypericin and 5.8 ng/mL for pseudohypericin (76). Kinetic parameters after i.v. administration of SJW extract (115 and 38 μg for hypericin and pseudohypericin, respectively) in two subjects correspond to those estimated after an oral dosage (Table 3) (74). Both hypericin and pseudohypericin were initially distributed into a central volume of 4.2 and 5.0 L, respectively. The mean distribution volumes at steady state were 19.7 L for hypericin and 39.3 L for pseudohypericin, and the mean total clearance rates were 9.2 mL/min for hypericin and 43.3 mL/min for pseudohypericin. The systemic availability of hypericin and pseudohypericin were roughly estimated to be 14% and 21%, respectively (Table 3) (74). In spite of their structural similarities, there were substantial pharmacokinetic differences between hypericin and pseudohypericin, which is not surprising considering the differences in the planarity of both molecules.

A placebo-controlled, randomized clinical trial with monitoring of hypericin and pseudohypericin plasma concentrations was performed to evaluate the increase in dermal photosensitivity in humans after application of high doses of SJW extract (Table 2) (73). The study was divided into a single-dose and a multiple-dose part. In the single dose crossover study, each of the 13 volunteers received either placebo or 900, 1800, or 3600 mg of the SJW extract LI 160. Maximum total hypericin plasma concentrations were observed about four hours after dosage and were 0, 28, 61, and 159 ng/mL, respectively. Pharmacokinetic parameters had a dose relationship that appeared to follow linear kinetics (73).

In another study, the concentrations of hypericin and pseudohypericin in serum and skin blister fluid after oral intake (single and steady state) of

Table 2 Data of *Hypericum perforatum* (SJW) Extracts and Pure Compounds in Animals and Humans After Oral Administration

Compound(s)	Hypericin (pure)			Hyperforin		Hypericin			Pseudohypericin		
Subject	Monkeys	Humans		Humans		Humans			Humans		
N	3	12		6		13			13		
Application	i.v.	Oral		Oral[a]		Oral[b]			Oral[b]		
Dose	5 mg/kg	0.05 mg/kg	300 mg	600 mg	1200 mg	900 mg	1800 mg	3600 mg	900 mg	1800 mg	3600 mg
C_{max} (ng/mL)	–	30.6±12.6	153.2±22	301±47	437.3±101	14–22	29–44	71–111	7–12	20–30	52–83
t_{max} (hr)		4.4±2.7		3.5±0.3	2.8±0.3	4.0–10	5.9–6.1	5.8–7.1	3.0–3.6	3.0–3.4	3.1–3.8
$t_{1/2(\alpha)}$ (hr)	2.8±0.3	–	3.2±10.6	2.6±0.7	2.5±0.9	–	–	–	–	–	–
$t_{1/2(\beta)}$ (hr)	26.0±14.0	36.1±22.6	9.5±1.1	8.6±0.7	9.6±0.8	25–31	26–33	25–30	16–24	14–18	14–22
CL (L/hr)	0.06±0.02	5.8±2.3	11.9±1.7	14.3±1.5	20.4±2.9	2.3–3.1	1.9–2.9	1.2–3.1	10.8–17.4	7.7–16.9	4.7–18.1
References	Fox et al.	Jacobson et al.		Biber et al.		Brockmöeller et al.			Brockmöeller et al.		

[a]WS 5572 extract containing 5% hyperforin.
[b]LI 360 tablets containing 0.25 mg hypericin and 0.52 mg pseudohypericin.
Abbreviations: SJW, St. John's wort; i.v., intravenous; N, number of subjects; C_{max}, maximum plasma concentration; t_{max}, time at C_{max}; $t_{1/2(\alpha,\beta)}$, elimination half-life; CL, clearance with regard to bioavailability.
Source: From Refs. 70–73.

Table 3 Data of *Hypericum perforatum* (SJW) Extracts in Humans After Oral and IV Administration

Compound(s)	Hypericin	Pseudohypericin	Hypericin			Pseudohypericin		
Subject	Humans	Humans	Humans			Humans		
N	3	12	6			13		
Application	IV[a]	IV[a]	Oral[b]			Oral[b]		
Dose	0.115 mg	0.038 mg	300 mg	900 mg	1800 mg	300 mg	900 mg	1800 mg
C_{max} (ng/mL)	29.5	6.8	0.9–3.3	4.1–17.3	4.1–66.3	1.1–7.1	6.8–28.4	8.9–48.0
t_{lag}	—	—	1.4–2.5	1.8–2.4	1.5–2.0	0.2–0.9	0.3–1.0	0.3–0.5
t_{max} (hr)	—	—	4.0–8.0	4.1–8.1	3.5–6.1	2.0–5.0	2.5–3.5	1.5–4.0
$t_{1/2(\alpha)}$ (hr)	3.8	0.79	1.4–8.3	2.8–8.0	2.1–11.5	1.2–4.5	1.2–4.7	1.2–2.0
$t_{1/2(\beta)}$ (hr)	39.9	22.8	14.7–57.8	28.2–57.8	22.9–57.8	13.9–27.9	13.9–69.3	13.9–41.9
V_{ss}/F (L)	18.5	44	32.3–280	41.0–147	18.5–297	40.6–519	24.1–134	28.8–209
CL/F (L/hr)	0.06 ± 0.02	5.8 ± 2.3	34.7–238	27.7–98.3	30.3–180	89.2–511	54.7–302	106–586
Reference			Kerb et al.					

[a]SJW extract for parenteral application (Hyperforat®).
[b]LI 160 tablets containing 300 mg extract (0.25 mg hypericin and 0.52 mg pseudohypericin per tablet).

Abbreviations: SJW, St. John's wort; IV, intravenous; N, number of subjects; C_{max}, maximum plasma concentration; t_{max}, time at C_{max}; AUC_{0-24}, area under the concentration time curve from time 0 to 24 hours; $t_{1/2(\alpha,\beta)}$, elimination half-life; CL/F, clearance with regard to bioavailability; V_{ss}, volume of distribution at steady state.

Source: From Ref. 74.

relatively high doses of LI 160 were determined in 12 healthy volunteers (75). After a single oral administration of SJW extract (1800 mg), the mean serum level of total hypericin (hypericin + pseudohypericin) was 43 ng/mL and the mean skin blister fluid level was 5.3 ng/mL. After steady-state administration (900 mg/day for seven days), the mean serum level of total hypericin was 12.5 ng/mL and the mean skin blister fluid level was 2.8 ng/mL. Serum levels of total hypericin were always higher than skin levels. However, the skin levels observed in this study are far below the hypericin skin levels that are estimated to be phototoxic (greater than 100 ng/mL) (75).

Pharmacokinetics, safety, and antiviral effects of hypericin were studied in patients with chronic hepatitis C infection (Fig. 4) (71). The patients received an eight-weeks course of 0.05 and 0.10 mg/kg hypericin orally once a day. The pharmacokinetic data revealed a long elimination half-life (mean values of 36.1 and 33.8 hours, respectively, for the doses of 0.05 and 0.10 mg/kg) and mean AUC determinations of 1.5 and 3.1 μg/mL/hr, respectively. Because relatively high doses of 0.05 and 0.10 mg/kg/day were given, which will probably be not reached after oral intake of recommended doses of SJW extract preparations, it is not surprising that hypericin caused a considerable phototoxicity in this study.

Animal studies: Early pharmacokinetic studies in mice report that maximum plasma concentrations of hypericin and pseudohypericin were reached at six hours and were maintained for at least eight hours. The aqueous-ethanolic SJW extract used in this study contained 1.0 mg of hypericin (77).

Pharmacokinetics and cerebrospinal fluid penetration of hypericin were studied after i.v. dose of 2 mg/kg in monkeys (Table 2) (70). Mean peak plasma concentration of hypericin following this dose was 71.7 μg/mL (142 μM). Elimination of hypericin from plasma was biexponential, with an average terminal half-life of 26 ± 14 hours. The 2 mg/kg dose in non-human primates was sufficient to maintain plasma concentrations above 5.1 μg/mL (10 μM) for up to 12 hours (the in vitro concentration required for growth inhibition of human glioma cell lines is greater than 10 μM).

In general, the biological evaluation of hypericin in various test models is limited by its poor water solubility. It was shown in in vitro as well as in vivo studies (18,78) that the water solubility of hypericin was remarkably enhanced in the presence of procyanidins or flavonol glycosides of SJW extract. In a recent pharmacokinetic study in rats, it was shown that procyanidin B2 as well as hyperoside increased the oral bioavailability of hypericin by approximately 58% (B2) and 34% (hyperoside) (Fig. 5) (19). Procyanidin B2 and hyperoside had a different influence on the plasma kinetics of hypericin; median maximal plasma levels of hypericin were detected after 360 minutes (C_{max}: 8.6 ng/mL) for B2, and after 150 minutes

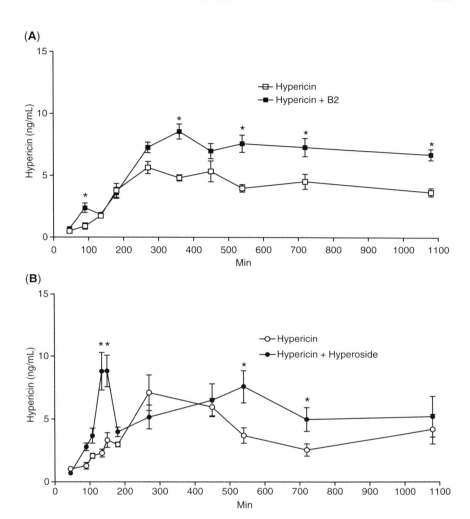

Figure 4 (**A**) Plasma levels of hypericin in the presence (■) and absence (□) of procyanidin B2. (**B**) Plasma levels of hypericin in the presence (●) and absence (○) of hyperoside. *Source*: From Ref. 19.

(C_{max}: 8.8 ng/mL) for hyperoside. The authors suggest that treatment of patients with the entire SJW extract, depending on its composition, should be superior to the treatment with isolated compounds, because the extract provides not only different classes of active compounds, but also constituents that influence their bioavailability (19).

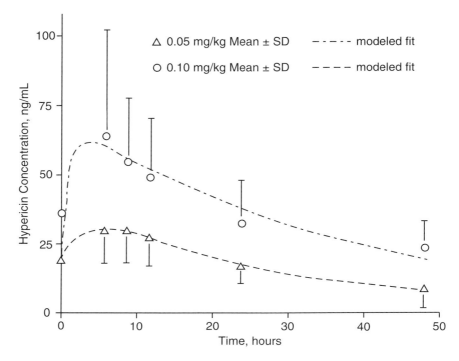

Figure 5 Plasma concentrations of hypericin after oral administration of hypericin (0.05 and 0.1 mg/kg) to hepatitis C patients. *Source*: From Ref. 71.

Hyperforin

Human clinical studies: Plasma levels of hyperforin were followed for 24 hours in two studies with healthy volunteers after administration of film-coated tablets containing 300 mg SJW extract representing 14.8 mg hyperforin (Table 2) (72). In the first crossover study, six male volunteers received 300, 600, or 1200 mg of a SJW extract preparation (WS 5572, Dr. Willmar Schwabe Arzneimittel, Karlsruhe, Germany) after a 10-hour fasting time. Maximum plasma levels of 150 ng/mL (approximately 280 nM) were reached after 3.5 hours after intake of 300 mg SJW extract. Half-life and MRT were 9 and 12 hours, respectively. Hyperforin pharmacokinetics were linear up to 600 mg of the extract. Increasing the doses to 900 or 1200 mg resulted in lower C_{max} and AUC values than those expected from linear extrapolation of data from lower doses. In a repeated dose study with seven healthy volunteers, no accumulation of hyperforin in plasma was observed after intake of 900 mg/day SJW extract for seven days. The estimated steady-state plasma concentrations of hyperforin after intake of 3×300 mg/day was approximately 100 ng/mL (approximately 180 nM) (Table 2) (72).

The bioavailability of compounds of SJW was found to be influenced by the formulation characteristics (79). An ethanolic SJW extract containing 5% hyperforin and 0.3% hypericin was administered as softgel capsules to 12 healthy volunteers. A second standard formulation in a two-piece hard gelatin capsule was also used for comparison purposes. C_{max} of hyperforin was 168.4 ng/mL for the soft gelatin formulation and 84.3 ng/mL for the hard gelatin capsule. The t_{max} values for hyperforin were 2.5 hours for the soft gelatin capsule compared to 3.1 hours for the reference formulation, whereas the total AUCs were 1483 and 583.7 hr ng/mL, respectively. Taken together, the soft gelatin capsules exhibited a higher individual absorption when compared with the corresponding data for the hard gelatin capsule. This finding confirms former results, which show that the absorption from soft gelatin capsules is in general higher if compared to hard gelatin capsules.

Animal studies: Pharmacokinetics of hyperforin after administration of an ethanolic SJW extract (WS 5572, Dr. Willmar Schwabe, Karlsruhe, Germany) to rats were investigated by Biber et al. (72). Maximum plasma levels of approximately 370 ng/mL (approximately 690 nM) were reached after three hours. Estimated half-life and clearance values were six hours and 70 mL/min/kg, respectively.

GARLIC

Garlic (*Allium sativum* L., Alliaceae) is a commonly used food and botanical supplement. Garlic is stated to possess diaphoretic, expectorant, antispasmodic, antiseptic, bacteriostatic, antiviral, hypotensive, and anthelmintic properties. Traditionally, it has been used to treat chronic bronchitis, respiratory catarrh, recurrent colds, bronchitic asthma, influenza, and chronic bronchitis. Modern use of garlic and garlic preparations is focused on their reputed antihypertensive, antiatherogenic, antithrombotic, antimicrobial, fibrinolytic, cancer preventive, and lipid-lowering effects (80–82). Garlic contains a large number of biologically active constituents. The constituents of garlic can be simply divided into two groups: sulfur-containing and non–sulfur-containing compounds. Most of the medicinal effects of garlic are referable to the sulfur compounds and the alliin-splitting enzyme alliinase, which converts alliin into allicin. This enzymatic reaction occurs when fresh garlic is chopped or crushed and alliin comes into contact with alliinase (enzyme and substrate are located in different compartments in the garlic bulb). Allicin is responsible for the characteristic garlic odor but it is unstable in aqueous and oily solution, and within a few hours it degrades into vinyldithiins and ajoenes (Fig. 6). Depending on the chemical nature of the solvent, the extract can contain a spectrum of different compounds. As a result, garlic is available in the form of different pharmaceutical preparations, such as dry powder products, oil-macerates, volatile

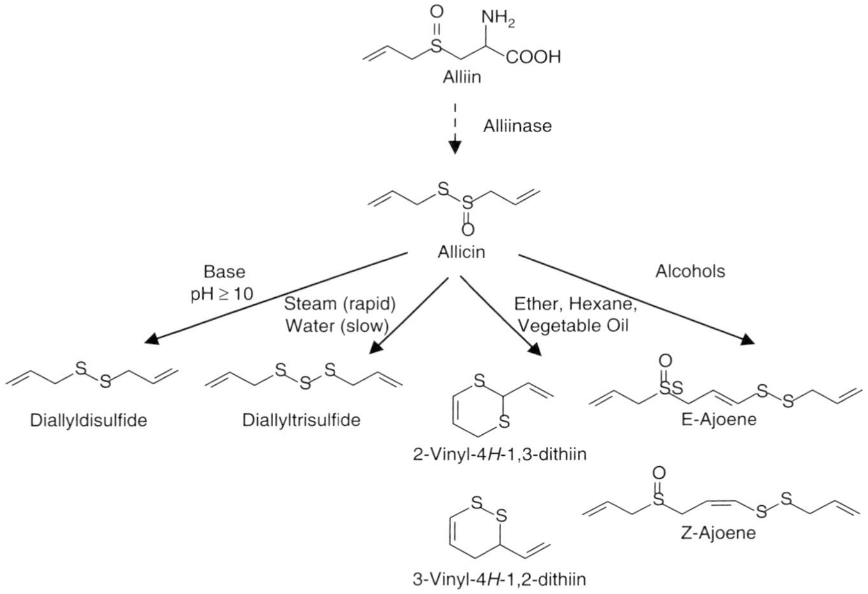

Figure 6 Typical garlic compounds. Transformation into different compounds depends on the chemical nature of the solvent.

garlic oil (obtained by water vapor distillation), or juices of fresh garlic. Most clinical studies have been mainly performed with the dry powder preparations (Kwai®, Lichtwer Pharma, Berlin, Germany) and some volatile oil macerates (80–82).

Pharmacokinetics

There are only a few reports on the absorption, metabolism, and excretion of garlic's sulfur compounds available. Further, until now it is not known what metabolic form of allicin actually reaches the target cells, and it is still unknown how garlic compounds might function in the body.

Allicin

Human clinical studies: Allicin is well absorbed, as indicated by a persistent garlicky odor on the breath, skin, and amniotic fluid of persons after consumption of fresh garlic (83). Because oral comsumption of pure allicin has been shown to significantly increase overall body catabolism of triglycerides, a substantial absorption of allicin is assumed to occur (84). However, the metabolic fate of allicin in the body is not well understood.

Neither allicin nor its common transformation products diallyl sulfides, vinyldithiins, or ajoene can be found in the blood or urine, nor can their odor be detected in the stool after consuming large amounts of garlic (up to 25 g) or pure allicin (85), indicating that it is rapidly metabolized to new compounds. In a recent study, Rosen et al. (86) used GC–MS/MS as major techniques to determine various metabolites after consumption of dehydrated granular garlic and an enteric-coated garlic preparation, in breath and plasma. The authors found that methyl allyl sulfide is the main volatile metabolite on the consumption of dehydrated dry garlic and enteric-coated garlic formulations. Hydrogen sulfide was observed but not quantified due to its extremely low levels. The non–sulfur-containing compounds limonene and *p*-cymene were also observed in the breath in those consuming garlic preparations. *S*-Allylcysteine can be observed in the blood of those who consume aged garlic preparations (so-called "Kyolic") (86).

Animal studies: The pharmacokinetic behavior of vinyldithiins, the main constituents of oily preparations of garlic, was investigated after oral administration of 27 mg 1,2-vinyldithiin and 9 mg 1,3-vinyldithiin to rats (87). In serum both forms of vinyldithiins could be detected. The serum concentration–time profile of 1,2-vinyldithiin can be characterized by an one-compartment model, whereas a two-compartment model is used as a best fit of the serum concentration of 1,3-vinyldithiin (87).

In rats, alliin and allicin were administered orally at doses of 8 mg/kg (88). Absorption of alliin and allicin was complete after 10 minutes and 30 to 60 minutes, respectively. The mean total urinary and fecal excretion of allicin after 72 hours was 85.5% of the dose. Pharmacokinetic studies of the garlic constituent *S*-allyl-L-cysteine administered orally in large doses to three different species (rat, mouse, and dog) showed that it is rapidly absorbed and is more abundant initially in several tissues, especially kidney, than it is in the blood (89). Its half-life in blood plasma (0.8–10.3 hours) and distribution among urinary metabolites varied greatly among the types of animals. The study showed that the bioavailability of *S*-allylcysteine decreased linearly with decreased dose, from 98% at 50 mg/kg body weight to 77% at 25 mg/kg and 64% at 12 mg/kg (89).

Recently, Germain et al. (90) studied the in vivo metabolism of diallyl disulfide (DADS), a garlic compound claimed to have anticarcinogenic effects. After oral administration of a single dose of 200 mg/kg, metabolites were measured in the stomach, liver, plasma, and urine by GC coupled with MS over 15 days. DADS was detected in almost all analyzed tissues within the first hours. In addition, the metabolites allylmercaptan (AM) and allyl methyl sulfide (AMS) were detected. The C_{max} of the metabolites were higher than that of DADS (1.46 μg/mL). The t_{max} for DADS was estimated to be less than one hour, whereas this time increased to 24 hours for AM and AMS (90).

WILLOW BARK

The willow family includes a number of different species of deciduous trees and shrubs native to Europe, Asia, and some parts of North America. Some of the more commonly known are white willow/European willow (*Salix alba*), black willow (*Salix nigra*), crack willow (*Salix fragilis*), purple willow (*Salix purpurea*), and weeping willow (*Salix babylonica*) (5). The willow bark sold in Europe and the United States usually includes a combination of the bark from white, purple, and crack willows. Willow bark's most important medicinal qualities are its ability to ease pain and reduce inflammation (80). Salicin is probably the most active anti-inflammatory compound in willow; it is metabolized to salicylic acid (91). The enzymatic degradation of salicin, salicortin, and tremulacin by β-glucosidase and by esterase has been investigated (92). Salicin and its conversion products are illustrated in Figure 7. Studies have identified several other components of willow bark that have antioxidant, fever-reducing, antiseptic, and immune-boosting effects (80).

The pharmacological actions of salicylates in humans are well documented and are applicable to willow. In recent clinical studies, willow bark extract had moderate analgesic effects in osteoarthritis and low back pain (93–96).

Pharmacokinetics

There are only a limited number of studies available evaluating the pharmacokinetics of salicin and its major metabolites in humans after oral administration.

Salicin

Human clinical studies: Two early studies have been published on the oral bioavailability of salicin in humans, but they showed different results. Oral ingestion of 4000 mg (13.97 mmol) of pure salicin by a single volunteer resulted in high serum concentrations of salicylic acid, with a peak level of 110 µg/mL (97). The peak level of salicylic acid in the serum after ingestion of salicin was reached somewhat later than after ingestion of an equimolar dose of sodium salicylate, with the fact that salicin must be first metabolized to salicylic acid. Eighty-six percent of the total ingested salicin was found in the 24-hour urine in the form of the usual salicylic acid metabolites, indicating a good oral bioavailability of pure salicin.

In contrast, oral administration of a willow bark extract showed a low bioavailability of salicin (98). After ingestion of commercial sugar-coated tablets containing willow bark extract corresponding to a total amount of 54.9 mg (0.192 mmol) salicin, the serum of 12 volunteers showed a peak concentration of only 0.13 µg/mL salicylic acid; this is only 5% of the serum

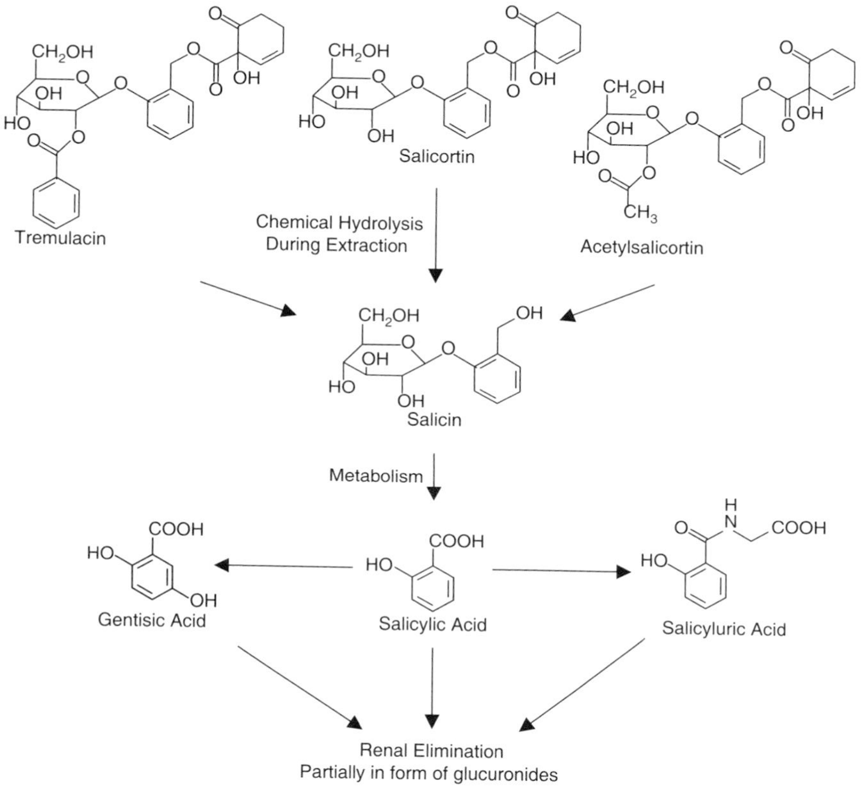

Figure 7 Main constituents of willow bark and pharmacokinetics of salicin in humans.

level expected after oral intake of an equimolar amount of synthetic salicylates. In a recent pharmacokinetic study of willow bark, Schmid et al. (99) carried out a pharmacokinetic study on the oral bioavailability of salicylates from willow bark extract in 10 healthy volunteers (Fig. 8). A chemically standardized willow bark extract was used in the form of coated tablets. Willow bark extract was given in two equal doses corresponding to 240 mg salicin at times zero and three hours. Over a period of 24 hours, urine and serum levels of salicylic acid and its metabolites, gentisic acid and salicyluric acid, were determined. Peak plasma levels of salicylic acid were on average 1.2 µg/mL and were reached less than two hours after oral administration. Salicylic acid was the major metabolite of salicin in the serum (86% of total salicylates), besides salicyluric acid (10%) and gentisic

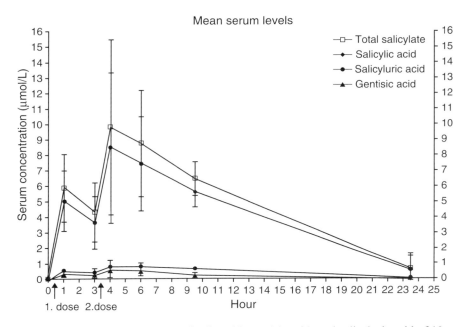

Figure 8   Mean serum levels of salicylic acid, gentisic acid, and salicyluric acid of 10 volunteers. "Total salicylate" represents the sum of the three individual compounds. Error bars indicate 95% confidence interval of the mean. *Source*: From Ref. 99.

acid (4%). After 24 hours, 15.8% of the orally ingested dose of salicin was detected in the urine on average. The AUC of salicylate obtained in this study was equivalent to that expected from an intake of 87 mg of acetylsalicylic acid. Taken together, in the study by Schmid et al. (99), willow bark in the dosage of 240 mg led to much lower serum salicylate levels than observed after analgesic doses of synthetic salicylates. The authors conclude that the formation of salicylic acid alone is therefore unlikely to explain analgesic or antirheumatic effects of willow bark.

HORSE CHESTNUT

The horse chestnut, *Aesculus hippocastaneum* (Hippocastanaceae), was introduced into the northern Europe from the Near East in the 16th century. Extracts from horse chestnut seeds were already being used therapeutically in France in the early 1800s. Several French works published between 1896 and 1909 reported successful outcomes in the treatment of hemorrhoidal ailments (100). Traditionally, horse chestnut has been used for the treatment of varicose veins, hemorrhoids, phlebitis, diarrhea, fever, and enlargement

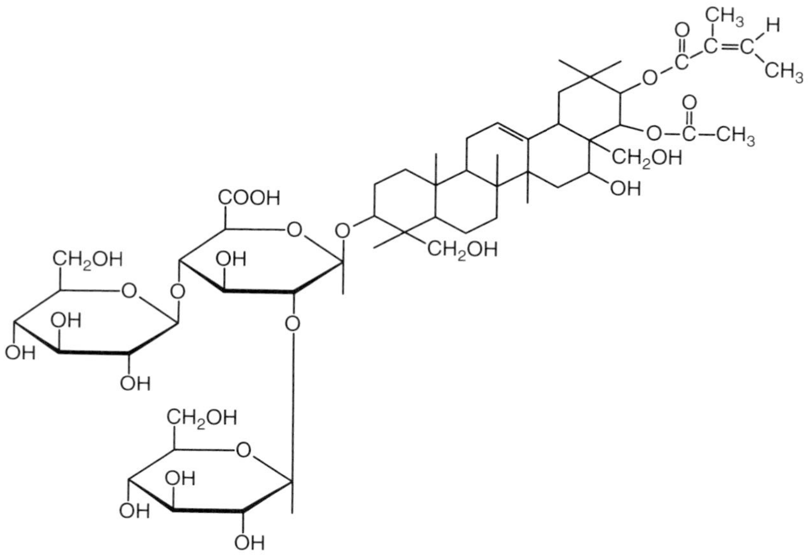

Figure 9 Chemical structure of aescin.

of the prostate gland. The German Commission E approved its use in the treatment of chronic venous insufficiency in the legs (5). The seeds of horse chestnut contain mainly aescin, which is a complex mixture of various chemically very similar triterpene glycosides having saponifying activities. The aglycones of these saponins are barringtogenol C and protoescigenin. Former investigations of the saponin mixture differentiated between three aescin subtypes, including the slightly soluble β-aescin, a C-21 and C-22 diester, readily water soluble crypto-aescin, which is created by spontaneous migration of the acetyl group from C-22 to C-28, and α-aescin, an equilibrium mixture of these two isomer diesters (Fig. 9) (101,102). A number of other compounds have been isolated from the chestnut seeds, i.e., flavonols (kaempferol and quercetin), flavonol glycosides (astragalin, isoquercitrin, and rutin), and coumarins (aesculetin, fraxin, and scopolin) (5). However, all of these compounds can be found in larger amounts from other sources and, furthermore, during 1960, Lorenz and Marek concluded that the anti-edemigenous, antiexudative, and vasoprotective activities of horse chestnut extracts are mainly due to aescin (103).

Pharmacokinetics

Pharmacokinetic studies with horse chestnut focus on the absorption, metabolism, and excretion of the main constituent—β-aescin.

Aescin

Human clinical studies: The significant advances in understanding of bioavailability and kinetics of β-aescin should be attributed to the development of a highly specific radioimmunoassay (RIA) allowing the detection of concentrations in the nanogram per milliliter range (10-6) (104). The relative oral bioavailability of beta-aescin from a sugar-coated tablet formulation was compared to a reference preparation available in capsule form to 18 healthy, male volunteers over a 48 h period. A large variation in absorption parameters for beta-aescin was measured. Maximum concentration (C_{max}) after a dose containing 50 mg aescin varied from 0.19 to 45.1 ng/mL, time for maximum concentration (t_{max}) varied from 0.73 to 8.5 hours, and the AUC varied from 24.6 to 389 ng/hr/mL (105). The second study, also on two solid-dose preparations (one with sustained release), using 24 volunteers found more consistent results (106). Parameters of the sustained-release tablet were superior. For example, after a dose containing 50 mg aescin, C_{max} for the sustained-release tablet 9.81 ± 8.9 ng/mL, t_{max} was 2.23 ± 0.9 hours, and AUC averaged 187.1 ng/hr/mL. The half-life time for both preparations was about 20 hours (106). However, the data of both studies have to be evaluated with care, because the RIA used for the determination is highly specific and its potential of cross-reactivity with different types of β-aescin is not known for the different extracts used in the different preparations. Thus, absolute plasma concentration values of β-aescin from a single preparation cannot be compared with other preparations (107). Further, saponins are large molecules containing highly polar groups and their intact bioavailability can be expected to be low after oral doses. This was confirmed in the above-mentioned studies, because the pharmacokinetic parameters indicate an absorption less than 10% of the administered dose. However, saponins can be hydrolyzed by intestinal flora, leaving the less polar aglycone or sapogenin available for absorption. These sapogenins, or their hepatic metabolites, may in fact be the main active form of aescin following oral doses. Further studies are needed to clarify this issue.

Animal studies: Pharmacokinetics and bioavailability of aescin was studied after oral and i.v. administration of tritiated aescin (108,109). About 66% and 33% of the dose was excreted in bile and urine, respectively, after i.v. administration. The oral bioavailability of aescin was about 12.5%. Percutaneous absorption of aescin was studied in mice and rats (110). The amounts of aescin in muscle were greater than in other organs. These results indicate that percutaneous administration of aescin could be beneficial.

GINSENG

Ginseng, a commonly used natural product, has a reputation as a "herb of eternal life." A survey of herbal-based over-the-counter products indicates that 28% of them contain ginseng. It has been estimated that ginseng comprises 15% to 20% of the total annual sales of botanical products in the United States (111).

Botanical remedies known as "ginseng" are based on the roots of several distinct species of plants, mainly Korean or Asian ginseng (*Panax ginseng*), Siberian ginseng (*Eleutherococcus senticosus*), and American ginseng (*Panax quinquefolius* and *Panax notoginseng*). All of these species belong to the Araliaceae family, but each of these different species has specific pharmacological effects. *P. ginseng* is the most commonly used and highly researched species of ginseng. This species, which is native to China, Korea, and Russia, has been an important botanical remedy in traditional Chinese medicine for thousands of years, where it has been used primarily as a treatment for weakness and fatigue (112). The main constituents of *P. ginseng* are the so-called ginsenosides, a complex mixture of saponins from the tetracyclic dammarane type (sapogenins protopanaxadiol and protopanaxatriol) and a pentacyclic triterpene from the oleanolic acid type. The ginsenosides can be divided into two classes: the protopanaxatriol class, consisting mainly of Rg_1, Rg_2, Rf, and Re, and the protopanaxadiol class, consisting mainly of Rc, Rd, Rb_1, and Rb_2 (Fig. 10).

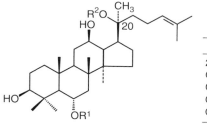

Protopanaxatriol Class

	R^1	R^2
20(S)-Protopanaxatriol	H	H
Ginsenoside Re	glc(2-1)rha	glc
Ginsenoside Rf	glc(2-1)glc	H
Ginsenoside Rg_1	glc	glc
Ginsenoside Rg_2	glc(2-1)rha	H

Protopanaxadiol Class

	R^1	R^2
20(S)-Protopanaxadiol	H	H
Ginsenoside Re	glc(2-1)glc	glc(6-1)glc
Ginsenoside Rf	glc(2-1)glc	glc(6-1)ara *p*
Ginsenoside Rg_1	glc(2-1)glc	glc(6-1)ara *f*
Ginsenoside Rg_2	glc(2-1)glc	glc

Figure 10 Chemical structures of ginsenosides. *Abbreviations*: glc, β-D-glucose; rha, α-L-rhamnose; ara, α-L-arabinose; *p*, pyranose; *f*, furanose.

Further, ginseng constituents are polysaccharides, essential oil constituents, polyacetylenes, peptides, and other lipids (7). Ginseng is included in the pharmacopeias of several countries such as China, Germany, and the United Kingdom (113). Modern therapeutic claims refer to vitality, immune function, cancer, cardiovascular diseases, and sexual function (114,115). More than 500 studies have been published on the pharmacological activity of ginseng (7,80).

Pharmacokinetics

Although ginseng is commonly used as an adaptogenic and immunomodulatory drug, and its efficacy has been shown in pharmacologic assays as well as in clinical trials, the number of pharmacokinetic studies is limited. This might be due to the chemical nature of the ginsenosides—as saponins, they are large molecules containing highly polar groups. Thus, their intact bioavailability can be expected to be low after oral intake.

Ginsenoside

Human clinical studies: Analysis of urine samples from Swedish athletes who had consumed ginseng preparations within 10 days before urine collection showed that out of 65 samples analyzed, 60 were found to contain the sapogenin 20(S)-protopanaxatriol. The concentrations of 20(S)-protopanaxatriol varied from 2 to 35 ng/mL urine (116). The results after intake of oral doses of ginseng preparations demonstrated a linear relationship between the amounts of ginsenosides consumed and the 20(S)-protopanaxatriol glycosides excreted in the urine. About 1.2% of the dose was recovered in the glycosidic form over five days (117). The main metabolites of ginsenosides Rb_1, Rb_2, Rc, Re, and Rg_1 after anaerobic incubation with fecal flora were identified as prosapogenins and sapogenins, although the metabolic rate and mode were affected by fermentation media. Further, prosapogenins and sapogenins were detected in blood (0.3–5.1 µg/mL) and in urine (2.2–96 µg/day) after the oral administration of ginseng extract (150 mg/day) to humans (118). One organism in the human fecal flora hydrolyzing ginsenosides was *Prevotella oris* (119).

Animal studies: Studies in rats focus on the pharmacokinetics of ginsenosides Rg_1, Rb_1, and Rb_2. Ginsenoside Rg_1 was absorbed rapidly from the upper parts of the digestive tract (accounting for 1.9–20.0% of the dose of Rg_1 administered orally, 100 mg/kg) (120). The serum level of ginsenoside Rg1 reached its peak at 30 minutes, and the maximum levels of ginsenosides Rg_1 in tissues were attained within 1.5 hours. However, Rg_1 was not found in the brain. About 80% of the dose of Rg_1 was excreted into urine and bile after i.v. administration to rats, showing that Rg_1 is hardly metabolized in rat liver. The authors could further show that degradation and/or metabolism of Rg_1 occurs in the stomach and large intestine of rats (120).

Only a small amount of Rb_1 was absorbed from the digestive tract after oral administration (100 mg/kg) to rats (121). The serum level of Rb_1 in rats after i.v. injection (5 mg/kg) declined biexponentially, a rapid decline (α-phase) followed by a slow decline (β-phase). The half-lives of Rb_1 were 11.6 minutes for the α-phase and 14.5 hours for the β-phase. The persistence of Rb_1 in serum and tissues in rats for long after i.v. administration was assumed to correlate with the high activity of plasma protein binding (121).

In one study, the degradation of ginsenoside Rg_1, Rb_1, and Rb_2 was studied in further detail (122). Rg_1 was decomposed to its prosapogenin in both the rat stomach and diluted hydrochloric acid, whereas Rb_1 and Rb_2 were little degraded in rat stomach but were easily converted to their prosapogenins by diluted hydrochloric acid. The ginsenosides were also metabolized to several prosapogenins by gut bacteria and enteric enzymes. The amount of Rg_1, Rb_1, and Rb_2 absorbed from the gastrointestinal tract (GI) of the rat were 1.9%, 0.1%, and 3.7%, respectively. Ginsenoside Rg_1 was excreted into rat urine bile in a ratio of 2:5. Rb_1 and Rb_2 were mainly excreted into the urine (122).

MILK THISTLE

Milk thistle (*Silybum marianum*) is an annual to biennial plant of the Asteraceae family. It is native principally to southern Europe and northern Africa. The crude drug consists of the ripe fruits from which the pappus has been removed. Milk thistle fruits contain 15% to 30% proteins. The main active compounds constitute only about 2% to 3% of the dried fruits. The active principle is a mixture of flavolignans called silymarin. Silymarin, a polyphenolic extract isolated from the seeds of milk thistle, is composed mainly of silybin (50–70%), with small amounts of other silybin structural isomers, namely isosilybin, silydianin, and silychristin (Fig. 11) (123–125). The highest concentration of silymarin is found in the ripe fruits (126). Silibinin is the main compound, also considered to be the most active one in several paradigms (127).

Traditionally, milk thistle fruits have been used for disorders of the liver, spleen, and gall bladder, such as jaundice and gall bladder colic. Milk thistle has also been used for nursing mothers for stimulating milk production, as a bitter tonic, for hemorrhoids, for dyspeptic complaints, and as a demulcent in catarrh and pleurisy. It is stated to possess hepatoprotective, antioxidant, and choleretic properties (128). Current interest is focused on the hepatoprotective activity of milk thistle and its use for the treatment of liver, spleen, and gall bladder disorders (129). Recently it has been shown that silibinin reduced prostate-specific antigen levels in prostate carcinoma cells lines, indicating a possible role of silibinin in human prostate cancer (130,131).

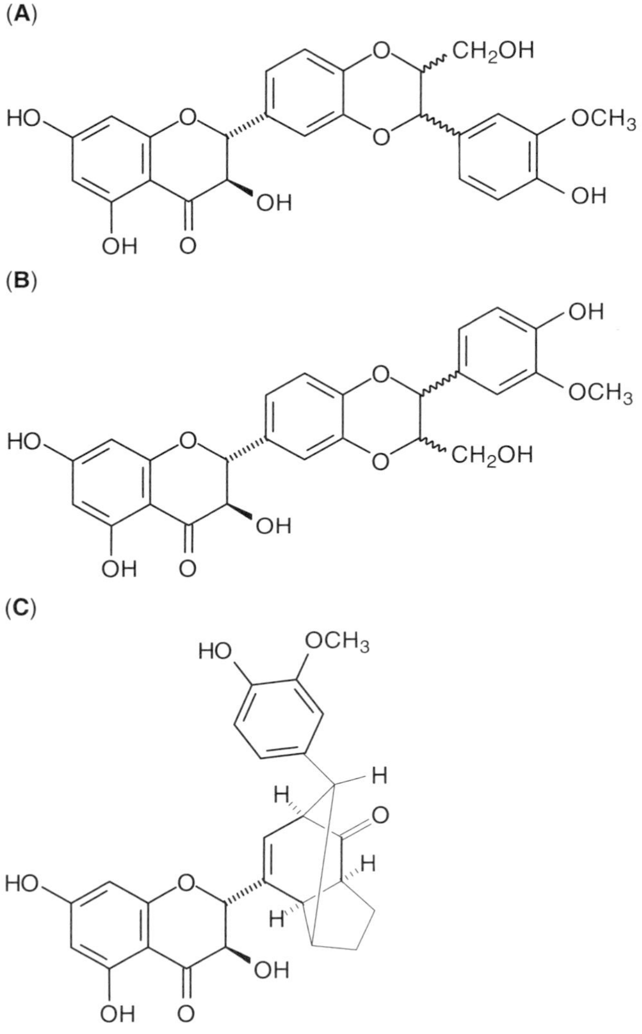

(**A**)

(**B**)

(**C**)

Figure 11   Structures of (**A**) silibinin, (**B**) isosilibinin, and (**C**) silidianin.

Pharmacokinetics

Studies of the pharmacokinetics of silymarin and of a silibinin–phosphatidyl-choline complex preparation (IdB 1016; silipide) in humans as well as rodents have been performed. Because silibinin is the main compound, pharmacokinetic parameters of silymarin and the active principle of any silymarin-containing products are always referred to, and standardized, as silibinin.

The bioavailability of silibinin from the extract is low and seems to depend on several factors such as (i) the content of accompanying substances with a solubilizing character such as other flavonoids, phenol derivatives, aminoacids, proteins, tocopherol, fat, cholesterol, and others found in the extract and (ii) the concentration of the extract itself (132,133). The systemic bioavailability can be enhanced by adding solubilizing substances to the extract (11,134). The bioavailability of silibinin can also be enhanced by the complexation with phosphatidylcholine or β-cyclodextrin, and possibly by the choice of the capsule material (135–137). The variations in content, dissolution, and (oral) bioavailability of silibinin between different commercially available silymarin products—despite the same declaration of content—are significant (138).

Therefore, comparisons between studies should be carried out with caution and consider the differences between the analytical methods used and whether free, conjugated, or total silibinin is the object of measurement (129). Systemic plasma concentrations are usually measured, even though the site of action of silymarin is the liver, because they provide an estimate on the quantity of the drug being absorbed from the GI tract.

Silibinin

Human clinical studies: In male volunteers, after single oral administration of a standardized dose of silibinin 100 to 360 mg, plasma silibinin C_{max} is reached after approximately two hours and ranges between 200 and 1400 ng/mL (Table 4), of which approximately 75% is presented in the conjugated form (139,140). For total silibinin, an elimination half-life of approximately six hours is estimated (141). Between 3% and 8% of an oral dose is excreted in the urine, while 20% to 40% is recovered from the bile as glucuronide and sulfate conjugates (142–144). The remaining part is excreted via the feces (unchanged, not absorbed). Silibinin concentrations in bile reach approximately 100 times those found in serum, with peak concentrations reached within two to nine hours. Biliary excretion continues for 24 hours after a single dose. After multiple dose administration, no accumulation is observed (143).

In patients with cirrhosis, the plasma C_{max} of silibinin after a single dose of silibinin 360 mg was lower (120 ng/mL) and time to C_{max} (t_{max}; 2.6 hours) slightly delayed compared with healthy volunteers (145,146).

Animal studies: The comparative pharmacokinetics of silipide (IdB 1016, a silybin–phosphatidylcholine complex) and silybin were investigated by measuring unconjugated and total plasma silybin levels as well as total biliary and urinary silybin excretion in rats following administration of a single dose (200 mg/kg as silybin) (136). Mean peak levels of unconjugated and total silybin after IdB 1016 were 8.17 and 74.23 μg/mL, respectively. Mean AUC (0–6) values were 9.78 and 232.15 μg/hr/mL, indicating that

Table 4 Data of *Carduus marianus* (Milk Thistle) Extract and Purified Compounds in Humans After Oral Administration

Compound	Unconjugated silybin	Conjugated silybin	Total silybin				Unconjugated silybin			
Subject	Humans	Humans	Humans				Humans			
N	12	12	6				6			
Dose	80 mg	80 mg	101.7 mg	152.6 mg	203.4 mg	254.3 mg	101.7 mg	152.6 mg	203.4 mg	254.3 mg
Application	Oral[a]	Oral[a]	Oral[b]	Oral[b]	Oral[b]	Oral[b]	Oral[b]	Oral[b]	Oral[b]	Oral[b]
C_{max} (ng/mL)	141 ± 31	255 ± 35	523.7 ± 292	961.5 ± 421	1018 ± 375	1383 ± 512	116.8 ± 111	250.8 ± 145	239.5 ± 103	317.2 ± 204
t_{max} (hr)	2.4 ± 0.3	3.8 ± 0.5	0.6–4.6	0.6–4.6	0.6–4.6	0.6–4.6	0.6–4.6	0.6–4.6	0.6–4.6	0.6–4.6
$t_{1/2}$ (hr)	1.62 ± 0.18	3.44 ± 0.42	–	–	–	–	–	–	–	–
MRT (hr)	3.36 ± 0.23	6.72 ± 0.60	–	–	–	–	–	–	–	–
References	Gatti et al.	Gatti et al.	Weyhenmeyer et al.				Weyhenmeyer et al.			

[a] After administration of silipide (lipophilic silybin-phosphatidylcholine complex) containing 80 mg equivalent silibinin.
[b] After administration of silybin (Legalon[R] 140 capsules).
Abbreviations: SJW, St. John's wort; i.v., intravenous; N, number of subjects; C_{max}, maximum plasma concentration; t_{max}, time at C_{max}; $t_{1/2}$, elimination half life; MRT, mean residence time.
Source: From Refs. 139, 140.

about 94% of the plasma silybin is present in a conjugated form. Cumulative biliary (zero to two hours) and urinary (0 to 72 hours) excretion values after administration of IdB 1016 accounted for 3.73% and 3.26% of the administered dose, respectively. After silybin administration, the biliary and urinary excretion accounted for only 0.001% and 0.032% of the dose, respectively (136).

CONCLUSION

The use of HMPs, including their use in addition or instead of conventional drugs, is continuing to increase. Unfortunately, only limited information is available regarding the pharmacokinetics and bioavailability of herbal medicines but the awareness of this issue is increasing. In the present chapter, we focused on the bioavailability and pharmacokinetics of some of the top selling botanical products on the U.S. and European market. However, some of the most popular medicinal plants were not further discussed in this chapter, because pharmacokinetic data are not available yet (e.g., Chasteberry, Saw palmetto, or Feverfew). A reason for the lack of pharmacokinetic data could be that the active compounds of these plants are still unknown. This issue points to the fact that the determination of herbal pharmacokinetics is a unique field, which is extremely complex. Thus, the question arises—Is studying herbal pharmacokinetics of any value in the therapeutic use of the plant, especially when the drug has been used therapeutically without this information for centuries?

However, the information derived from a detailed pharmacokinetic study will help to anticipate potential botanical product–drug interactions, to optimize the bioavailability, the quality, and hence the efficacy of herbal medicines, to support evidence for the synergistic nature of herbal medicines, and to better appreciate the safety and toxicity of the plant. Because pharmacokinetic studies with herbal medicines are often complicated by their chemical complexity and by the fact that the active compounds are often unknown, it could be one future issue to assess bioavailability by measuring surrogate parameters in plasma or tissue instead of directly assaying putative active compounds in the blood. In summary, to use HMPs in an evidence-based approach and to achieve the status "rational phytomedicine," more experimental studies are needed to characterize the bioavailability and pharmacokinetics of botanical products.

REFERENCES

1. Brevoort P. The U.S. botanical market—an overview. Herbalgram 1996; 36:49–57.
2. Brevoort P. The booming US botanical market. A new overview. Herbalgram 1998; 44:33–46.
3. De Smet PA, Bonsel G, Van der Kuy A, et al. Introduction of the pharmacoeconomics of herbal medicines. Pharmacoeconomics 2000; 32:427–436.

4. Kessler RC, Davis RB, Foster DF, et al. Long-term trends in the use of complementary and alternative medical therapies in the United States. Ann Intern Med 2001; 135:262–268.

5. Blumenthal M. Herbs and phytomedicines in the European Community. In: Blumenthal M, ed. The Complete German Commission E Monographs. Therapeutic Guide to Herbal Medicines. Austin, Texas: American Botanical Council, 1998.

6. Bhattaram VA, Graefe U, Kohlert C, Veit M, Derendorf H. Pharmacokinetics and bioavailability of herbal medicinal products. Phytomedicine 2002; 9:1–33.

7. Mills S, Bone K. Principles of herbal pharmacology. In: Mills S, Bone K, eds. Principles and Practice of Phytotherapy. London, New York: Harcourt Publishers, 2000:23–79.

8. Derendorf H, Gramatte T, Schaefer HG. Pharmakokinetik-Einfuehrung in die Theorie und Relevanz fuer die Arzneimitteltherapie. Stuttgart: Wissenschaftliche Verlagsgesellschaft mbH, 2002.

9. Schilcher H. Standardisierung, Kontrolle und Qualitätsprüfung von nichttoxischen flüssigen Arzneipflanzenzubereitungen. Arzneimittelstandardisierung 1965; 6:649–655.

10. Menßen HG. Standardisierte Arzneien aus Heilpflanzen und ihre Bedeutung für die moderne Phytotherapie. Therapiewoche 1968; 18:1432–1433.

11. Eder M, Mehnert W. Pflanzliche Begleitstoffe-wertvolle Hilfsstoffe oder überflüssiger Ballast? Pharmazie in unserer Zeit 2000; 29:377–384.

12. Yata N, Sugihara N, Yamajo R, et al. Enhanced small intestinal absorption of β-lactam antibiotics in rats in presence of monodesmosides from pericaps of *Sapindus mukurossi* (Ennmei-hi). J Pharmacobio-Dyn 1986; 9:211–217.

13. Hänsel R, Sticher O, Steinegger E. Pharmakognosie-Phytopharmazie. Berlin, Heidelberg: Springer-Verlag, 1999.

14. Keledjian J, Duffield PH, Janieson DD, Lidgard RO, Duffield AM. Uptake into mouse brain of four compounds present in the psychoactive beverage Kava. J Pharm Sci 1988; 77:1003–1006.

15. Biber A, Nöldner M, Schlegelmilch R. Development of a formulation of Kava-Kava extract through pharmacokinetic experiments in animals. Naunyn Schmiedeberg's Arch Pharmacol 1992; 345:R24.

16. Vinson JA, Bose P. Comparative bioavailability to humans of ascorbic acid alone or in a citrus extract. Am J Clin Nutr 1988; 48:601–604.

17. List PH, Schmid W, Weil E. Reinsubstanz oder galenische Zubereitung. Arzneim Forsch/Drug Res 1969; 19:181–185.

18. Butterweck V, Petereit F, Winterhoff H, Nahrstedt A. Solubilized hypericin and pseudohypericin from *Hypericum perforatum* exert antidepressant activity in the forced swimming test. Planta Med 1998; 64:291–294.

19. Butterweck V, Lieflaender-Wulf U, Winterhoff H, Nahrstedt A. Plasma levels of hypericin in presence of procyanidin B2 and hyperoside: a pharmacokinetic study in rats. Planta Med 2003; 69:189–192.

20. Reuter HD. *Ginkgo biloba*—botany, constituents, pharmacology and clinical trials. Br J Phytother 1995/6; 4:3–20.

21. Bensky D, Gamble A. Chinese Herbal Medicine Materia Medica. Seattle: Eastland Press, 1986:560–561.

22. Ahlemeyer B, Krieglstein J. Neuroprotective effects of *Ginkgo biloba* extract. Cell Mol Life Sci 2003; 60:1779–1792.
23. DeFeudis FV. A brief history of EGb 761 and its therapeutic uses. Pharmacopsychiatry 2002; 35:1–6.
24. DeFeudis FV, Papadopoulos V, Drieu K. *Ginkgo biloba* extracts cancer: a research area in its infancy. Fundam Clin Pharmacol 2003; 17:405–417.
25. Ponto LL, Schultz SK. *Ginkgo biloba* extract: review of CNS effects. Ann Clin Psychiatr 2003; 15:109–119.
26. Sierpina VS, Wollschlaeger B, Blumenthal M. *Ginkgo biloba*. Am Fam Physician 2003; 68:923–926.
27. Van Beek TA, Bombardelli E, Morazzoni P, Peterlongo F. *Ginkgo biloba* L. Fitoterapia 1998; 69:195–244.
28. Monograph of the Commission E. *Ginkgo biloba*. Bundesanzeiger No. 133, 1994.
29. Baron-Ruppert G, Luepke NP. Evidence for toxic effects of alkylphenols from *Ginkgo biloba* in the hen's egg test. Phytomedicine 2001; 8:133–138.
30. Becker LE, Skipworth GB. Ginkgo-tree dermatitis, stomatitis and proctitis. JAMA 1975; 231:1162–1163.
31. Jaggy H, Koch E. Chemistry and biology of alkylphenols from *Ginkgo biloba* L. Pharmazie 1997; 52:735–738.
32. Hausen BM. The sensitizing capacity of ginkgolic acids in guinea pigs. Am J Contact Derm 1998; 9:146–148.
33. Pietta PG, Mauri PL, Gardana C, Benazzi L. Assay of soluble guanylate cyclase activity by isocratic high-performance liquid chromatography. J Chromatogr B Biomed Sci Appl 1997; 690:343–347.
34. Nieder M. Pharmakokinetik der Ginkgo Flavonole im Plasma. Muench Med Wschr 1991; 133:S61–S62.
35. Wocjcicki J, Gawronska-Szklarz B, Bieganowski W, et al. Comparative pharmacokinetics and bioavailability of flavonoid glycosides of *Ginkgo biloba* after a single oral administration of three formulations to healthy volunteers. Mat Med Pol 1995; 27:141–146.
36. Kressmann S, Biber A, Wonnemann M, Schug B, Blume HH, Mueller WE. Influence of pharmaceutical quality on the bioavailability of active components from *Ginkgo biloba* preparations. J Pharm Pharmacol 2002; 54:1507–1514.
37. Kressmann S, Mueller WE, Blume HH. Pharmaceutical quality of different *Ginkgo biloba* brands. J Pharm Pharmacol 2002; 54:661–669.
38. Watson DG, Oliviera EJ. Solid-phase extraction and gas chromatography-mass spectrometry determination of kaempferol and quercetin in human urine after consumption of *Ginkgo biloba* tablets. J Chromatogr B Biomed Sci Appl 1999; 723:203–210.
39. Pietta PG, Gardana C, Mauri PL, Maffei-Facino R, Carini M. Identification of flavonoid metabolites after oral administration to rats of a *Ginkgo biloba* extract. J Chromatogr B Biomed Appl 1995; 673:75–80.
40. Watanabe CM, Woffram S, Ader PR, et al. The *in vivo* neuromodulatory effects of the herbal medicine *Ginkgo biloba*. Proc Natl Acad Sci USA 2001; 98:6577–6580.

41. Mauri PL, Simonetti P, Gardana C, et al. Liquid chromatography/ atmospheric pressure chemical ionization mass spectrometry of terpene lactones in plasma of volunteers dosed with *Ginkgo biloba* L. extracts. Rapid Commun Mass Spectrom 2001; 15:929–934.

42. Fourtillan JB, Brisson AM, Girault J, et al. Pharmacokinetic properties of bilobalide and ginkgolides A and B in healthy subjects after intravenous and oral administration of *Ginkgo biloba* extract (EGb 761). Therapie 1995; 50: 137–144.

43. Drago F, Floriddia ML, Cro M, Giuffrida S. Pharmacokinetics and bioavailability of a *Ginkgo biloba* extract. J Ocul Pharmacol Ther 2002; 18:197–202.

44. Biber A, Koch E. Bioavailability of ginkgolides and bilobalide from extracts of *Ginkgo biloba* using GC/MS. Planta Med 1999; 65:192–193.

45. Li CL, Wong YY. The bioavailability of ginkgolides in *Ginkgo biloba* extracts. Planta Med 1997; 63:563–565.

46. Brenner R, Azbel V, Madhusoodanan S, Pawlowska M. Comparison of an extract of *Hypericum* (LI 160) and sertraline in the treatment of depression: a double-blind, randomized pilot study. Clin Ther 2000; 22:411–419.

47. Harrer G, Schulz V. Clinical investigation of the antidepressant effectiveness of *Hypericum*. J Geriatr Psychiatr Neurol 1994; 7:S6–S8.

48. Philipp M, Kohnen R, Hiller K. *Hypericum* extract versus imipramine or placebo in patients with moderate depression: randomised multicentre study of treatment for eight weeks. Br Med J 1999; 319:1534–1538.

49. Schrader E. Equivalence of St John's wort extract (Ze 117) and fluoxetine: a randomized, controlled study in mild-moderate depression. Int Clin Psychopharmacol 2000; 5:61–68.

50. Volz HP. Controlled clinical trials of *Hypericum* extracts in depressed patients: an overview. Pharmacopsychiatry 1997; 30:72–76.

51. Woelk H. Comparison of St John's wort and imipramine for treating depression: randomised controlled trial. Br Med J 2000; 321:536–539.

52. Bombardelli E, Morazzoni P. *Hypericum perforatum*. Fitoterapia 1995; 66: 43–68.

53. Nahrstedt A, Butterweck V. Biologically active and other chemical constituents of the herb of *Hypericum perforatum* L. Pharmacopsychiatry 1997; 30: 129–134.

54. Nahrstedt A. Antidepressant constituents of *Hypericum perforatum*. In: Chrubasik S, Roufogalis BD, eds. Herbal Medicinal Products for the Treatment of Pain. Lismore: Southern Cross University Press, 2000:144–153.

55. Butterweck V. Mechanism of action of St. John's wort in depression: what is known? CNS Drugs 2003; 17:539–562.

56. Greeson JM, Sanford B, Monti DA. St. John's wort (Hypericum perforatum): a review of the current pharmacological, toxicological, and clinical literature. Psychopharmacology 2001; 153:402–414.

57. Mueller WE. Current St John's wort research from mode of action to clinical efficacy. Pharmacol Res Commun 2003; 47:101–109.

58. Nathan PJ. The experimental and clinical pharmacology of St. John's wort (Hypericum perforatum L.). Mol Psychiatr 1999; 4:333–338.

59. Mueller WE, Singer A, Wonnemann M, Hafner U, Rolli M, Schaefer C. Hyperforin represents the neurotransmitter reuptake inhibiting constituent of *Hypericum* extract. Pharmacopsychiatry 1998; 31:16–21.
60. Mueller WE, Singer A, Wonnemann M. Hyperforin—antidepressant activity by a novel mechanism of action. Pharmacopsychiatry 2001; 34:S98–S102.
61. Singer A, Wonnemann M, Mueller WE. Hyperforin, a major antidepressant constituent of St. John's Wort, inhibits serotonin uptake by elevating free intracellular Na$^+$. J Pharmacol Exp Ther 1999; 290:1363–1368.
62. Wonnemann M, Singer A, Siebert B, Mueller WE. Evaluation of synaptosomal uptake inhibition of most relevant constituents of St. John's wort. Pharmacopsychiatry 2001; 41:S148–S151.
63. Butterweck V, Wall A, Lieflander-Wulf U, Winterhoff H, Nahrstedt A. Effects of the total extract and fractions of *Hypericum perforatum* in animal assays for antidepressant activity. Pharmacopsychiatry 1997; 30:117–124.
64. Butterweck V, Korte B, Winterhoff H. Pharmacological and endocrine effects of *Hypericum perforatum* and hypericin after repeated treatment. Pharmacospychiatry 2001; 34:S2–S7.
65. Butterweck V, Winterhoff H, Herkenham M. St. John's wort, hypericin, and imipramine: a comparative analysis of mRNA levels in brain areas involved in HPA axis control following short-term and long-term administration in normal and stressed rats. Mol Psychiatr 2001; 6:547–564.
66. Butterweck V, Jürgenliemk G, Nahrstedt A, Winterhoff H. Flavonoids from *Hypericum perforatum* show antidepressant activity in the forced swimming test. Planta Med 2000; 66:3–6.
67. Butterweck V, Christoffel V, Nahrstedt A, Petereit F, Spengler B, Winterhoff H. Step by step removal of hyperforin and hypericin: activity profile of different *Hypericum* preparations in behavioral models. Life Sci 2003; 73:627–639.
68. Calapai G, Crupi A, Firenzuoli F, et al. Effects of *Hypericum perforatum* on levels of 5-hydroxytryptamine, noradrenaline and dopamine in the cortex, diencephalon and brainstem of the rat. J Pharm Pharmacol 1999; 51:723–728.
69. Noeldner M, Schotz K. Rutin is essential for the antidepressant activity of *Hypericum perforatum* extracts in the forced swimming test. Planta Med 2002; 68:577–580.
70. Fox E, Murphy RF, McCully CL, Adamson PC. Plasma pharmacokinetics and cerebrospinal fluid penetration of hypericin in nonhuman primates. Cancer Chemother Pharmacol 2001; 47:41–44.
71. Jacobson JM, Feinman L, Liebes L, et al. Pharmacokinetics, safety, and antiviral effects of hypericin, a derivative of St. John's wort plant, in patients with chronic hepatitis C virus infection. Antimicrob Agents Chemother 2001; 45:517–524.
72. Biber A, Fischer H, Romer A, Chatterjee SS. Oral bioavailability of hyperforin from *Hypericum* extracts in rats and human volunteers. Pharmacopsychiatry 1998; 31:36–43.
73. Brockmoeller J, Reum T, Bauer S, Kerb R, Huebner WD, Roots I. Hypericin and pseudohypericin and effects on sensitivity in humans. Pharmacopsychiatry 1997; 30:94–101.

74. Kerb R, Brockmoeller J, Staffeldt B, Ploch M, Roots I. Single-dose and steady state pharmacokinetics of hypericin and pseudohypericin. Antimicrob Agents Chemother 1996; 40:2087–2093.
75. Schempp CM, Winghofer B, Langheinrich M, Schopf E, Simon JC. Hypericin levels in human serum and interstitial skin blister fluids after oral single-dose and steady-state administration of *Hypericum perforatum* extract (St. John's wort). Skin Pharmacol Appl Skin Physiol 1999; 12:299–304.
76. Staffeldt B, Kerb R, Brockmoeller J, Ploch M, Roots I. Pharmacokinetics of hypericin and pseudohypericin after oral intake of the *Hypericum perforatum* extract LI 160 in healthy volunteers. J Geriatr Psychiatr Neurol 1994; 7:S47–S53.
77. Stock S, Hoelzl J. Pharmacokinetic tests of (14C)-labeled hypericin and pseudohypericin from *Hypericum perforatum* and serum kinetics of hypericin in man. Planta Med 1991; 57:A61.
78. Juergenliemk G, Nahrstedt A. Dissolution, solubility and cooperativity of phenolic compounds from *Hypericum perforatum* L. in aqueous systems. Pharmazie 2003; 58:200–203.
79. Agrosi M, Mischiatti S, Harrasser PC, Savio D. Oral bioavailability of active principles from herbal products in humans. A study on Hypericum perforatum extract using the soft gelatin capsule technology. Phytomedicine 2000; 7:455–462.
80. Barnes J, Anderson LA, Phillipson JD. Herbal Medicines. Bath: The Bath Press, 2002.
81. Koch HP, Reuter HD. Garlic. The Science and Therapeutic Application of *Allium sativum* L. and Related Species. Baltimore: Williams and Wilkins, 1996.
82. Reuter HD. *Allium sativum* and *Allium ursinum*: Part 2—pharmacology and medicinal application. Phytomedicine 1995; 2:73–91.
83. Mennella JA, Johnson A, Beauchamp GK. Garlic ingestion by pregnant women alters the odor of amniotic fluid. Chem Senses 1995; 20:207–209.
84. Lawson LD. Garlic: a review of its medicinal effects and indicated active compounds. In: Lawson DL, Bauer R, eds. Phytomedicines of Europe—Chemistry and Biological Activity. Washington, D.C.: American Chemical Society, 1998:176–209.
85. Lawson LD, Ranson DK, Hughes BG. Inhibition of whole blood platelet-aggregation by compounds in garlic extracts and commercial garlic products. Thromb Res 1992; 65:141–156.
86. Rosen RT, Hiserodt RD, Fukuda EK, et al. The determination of metabolites of garlic preparations in breath and human plasma. Bio Factors 2000; 13:241–249.
87. Egen-Schwind C, Eckard R, Jekat FW, Winterhoff H. Pharmacokinetics of vinyldithiins, transformation products of allicin. Planta Med 1992; 58:8–13.
88. Lachmann G, Lorenz D, Radeck W, Steiper M. The pharmacokinetics of the S35 labeled garlic constituents alliin, allicin and vinyldithiine. Arzneimittelforschung 1994; 44:734–743.
89. Nagae S, Ushijima M, Hatono S, et al. Pharmacokinetics of the garlic compound S-allylcysteine. Planta Med 1994; 60:214–217.
90. Germain E, Auger J, Ginies C, Siess MH, Teyssier C. *In vivo* metabolism of diallyl disulphide in the rat: identification of two new metabolites. Xenobiotica 2002; 32:1127–1138.

91. Meier B, Liebi M. Salicinhaltige pflanzliche Arzneimittel: Ueberlegungen zur WIrksamkeit und Unbedenklichkeit. Z Phytother 1990; 11:50–58.
92. Julkunen-Tiitto R, Meier B. The enzymatic decomposition of salicin and its derivatives obtained from salicaceae species. J Nat Prod 1992; 55:1204–1212.
93. Chrubasik S, Eisenberg E, Balan E, Weinberger T, Luzzati R, Conradt C. Treatment of low back pain exacerbations with willow bark extract: a randomized double-blind study. Am J Med 2000; 109:9–14.
94. Chrubasik S, Kunzel O, Model A, Conradt C, Black A. Treatment of low back pain with a herbal or synthetic anti-rheumatic: a randomized controlled study. Willow bark extract for low back pain. Rheumatology 2001; 40:1388–1393.
95. Chrubasik S, Kunzel O, Black A, Conradt C, Kerschbaumer F. Potential economic impact of using a proprietary willow bark extract in outpatient treatment of low back pain: an open non-randomized study. Phytomedicine 2001; 8:241–251.
96. Schmid B, Ludtke R, Selbmann HK, et al. Effectiveness and tolerance of standardized willow bark extract in arthrosis patients. Randomized, placebo controlled double-blind study. Z Rheumatol 2000; 59:314–320.
97. Steinegger E, Hövel H. Analytische und biologische Untersuchungen an Saliceen-Wirkstoffen, insbesondere an Salicin: I. Identifizierungs-, Isolierungs- und Bestimmungsmethoden. Pharm Acta Helv 1972; 47:133–141.
98. Pentz R, Busse HG, König R, Siegers CP. Bioverfügbarkeit von Salicylsäure und Coffein aus einem phytoanalgetischen Kombinationspräparat. Z Phytother 1989; 10:92–96.
99. Schmid B, Koetter I, Heide L. Pharmacokinetics of salicin after oral administration of a standardised willow bark extract. J Clin Pharmacol 2001; 57:387–391.
100. Fournier P. Le livres des plantes medicinales et veneneuses de France. Paris: P. Lechevalier, 1948:475–479.
101. Beck M, Haensel R, Keller K, Rimpler H, Schneider G, eds. Hagers Handbuch der Pharmazeutischen Praxis. Berlin: Springer, 1992:108–122.
102. Sticher O. Triterpensaponine. In: Haensel R, Sticher O, Steinegger E, eds. Pharmakognosie-Phytopharmazie. Berlin: Springer, 1999.
103. Lorenz D, Marek ML. Das therapeutische wirksame Prinzip der Rosskastanie (*Aesculus hippocastaneum*). Arzneim Forsch/Drug Res 1960; 10:263–272.
104. Lehtola T, Huhtikangas A. Radioimmunoassay of aescine, a mixture of triterpene glycosides. J Immunoassay 1990; 11:17–30.
105. Schrader E, Schwankl W, Sieder C, Christoffel V. Comparison of the bioavailability of beta-aescin after single oral administration of two different drug formulations containing an extract of horse-chestnut seeds. Pharmazie 1995; 50:623–627.
106. Oschmann R, Biber A, Lang F, Stumpf H, Kunz K. Pharmacokinetics of beta-escin after administration of various *Aesculus* extract containing formulations. Pharmazie 1996; 51:577–581.
107. Loew D, Schrodter A, Schwankl W, Marz RW. Measurement of the bioavailability of aescin-containing extracts. Methods Find Exp Clin Pharmacol 2000; 22:537–542.

108. Lang W, Mennicke WH. Pharmacokinetic studies on tritiated aescin in the mouse and rat. Arzneim Forsch/Drug Res 1972; 22:1928–1932.
109. Meyer-Bertenrath J, Kaffarnik H. Enteral resorption of aescin. Arzneim Forsch/Drug Res 1970; 20:147–148.
110. Lang W. Percutaneous absorption of 3H-aescin in mice and rats. Arzneim Forsch/Drug Res 1974; 24:71–76.
111. Murray MM. *Panax ginseng*. In: The Healing Power of Herbs. USA: Prima Publishing, 1995:265–279.
112. Mahady GB, Gyllenhall C, FIong HH, Farnsworth NR. Ginsengs: a review of safety and efficacy. Nutr Clin Care 2000; 3:90–101.
113. Martindale. British Pharmacopoeia Martindale. London: HMSO, 1996.
114. Li TSC, Harries D. Medicinal values of ginseng. Herb, Spice Medicinal Plant Digest 1996; 14:1–5.
115. Sonnenborn U, Proppert Y. Ginseng (*Panax ginseng* C. A. Meyer). Z Phytother 1990; 11:35–49.
116. Cui JF, Garle M, Bjorkhem I, Eneroth P. Determination of aglycones of ginsenosides in ginseng preparations sold in Sweden and in urine samples from Swedish athletes consuming ginseng. Scand J Clin Lab Invest 1996; 56: 151–160.
117. Cui JF, Bjorkhem I, Eneroth P. Gas chromatographic-mass spectrometric determination of 20(S)-protopanaxadiol and 20(S)-protopanaxatriol for study on human urinary excretion of ginsenosides after ingestion of ginseng preparations. J Chromatogr B Biomed Sci Appl 1997; 689:349–355.
118. Hasegawa H, Sung JH, Matsumiya S, Uchiyama M. Main ginseng saponin metabolites formed by intestinal bacteria. Planta Med 1996; 62:453–457.
119. Hasegawa H, Sung JH, Benno Y. Role of human intestinal *Prevotella oris* in hydrolyzing ginseng saponins. Planta Med 1997; 63:436–440.
120. Odani T, Tanizawa H, Takino Y. Studies on the absorption, distribution, excretion and metabolism of ginseng saponins. II. The absorption, distribution and excretion of ginsenoside Rg1 in the rat. Chem Pharm Bull 1983; 31: 292–298.
121. Odani T, Tanizawa H, Takino Y. Studies on the absorption, distribution, excretion and metabolism of ginseng saponins. III. The absorption, distribution and excretion of ginsenoside Rb1 in the rat. Chem Pharm Bull 1983; 31:1059–1066.
122. Takino Y. Studies on the pharmacodynamics of ginsenoside-Rg1, -Rb1 and -Rb2 in rats. Yakugaku Zasshi 1994; 114:550–564.
123. Arnone A, Merlini L, Zanarotti A. Constituents of *Silybum marianum*. Structure of isosilybin and stereochemistry of isosilybin. J Chem Soc (Chem Commun) 1979; 5:696–697.
124. Pelter A, Haensel R. The structure of silybib (Silybum substance E$_6$), the first flavonolignan. Tetrahedron Lett 1969; 25:2911–2916.
125. Wagner H, Seligman O, Seilz M, Abraham D, Sonnenbichler J. Silydanin und Silychristin, zwei isomere Silymarine aus *Silybum marianum*. Z Naturforsch 1976; 31b:876–884.
126. Quaglia MG, Bossu E, Donati E, Mazzanti G, Brandt A. Determination of silymarine in the extract from the dried *Silybum marianum* fruits by high

performance liquid chromatography and capillary electrophoresis. J Pharm Biomed Anal 1999; 19:435–442.

127. Leng-Peschlow E, Strenge-Hesse A. Die Mariendistel (*Silybum marianum*) und Silymarin als Lebertherapeutikum. Z Phytother 1991; 12:162–174.

128. Morazzoni P, Bombardelli E. *Silybum marianum* (*Carduus marianus*). Fitoterapia 1995; 66:3–42.

129. Saller R, Meier R, Brignoli R. The use of silymarin in the treatment of liver diseases. Drugs 2001; 61:2035–2063.

130. Zi X, Agarwal R. Silibinin decreases prostate-specific antigen with cell growth inhibition via G1 arrest, leading to differentiation of prostate carcinoma cells: implications for prostate cancer intervention. Proc Natl Acad Sci USA 1999; 96:7490–7495.

131. Sharma Y, Agarwal C, Singh AK, Agarwal R. Inhibitory effect of silibinin on ligand binding to erbB1 and associated mitogenic signaling, growth, and DNA synthesis in advanced human prostate carcinoma cells. Mol Carcinog 2001; 30:224–236.

132. Chasseaud LF. Zur biologischen Verfuegbarkeit und Verstoffwechselung von Silybin. Dtsch Apoth Ztg 1975; 115:1205–1206.

133. Koch H, Zinsberger G. Loeslichkeitsparameter von Silybin, Silydianin und Silychristin. Arch Pharm 1980; 313:526–533.

134. Froemming KH, Saller R, Waechter W. Silymarinhaltige Phytopharmaka. Biopharmazie als wesentliches therapeutisches Qualitaetskriterium. Z Arztl Fortbild Qualitaetssich 1999; 93:6–11.

135. Barzaghi N, Crema F, Gatti G, Pifferi G, Perucca E. Pharmacokinetic studies on IdB 1016, a silybin-phosphatidylcholine complex, in healthy human subjects. Eur J Drug Metab Pharmacokinet 1990; 15:333–338.

136. Morazzoni P, Magistretti MJ, Giachetti C, Zanolo G. Comparative bioavailability of Silipide, a new flavanolignan complex, in rats. Eur J Drug Metab Pharmacokinet 1992; 17:39–44.

137. Savio D, Harrasser PC, Basso G. Softgel capsule technology as an enhancer device for the absorption of natural principles in humans. Arzneim Forsch/Drug Res 1998; 48:1104–1106.

138. Schulz HU, Schurer M, Krumbiegel G, Wachter W, Weyhenmeyer R, Seidel G. The solubility and bioequivalences of silymarin preparations. Arzneim Forsch/Drug Res 1995; 45:61–64.

139. Gatti G, Perucca E. Plasma concentrations of free and conjugated silybin after oral intake of a silybin-phosphatidyl complex (silipide) in healthy volunteers. Int J Clin Pharmacol Ther 1994; 30:134–138.

140. Weyhenmeyer R, Mascher H, Birkmayer J. Study on dose-linearity of the pharmacokinetics of silibinin diastereomers using a new stereospecific assay. Int J Clin Pharmacol Ther Toxicol 1992; 30:134–138.

141. Lorenz D, Luecker PW, Mennicke WH, Wetzelsberger N. Pharmacokinetic studies with silymarin in human serum and bile. Methods Find Exp Clin Pharmacol 1984; 6:655–661.

142. Flory PJ, Krug G, Lorenz D, Mennicke WH. Studies on elimination of silymarin in cholecystectomized patients. I. Biliary and renal elimination after a single oral dose. Planta Med 1980; 38:227–237.

143. Lorenz D, Mennicke WH, Behrendt W. Elimination of silymarin by cholecystectomied patients. 2. Biliary elimination after multiple oral doses. Planta Med 1982; 45:216–223.
144. Schandalik R, Gatti G, Perucca E. Pharmacokinetics of silybin in bile following administration of silipide and silymarin in cholecystectomy patients. Arzneim Forsch/Drug Res 1992; 42:664–668.
145. Orlando R, Fragasso A, Lampertico M, et al. Pharmacokinetic study of silybin-phosphatidylcholin complex in liver cirrhosis after multiple doses. Med Sci Res 1990; 19:827–828.
146. Orlando R, Fragasso A, Lampertico M, et al. Silybin kinetics in patients with liver cirrhosis: comparative study between silybin-phosphatidylcholin complex and silymarin. Med Sci Res 1990; 18:861–863.

10

Drug–Drug, Drug–Dietary Supplement, Drug–Citrus Fruit, and Other Food Interactions—Labeling Implications

Shiew-Mei Huang and Lawrence J. Lesko

Office of Clinical Pharmacology and Biopharmaceutics, Center for Drug Evaluation and Research (CDER), Food and Drug Administration, Silver Spring, Maryland, U.S.A.

Robert Temple

Office of Medical Policy, Center for Drug Evaluation and Research (CDER), Food and Drug Administration, Silver Spring, Maryland, U.S.A.

INTRODUCTION

Serious drug–drug interactions have contributed to recent U.S. market withdrawals and nonapprovals of new molecular entities (NMEs) (1,2). In addition to coadministration of other drugs, concomitant ingestion of dietary supplement or citrus fruit or fruit juice could also alter systemic exposure, leading to adverse drug reactions or loss of drug efficacy (1,3). This chapter will discuss the labeling implications of these interactions.

METABOLISM OF NEW MOLECULAR ENTITIES AND INTERACTIONS WITH OTHER DRUGS

The interactions of concern can be divided into two types. First, other drugs can affect the blood levels of the NME by inhibiting or inducing its absorption, distribution, metabolism, or excretion pathways. Second, the NME can affect the blood levels of other drugs by inhibiting or inducing their absorption, distribution, metabolism, or excretion pathways. Of particular interest is the role of hepatic and intestinal cytochrome P450 (CYP) enzymes. Thus, "Is the drug a substrate for CYP enzymes?" and "Is the drug an inhibitor and/or an inducer of CYP enzymes?" are among the critical questions that need to be addressed when evaluating clinical pharmacology data of NMEs in new drug applications (4). Recognizing the importance of addressing these questions early in drug development, pharmaceutical companies routinely assess a NME's clearance pathways (5–11), including in vitro evaluation of a drug's metabolic pathways and its modulating effects on CYP1A2, CYP2C9, CYP2C19, CYP2D6, and CYP3A activities and subsequent clinical interaction studies based on in vitro data. In addition to CYP enzymes, other enzymes such as glucuronosyl transferases and various transporters also play important roles in drug interactions and changes in systemic exposure (1,6,10,12–16).

The clinical significance of altered systemic exposure of coadministered drugs depends on the concentration–response relationships for clinical effects, both effectiveness and toxicity (1,4,17–20). If the concentration–response relationship is well described, knowledge of the effects of interactions can lead to rational adjustment of dose or dosing interval, or to appropriate warnings and precautions. Table 1, from Food and Drug Administration's (FDA's) concept paper on drug interactions (20), suggests how metabolic and interaction information should become broadly integrated into many sections of labeling.

Table 1   Drug Interactions—Labeling Implications

All relevant information on the metabolic pathways, metabolites, and
pharmacokinetic interactions should be included in the "Pharmacokinetics"
subsection of the "Clinical Pharmacology" section of the labeling. The clinical
consequences of metabolism and interactions should be placed in "Drug
Interactions, Warnings and Precautions, Boxed Warnings, Contraindications, or
Dosage and Administration" sections, as appropriate. Such information related to
clinical consequences should not be included in detail in more than one section, but
rather referenced from one section to other sections as needed. When the metabolic
pathway or interaction data resulted in recommendations for dosage adjustments,
contraindications, and warnings (e.g., coadministration should be avoided), which
were included in the "Boxed Warnings, Contraindications, Warnings and
Precautions, or Dosage and Administration" sections, these recommendations
should also be included in "Highlights." Refer to the guidance for industry entitled
"Labeling for Human Prescription Drug and Biological Products—Implementing
the New Content and Format Requirements (21)" and "Drug Interaction Studies-
Study Design, Data Analysis, and Implications for Dosing and Labeling (22,23)"
for more information on presenting drug interaction information in labeling

Source: From Ref. 20.

    Labeling descriptions of drug–drug interactions can be based on interactions observed in clinical studies or projected interactions extrapolated from other studies. As shown in Figure 1, if a drug is shown not to inhibit a particular CYP enzyme based on in vitro data, labeling will indicate no interaction with substrates of that CYP. For example, the current ABILIFY® labeling (May 2004 labeling) states that "aripiprazole and dehydro-aripiprazole did not show potential for altering CYP1A2-mediated metabolism *in vitro*" (24).

    Table 2A shows labeling examples for drugs that are substrates of CYP enzymes, where the drug interaction data have implications for their dosing and administration. If a drug has been determined to be a sensitive CYP3A substrate (e.g., budesonide, buspirone, eletriptan, eplerenone, felodipine, lovastatin, midazolam, saquinavir, sildenafil, simvastatin, triazolam, and vardenafil) or a CYP3A substrate with a narrow therapeutic range (e.g., alfentanil, astemizole, cisapride, cyclosporine, diergotamine, ergotamine, fentanyl, pimozide, quinidine, sirolimus, tacrolimus, and terfenadine), it does not need to be tested with all strong or moderate inhibitors of CYP3A, to warn about an interaction with "strong" or "moderate" CYP3A

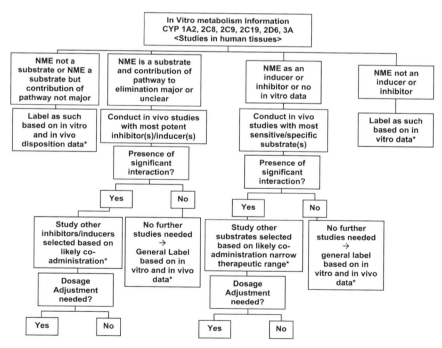

* Additional population pharmacokinetic analysis may assist the overall evaluation

Figure 1 CYP-based drug–drug interaction studies decision tree. *Source*: Adapted from Ref. 7. *Abbreviation*: NME, new molecular entity.

Table 2A Labeling Examples of Drug–Drug Interactions (Evaluation of Drugs as Substrates for CYP Enzymes)

Drug name	Labeling section	Labeling
RELPAX® (Pfizer) (eletriptan) tablets September 2003 labeling	*Warnings and Dosage and Administration*	Eletriptan should not be used within at least 72 hours of treatment with the following potent CYP3A4 inhibitors: ketoconazole, itraconazole, nefazodone, troleandomycin, clarithromycin, ritonavir, and nelfinavir. Eletriptan should not be used within 72 hours with drugs that have demonstrated potent CYP3A4 inhibition and have this potent effect described in the *"Contraindications, Warnings or Precautions"* sections of their labeling (see *"Clinical Pharmacology*: Drug Interactions and *Dosage and Administration"*)
LEVITRA® (Bayer) (vardenafil) tablets January 2004 labeling	*Dosage and Administration*	Concomitant medications: The dosage of LEVITRA may require adjustment in patients receiving certain CYP3A4 inhibitors (e.g., ketoconazole, itraconazole, ritonavir, indinavir, and erythromycin) (see *"Warnings, Precautions*: Drug Interactions"). For ritonavir, a single dose of 2.5 mg LEVITRA should not be exceeded in a 72-hr period. For indinavir, ketoconazole 400 mg daily, and itraconazole 400 mg daily, a single dose of 2.5 mg LEVITRA should not be exceeded in a 24-hr period. For ketoconazole 200 mg daily, itraconazole 200 mg daily, and erythromycin, a single dose of 5 mg LEVITRA should not be exceeded in a 24-hr period
INSPRA™ (Pfizer) (eplerenone) tablets October 2003 labeling	*Contraindications Dosage and Administration*: Hypertension	INSPRA is contraindicated in all patients with the following: Concomitant use with the following potent CYP3A4 inhibitors: ketoconazole, itraconazole, nefazodone, troleandomycin, clarithromycin, ritonavir, and nelfinavir. INSPRA should also not be used with other drugs noted in the

(Continued)

Table 2A Labeling Examples of Drug–Drug Interactions (Evaluation of Drugs as Substrates for CYP Enzymes) (*Continued*)

Drug name	Labeling section	Labeling
		"Contraindications, Warnings or Precautions" sections of their labeling as potent CYP3A4 inhibitors (see *"Clinical Pharmacology*: Drug–Drug Interactions; *Precautions*: Congestive Heart Failure Post-Myocardial Infarction and Hypertension, and Drug Interactions; and *Dosage and Administration*: Hypertension") For patients receiving weak CYP3A4 inhibitors, such as erythromycin, saquinavir, verapamil, and fluconazole, the starting dose should be reduced to 25 mg once daily (see *"Contraindications and Precautions*: Congestive Heart Failure Post-Myocardial Infarction and Hypertension, and Drug Interactions")

Abbreviation: CYP, cytochrome P450.
Source: From Refs. 24, 26, 27.

inhibitors (20,25). For example, the labeling of RELPAX® (Table 2A) indicates that it should not be taken with strong CYP3A inhibitors such as ketoconazole, itraconazole, nefazodone, troleandomycin, clarithromycin, ritonavir, and nelfinavir. The interactions with itraconazole, nefazodone, troleandomycin, clarithromycin, ritonavir, and nelfinavir have not been evaluated; the warnings are based on data from a clinical interaction study conducted with ketoconazole and on other relevant in vitro data.

Table 2B shows labeling examples of drugs that are inhibitors or inducers of CYP enzymes. Labeling of drugs as "strong" or "potent" CYP3A inhibitors can facilitate, for example, the projection of its interaction with other sensitive substrates. Examples of "strong CYP3A inhibitors" include atanazavir, clarithromycin, indinavir, itraconazole, ketoconazole, nefazodone, nelfinavir, ritonavir, saquinavir, telithromycin, etc. These are drugs that increase the area under the plasma concentration-time curve (AUC) of either orally administered midazolam or other CYP3A substrates by five-fold or greater (20,25). Examples of "moderate CYP3A inhibitors" include amprenavir, aprepitant, diltiazem, erythromycin, fluconazole, fosaprenavir, (grapefruit juice), verapamil, etc. These are drugs that increase the AUC of

Table 2B Labeling Examples of Drug–Drug Interactions (Drugs as Inhibitors or Inducers of CYP Enzymes)

Drug name	Labeling section	Labeling
KETEK™ (Aventis) (telithromycin) tablets March 2004 labeling	*Contraindications*	Concomitant administration of KETEK with cisapride or pimozide is contraindicated (see *"Clinical Pharmacology*: Drug–Drug Interactions and *Precautions"*)
	Precautions: Drug Interactions	Telithromycin is a strong inhibitor of the CYP3A4 system. Coadministration of KETEK tablets and a drug primarily metabolized by the CYP3A4 enzyme system may result in increased plasma concentration of the drug coadministered with telithromycin that could increase or prolong both the therapeutic and adverse effects. Therefore, appropriate dosage adjustments may be necessary for the drug coadministered with telithromycin
RIFADIN® (Aventis) (rifampin) capsules January 2004 labeling	*Precautions*: Drug Interactions	Enzyme induction: Rifampin is known to induce certain CYP enzymes. Administration of rifampin with drugs that undergo biotransformation through these metabolic pathways may accelerate elimination of coadministered drugs. To maintain optimum therapeutic blood levels, dosages of drugs metabolized by these enzymes may require adjustment when starting or stopping concomitantly administered rifampin
BIAXIN® (Abbott) (clarithromycin tablets, extended-release tablets, suspension) December 2003 labeling	*Contraindications*	Concomitant administration of clarithromycin with cisapride, pimozide, astemizole, or terfenadine is contraindicated. There have been postmarketing reports of drug interactions when clarithromycin and/ or erythromycin are coadministered with cisapride, pimozide, astemizole, or terfenadine resulting in cardiac arrhythmias (QT prolongation, ventricular tachycardia, ventricular fibrillation, and torsades de pointes),

(Continued)

Table 2B Labeling Examples of Drug–Drug Interactions (Drugs as Inhibitors or Inducers of CYP Enzymes) (*Continued*)

Drug name	Labeling section	Labeling
KALETRA® (Abbott) (lopinavir/ ritonavir) capsules or oral solution February 2004 labeling		most likely due to inhibition of metabolism of these drugs by erythromycin and clarithromycin. Fatalities have been reported
	Contraindications	Coadministration of KALETRA is contraindicated with drugs that are highly dependent on CYP3A for clearance and for which elevated plasma concentrations are associated with serious and/or life-threatening events. These drugs are listed in Table 7
	Warnings: Drug Interactions	KALETRA is an inhibitor of the P450 isoform CYP3A. Coadministration of KALETRA and drugs primarily metabolized by CYP3A may result in increased plasma concentrations of the other drug that could increase or prolong its therapeutic and adverse effects (see Pharmacokinetics: Drug–Drug Interactions, *Contraindications*—Table 7: Drugs That Are Contraindicated With KALETRA, *Precautions*—Table 8: Drugs That Should Not Be Coadministered With KALETRA and Table 9: Established and Other Potentially Significant Drug Interactions.)
	Precautions: Drug Interactions	Decrease indinavir dose to 600 mg b.i.d., when coadministered with KALETRA 400/100 mg b.i.d. (see "*Clinical Pharmacology*": Table 3A) Sildenafil: Use with caution at reduced doses of 25 mg every 48 hours with increased monitoring for adverse events

Abbreviation: CYP, cytochrome P450.
Source: From Refs. 24, 26, 27.

orally administered midazolam or other sensitive CYP3A substrates by two-fold or greater, but less than fivefold (20,25). The labeling of KETEK™ (Table 2B) indicates that telithromycin is a strong inhibitor of CYP3A, that its concomitant use with simvastatin, lovastatin, or atorvastatin should be avoided, and that its use is contraindicated with cisapride and pimozide.

Note that the warnings in the labeling about interactions with lovastatin, atorvastatin, and pimozide are based on extrapolation from clinical studies with simvastatin and cisapride.

EFFECT OF DIETARY SUPPLEMENTS ON NEW MOLECULAR ENTITIES AND INTERACTIONS

St. John's Wort

FDA has received adverse-event reports that suggested a role of St. John's wort in reducing the effectiveness of a number of drugs, such as cyclosporine (e.g., transplant rejection), oral contraceptives (e.g., breakthrough bleedings and pregnancy), and sildenafil (e.g., loss of efficacy) (28). Chapter 12 provides details of these observations. Chapter 4 discusses the results of studies to evaluate the effects of St. John's wort on various CYP enzymes and transporters, findings that St. John's wort is generally an inducer of CYP3A, P-glycoprotein (P-gp), and other CYP enzymes.

Impact on Drug Labeling

As the effect of an enzyme inducer is reasonably predictable, the current labeling recommendation is that, for drugs that are substrates of CYP3A or P-gp, and when the products' effectiveness would be reduced upon coadministration of St. John's wort, St. John's wort should be listed along with other known inducers, such as rifampin, rifabutin, rifapentin, dexamethasone, phenytoin, carbamazepine, phenobarbital, etc., in the labeling as possibly decreasing the plasma levels. Table 3A lists 17 examples of St. John's wort–drug interactions. Another 38 drug products with similar labeling languages are listed in the footnotes. Of these 55 labels, only two labels, CRIXIVAN® and INSPRA™, are based on actual clinical studies on these drug products. The others either indicate that there are reports of interactions (e.g., NEORAL® and TRIPHASIL®) or that there are mechanistic reasons and there is the potential for interactions (e.g., AGENERASE®, ALESSE®, and UNIPHIL). Several products with teratogenic potential (e.g., ACCU-TANE® and THALOMID®) list interactions not directly related to the drug products, but to the oral contraceptives that need to be taken. Except for ACCUTANE, whose warning about the interaction with St. John's wort is in the "Contraindications" section, all current labelings on St. John's wort appear either in the "Warnings" or the "Precautions" sections, the two sections that will be combined in one section "Warnings/Precautions" under the new labeling rule (21). A recently published guidance for industry entitled "Labeling for combined oral contraceptives" includes labeling language on drug interactions between oral contraceptives and St. John's wort, such as "Herbal products containing St. John's wort (*Hypericum perforatum*) may induce hepatic enzymes (cytochrome P450) and P-glycoprotein transporter and may reduce the effectiveness of contraceptive steroids. This may also

Table 3A St. John's Wort Interactions in Labeling of Drug Products

Drug name	Labeling section	Labeling
ACCUTANE® (Isotretinoin) Roche August 2003 labeling	*Contraindications and Warnings*	Patients should be prospectively cautioned not to self-medicate with the herbal supplement St. John's wort, because a possible interaction has been suggested with hormonal contraceptives based on reports of breakthrough bleeding on oral contraceptives shortly after starting St. John's wort. Pregnancies have been reported by users of combined hormonal contraceptives who also used some form of St. John's wort (see "*Precautions*")[a]
AGENERASE® (amprenavir) GSK February 2004 labeling	*Warnings*	Concomitant use of drug product and St. John's "wort" (*Hypericum perforatum*) or products containing St. John's wort" is not recommended. Coadministration of protease inhibitors with drug product and St. John's "wort" is expected to substantially decrease protease inhibitor concentrations and may result in suboptimal levels of drug product and may lead to loss of virologic response and possible resistance to the drug product or to the class of protease inhibitors[b]
ALESSE® 28 (levonorgestrel and ethinyl estradiol tablets) Wyeth April 2004 labeling	*Precautions*: Drug Interactions	Herbal products containing St. John's wort (*H. perforatum*) may induce hepatic enzymes (CYP) and P-gp transporter and may reduce the effectiveness of contraceptive steroids. This may also result in breakthrough bleeding[c]
AROMASIN® (Pharmacia & Upjohn) (exemestane tablets) March 2004	*Precautions*: Drug Interactions	Comedications that induce CYP3A4 (e.g., rifampicin, phenytoin, carbamazepine, phenobarbital, or St. John's wort) may significantly decrease exposure to exemestane. Dose modification is recommended for patients who are also receiving a potent CYP3A4 inducer (see "*Dosage and Administration* and *Clinical Pharmacology*")

(*Continued*)

Table 3A St. John's Wort Interactions in Labeling of Drug Products (*Continued*)

Drug name	Labeling section	Labeling
CENESTIN® (Duramed) (synthetic conjugated estrogens) February 2004 labeling	*Clinical Pharmacology*: Drug Interactions	Inducers of CYP3A4 such as St. John's wort preparations (*H. perforatum*), phenobarbital, carbamazepine, and rifampin may reduce plasma concentrations of estrogens, possibly resulting in a decrease in therapeutic effects and/or changes in the uterine bleeding profile[d]
COUMADIN® (Bristol-Myers Squibb) (warfarin) tablets, and for Injection June 2002 labeling	*Precautions—Exogenous Factors*	Botanical (herbal) medicines Coenzyme Q_{10}(ubidecarenone) and St. John's "wort" are associated most often with a *decrease* in the effects of COUMADIN[e]
	Information for patients	Do not take or discontinue any other medication, including salicylates (e.g., aspirin and topical analgesics), other over-the-counter medications, and botanical (herbal) products (e.g., bromelains, coenzyme Q_{10}, danshen, dong quai, garlic, *Ginkgo biloba*, ginseng, and St. John's "wort") except on advice of the physician
CRIXIVAN® (Merck) (indinavir sulfate) capsules May 2004 labeling	*Warnings*: Drug Interactions	Concomitant use of CRIXIVAN and St. John's "wort" (*H. perforatum*) or products containing St. John's "wort" is not recommended. Coadministration of CRIXIVAN and St. John's "wort" has been shown to substantially decrease indinavir concentrations (see "*Clinical Pharmacology*: Drug Interactions") and may lead to loss of virologic response and possible resistance to CRIXIVAN or to the class of protease inhibitors
NEORAL® (Novartis) (cyclosporine capsules, oral solution, USP) March 2004 labeling	*Precautions*: Drug Interactions	There have been reports of a serious drug interaction between cyclosporine and the herbal dietary supplement, St. John's "wort". This interaction has been reported to produce a marked reduction in the blood concentrations of cyclosporine, resulting in subtherapeutic levels, rejection of transplanted organs, and graft loss[f]

GLEEVEC® (Novartis) (imatinib mesylate) tablets July 2004 labeling	*Precautions*: Drug Interactions	Substances that are inducers of CYP3A4 activity may increase metabolism and decrease imatinib plasma concentrations. Comedications that induce CYP3A4 (e.g., dexamethasone, phenytoin, carbamazepine, rifampin, phenobarbital, or St. John's wort) may significantly reduce exposure to GLEEVEC. Pretreatment of healthy volunteers with multiple doses of rifampin followed by a single dose of GLEEVEC, increased GLEEVEC oral-dose clearance by 3.8-fold, which significantly ($P < 0.05$) decreased mean C_{max} and $AUC_{(0-\infty)}$. In patients where rifampin or other CYP3A4 inducers are indicated, alternative therapeutic agents with less enzyme induction potential should be considered (see "*Clinical Pharmacology and Dosage and Administration*")
INSPRA™ (Pfizer) (eplerenone tablets) October 2003	*Clinical Pharmacology*: Drug Interactions	St. Johns "wort" (a CYP3A4 inducer) caused a small (about 30%) decrease in eplerenone AUC
Mifepristone (Mifeprex ®) November 2004 labeling	*Precautions*: Drug Interactions	Although specific drug or food interactions with mifepristone have not been studied, on the basis of this drug's metabolism by CYP3A4, it is possible that ketoconazole, itraconazole, erythromycin, and grapefruit juice may inhibit its metabolism (increasing serum levels of mifepristone). Furthermore, rifampin, dexamethasone, St. John's wort, and certain anticonvulsants (e.g., phenytoin, phenobarbital, and carbamazepine) may induce mifepristone metabolism (lowering serum levels of mifepristone)
ORTHO TRI-CYCLEN®, ORTHO-CYCLEN® tablets (Ortho-McNeil) (norgestimate/ethinyl estradiol) March 2001 labeling	*Precautions*: Drug Interactions	A possible interaction has been suggested with hormonal contraceptives and the herbal supplement St. Johns "wort" based on some reports of oral contraceptive users experiencing breakthrough bleeding shortly after starting St. Johns "wort". Pregnancies have been reported by users of combined hormonal contraceptives who also used some form of St. Johns "wort". Healthcare prescribers are advised to consult the package inserts of medication administered concomitantly with oral contraceptives

(Continued)

Table 3A St. John's Wort Interactions in Labeling of Drug Products (*Continued*)

Drug name	Labeling section	Labeling
VRETTE® Tablets (Wyeth-Ayerst) (norgestrel tablets) October 2003 labeling	*Precautions*: Drug Interactions	The effectiveness of progestin-only pills is reduced by hepatic enzyme-inducing drugs such as the anticonvulsants, phenytoin, carbamazepine; barbiturates; the antituberculosis drug rifampin; protease inhibitors; and herbal preparations containing St. John's "wort" (*H. perforatum*)
PACERONE® (Upsher-Smith) (Amiodarone HCl) August 2003 labeling	*Precautions*: Drug Interactions	St. John's "wort" (*H. perforatum*) induces CYP3A4. Because drug product is a substrate for CYP3A4, there is the potential that the use of St. John's "wort" in patients receiving drug product could result in reduced amiodarone levels[g]
THALOMID® (Celgene) (thalidomide) capsules February 2004 labeling	*Precautions*: Important Non-Thalidomide Drug Interactions	Drugs That Interfere with Hormonal Contraceptives: Concomitant use of HIV-protease inhibitors, griseofulvin, modafinil, penicillins, rifampin, rifabutin, phenytoin, carbamazepine, or certain herbal supplements such as St. John's "wort" with hormonal contraceptive agents may reduce the effectiveness of the contraception and up to one month after discontinuation of these concomitant therapies. Therefore, women requiring treatment with one or more of these drugs must use two *other* effective or highly effective methods of contraception or abstain from heterosexual sexual contact while taking thalidomide
TRIPHASIL®-28 (Wyeth-Ayerst) Tablets (levonorgestrel and ethinyl estradiol tablets—triphasic regimen) June 2004 labeling	*Precautions*: Drug Interactions	Reduced ethinyl estradiol concentrations have been associated with concomitant use of substances that induce hepatic microsomal enzymes, such as rifampin, rifabutin, barbiturates, phenylbutazone, phenytoin sodium, griseofulvin, topiramate, some protease inhibitors, modafinil, and possibly St. John's "wort"

UNIPHYL® Tablets (Purdue Frederick) (theophylline, anhydrous) 400 and 600 mg UNICONTIN® Controlled-Release System March 2004 labeling	*Precautions*: Information for Patients	The dietary supplement St. John's "wort" (*H. perforatum*) should not be taken at the same time as theophylline, because it may result in decreased theophylline levels. If patients are already taking St. John's "wort" and theophylline together, they should consult their healthcare professional before stopping the St. John's "wort," because their theophylline concentrations may rise when this is done, resulting in toxicity

[a]Similar labeling language also in the labeling of AMNESTEEM (Isotretinoin) Mylan, May 2004 and SORIATANE® (Connetics) (acitretin) capsules, March 2004.

[b]Similar labeling language also in the labeling of JANTOVEN™ (Upsher-Smith) (warfarin sodium tablets, USP), July 2003; NORVIR® (Abbott) (ritonavir capsules) Soft Gelatin (ritonavir oral solution), October 2003; RESCRIPTOR® (Pfizer) brand of delavirdine mesylate tablets, August 2003; REYATAZ® (Bristol-Myers Squibb) (atazanavir sulfate) capsules, July 2004; SUSTIVA® (Bristol-Myers Squibb) (efavirenz) capsules and tablets Rx Only, June 2003; VIRACEPT® (Pfizer) (nelfinavir mesylate) tablets and oral powder, May 2004; VIRAMUNE® (Boehringer Ingelheim) (nevirapine) tablets VIRAMUNE (nevirapine) oral suspension, January 2004; and FORTOVASE® (Roche Laboratories) (saquinavir) soft gelatin capsules, December 2003.

[c]Similar labeling language also in the labeling of LO/OVRAL®-28 (Wyeth-Ayerst) tablets (norgestrel and ethinyl estradiol tablets), April 2004; LUNELLE™ Monthly (Pharmacia & Upjohn) Contraceptive Injection medroxyprogesterone acetate and estradiol cypionate injectable suspension, July 2001; NUVARING® (Organon, U.S.) (etonogestrel/ethinyl estradiol vaginal ring), October 2003; ORTHO EVRA® (Ortho-McNeil) (norelgestromin/ethinyl estradiol transdermal system), May 2003; ORTHO TRI-CYCLEN® LO tablets (Ortho-McNeil) 18 (norgestimate/ethinyl estradiol), August 2002; ORTHO-CEPT® (Ortho-McNeil) 18 (desogestrel and ethinyl estradiol) tablets, January 2004; OVRAL®-28 (Wyeth-Ayerst) tablets (norgestrel and ethinyl estradiol tablets) 0.15 mg/0.03 mg, September 2003; and YASMIN® 28 tablets (Berlex) (drospirenone and ethinyl estradiol), June 2003.

[d]Similar labeling language also in the labeling of CLIMARA® (Berlex) (estradiol transdermal system), continuous delivery for once-weekly application, January 2004; COMBIPATCH® (Novartis) (estradiol/norethindrone acetate transdermal system), July 2004; ESTRASORB® (Novavax), (estradiol topical emulsion), October 2003; ESTROGEL® 0.06% (Solvay) (estradiol gel), March 2004; CLIMARA PRO™ (Berlex) (estradiol/levonorgestrel transdermal system); November 2003; FEMTRACE® (Warner Chilcott) (estradiol acetate tablets), August 2004; MENOSTAR™ (Berlex) (estradiol transdermal system), June 2004; PREMARIN® (Wyeth-Ayerst) Intravenous (conjugated estrogens, USP) for injection specially prepared for intravenous and intramuscular use, July 2004; PREMARIN (Wyeth-Ayerst) (conjugated estrogen tablets, USP), August 2004; PREMARIN (Wyeth-Ayerst) (conjugated estrogens) vaginal cream in a nonliquefying base, July 2004; PREMPRO™ (Wyeth-Ayerst) (conjugated estrogens/medroxyprogesterone acetate tablets), August 2004; and PREMPHASE® (conjugated estrogens/medroxyprogesterone acetate tablets), August 2004; and VIVELLE-DOT® (Novartis) (estradiol transdermal system), Continuous delivery for twice-weekly application, February 2004.

Table 3A   St. John's Wort Interactions in Labeling of Drug Products (*Continued*)

eSimilar labeling language also in the labeling of INVIRASE® (Roche Laboratories) (saquinavir mesylate) capsules, December 2003; KALETRA® (Abbott) (lopinavir/ritonavir) capsules, (lopinavir/ritonavir) oral solution, February 2004; and LEXIVA® (GlaxoSmithKline) (fosamprenavir calcium) tablets, May 2004.

fSimilar labeling language also in the labeling of PROGRAF® (Fujisawa) tacrolimus capsules, tacrolimus injection (for intravenous infusion only), July 2001; RAPAMUNE® (Wyeth-Ayerst) (sirolimus) oral solution and tablets, August 2004; and GENGRAF® capsules (Abbott) (cyclosporine) capsules, USP, January 2003.

gSimilar labeling language also in the labeling of SANDIMMUNE® (Novartis) (cyclosporine capsules or oral solution, USP), SANDIMMUNE® injection (cyclosporine injection, USP). May 2004.

Abbreviations: AUC, area under the plasma concentration–time curve; CYP, cytochrome P450; P-gp, P-glycoprotein.
Source: From Refs. 24, 26, 27.

Table 3B St. John's Wort–Drug Interactions in Labeling of St. John's Wort
Products

Drug name	Labeling
Herbal outlook or similar product (Panda) St. John's Kava Kava (ForMor)	*Warning*: St. John's wort can have potentially dangerous interactions with some prescription drugs. Consult your physician before taking St. John's wort if you are currently taking anticoagulants, oral contraceptives, antidepressants, antiseizure medications, drugs to treat HIV or prevent transplant rejection, or any other prescription drug. This product is not recommended for use if you are or could be pregnant unless a qualified health care provider tells you to use it. The product may not be safe for your developing baby

Source: From Ref. 20.

result in breakthrough bleeding" (29). Several St. John's wort products also
carry warning language about potential interactions with various drug products (Table 3B) (30).

EFFECT OF CITRUS FRUIT/FRUIT JUICE ON NEW MOLECULAR ENTITIES

Grapefruit Juice Effects on CYP3A

FDA has received adverse-event reports that implicated grapefruit juice in
the observed exaggeration of pharmacological effects or adverse drug
reactions for calcium channel blockers (e.g., resulting in hypotension),
statins (e.g., leading to muscle pain), antihistamines (e.g., QT prolongation
and arrhythmias), and others (31–33). Chapter 13 describes details of these
reports. Clinical pharmacology studies have also clearly shown that concomitant grapefruit juice ingestion increased the systemic exposure of orally
administered drugs that are CYP3A substrates and have low oral bioavailability due to extensive presystemic extraction contributed by enteric
CYP3A. Chapter 7 discusses grapefruit juice's modulating effects on various
CYP enzymes and transporters.

Impact on Drug Labeling

The current labeling recommendation is that, for drugs that are primarily
substrates of CYP3A with low oral bioavailability due to extensive presystemic extraction, grapefruit juice should be listed along with other CYP3A
inhibitors in the labeling as possibly increasing the plasma levels of coadministered drugs. Table 4 lists 28 labeling examples of grapefruit juice–drug

Table 4 Labeling Examples of Drug–Grapefruit Juice Interactions

Drug name	Labeling section	Labeling
ABILIFY® (Otsuka America; Bristol-Myers Squibb) (aripiprazole) May 2004 labeling	*Precautions*: Drug–drug interactions	When concomitant administration of ketoconazole with aripiprazole occurs, aripiprazole dose should be reduced to one-half of its normal dose. Other strong inhibitors of CYP3A4 (itraconazole) would be expected to have similar effects and need similar dose reductions; weaker inhibitors (erythromycin, "grapefruit" "juice") have not been studied
ALLEGRA-D® 24 HOUR (Aventis) (fexofenadine HCl 180 mg and pseudoephedrine HCl 240 mg) extended-release tablets October 2004 labeling	*Dosage and Administration*	The recommended dose of ALLEGRA-D 24 HOUR extended-release tablets is one tablet once daily administered with water on an empty stomach, for adults and children 12 years of age and older
	Precautions: Drug Interactions	Fruit juices such as grapefruit, orange, and apple may reduce the bioavailability and exposure of fexofenadine. This is based on the results from three clinical studies using histamine-induced skin wheals and flares coupled with population pharmacokinetic analysis. Therefore, to maximize the effects of fexofenadine, it is recommended that ALLEGRA-D 24 HOUR *should be taken with water*
ADALAT® CC (Bayer) (nifedipine) January 2004 labeling	*Dosage and Administration*	Coadministration of nifedipine with "grapefruit" "juice" is to be avoided (see "*Clinical Pharmacology* and *Precautions*")
	Precautions: Other interactions	Grapefruit juice: Coadministration of nifedipine with "grapefruit" "juice" results in up to a twofold increase in AUC and C_{max}, due to inhibition of CYP3A4-related first-pass metabolism. This effect of "grapefruit" "juice" may last for at least three days. Administration of nifedipine with "grapefruit" "juice" is to be avoided

ADVICOR® (Kos) (niacin extended-release/lovastatin tablets) November 2003 labeling	*Warnings*	The risk of myopathy appears to be increased by high levels of HMG-CoA reductase inhibitory activity in plasma. Lovastatin is metabolized by the CYP isoform 3A4. Certain drugs, that share this metabolic pathway can raise the plasma levels of lovastatin and may increase the risk of myopathy. These include cyclosporine, itraconazole, ketoconazole and other antifungal azoles, the macrolide antibiotics erythromycin and clarithromycin, HIV protease inhibitors, the antidepressant nefazodone, or large quantities of "grapefruit" "juice" (greater than 1 quart daily)
	Precautions *Clinical Pharmacology:* Pharmacokinetics absorption	Should not be administered with "grapefruit" "juice" Lovastatin absorption appears to be increased by at least 30% by "grapefruit" "juice"; however, the effect is dependent on the amount of "grapefruit" "juice" consumed and the interval between "grapefruit" "juice" and lovastatin ingestion
MEVACOR® (Merck) (Lovastatin) tablets June 2002 labeling	*Clinical Pharmacology:* Absorption	Lovastatin is a substrate for CYP3A4 (see "*Precautions*: Drug Interactions"). "Grapefruit" "juice" contains one or more components that inhibit CYP3A4 and can increase the plasma concentrations of drugs metabolized by CYP3A4. In one study (1), 10 subjects consumed 200 mL of double-strength "grapefruit" "juice" (one can of frozen concentrate diluted with one rather than three cans of water) three times daily for two days and an additional 200 mL double-strength "grapefruit" "juice" together with and 30 and 90 min following a single dose of 80 mg lovastatin on the third day. This regimen of "grapefruit" "juice" resulted in mean increases in the concentration of lovastatin and its beta-hydroxyacid metabolite

(Continued)

Table 4 Labeling Examples of Drug–Grapefruit Juice Interactions (*Continued*)

Drug name	Labeling section	Labeling
		(as measured by the area under the concentration-time curve) of 15-fold and fivefold respectively (as measured using a chemical assay—liquid chromatography/tandem mass spectrometry). In a second study, 15 subjects consumed one 8 oz glass of single-strength "grapefruit" "juice" (one can of frozen concentrate diluted with three cans of water) with breakfast for three consecutive days and a single dose of 40 mg lovastatin in the evening of the third day. This regimen of "grapefruit" "juice" resulted in a mean increase in the plasma concentration (as measured by the area under the concentration-time curve) of active and total HMG-CoA reductase inhibitory activity [using a validated enzyme inhibition assay different from that used in the first study, both before (for active inhibitors) and after (for total inhibitors) base hydrolysis] of 1.34-fold and 1.36-fold, respectively, and of lovastatin and its (beta)-hydroxyacid metabolite (measured using a chemical assay—liquid chromatography/tandem mass spectrometry) of 1.94-fold and 1.57-fold, respectively. The effect of amounts of "grapefruit" "juice" between those used in these two studies on lovastatin pharmacokinetics has not been studied
	Warnings	The risk of myopathy/rhabdomyolysis is increased by concomitant use of lovastatin with the following: Potent inhibitors of CYP3A4: Cyclosporine, itraconazole, ketoconazole, erythromycin, clarithromycin, HIV protease inhibitors, nefazodone, or large quantities of "grapefruit" "juice" (greater than 1 quart daily), particularly with higher

Drug	Labeling section	Description
BILTRICIDE® (Bayer) (praziquantel) tablets August 2004 labeling	*Clinical Pharmacology*	doses of lovastatin (see below: *"Clinical Pharmacology:* Pharmacokinetics; *Precautions:* Drug Interactions, CYP3A4 Interactions")
	Drug–drug interactions	"Grapefruit" "juice" was reported to produce a 1.6-fold increase in the C_{max} and a 1.9-fold increase in the AUC of praziquantel. However, the effect of this exposure increase on the therapeutic effect and safety of praziquantel has not been systematically evaluated
CENESTIN® (Duramed) (synthetic conjugated estrogens, A) February 2004 labeling	*Clinical Pharmacology:* Drug–drug interactions	Inhibitors of CYP3A4 such as erythromycin, clarithromycin, ketoconazole, itraconazole, ritonavir and "grapefruit" "juice" may increase plasma concentrations of estrogens and may result in side effects[c]
CIALIS® (Lilly ICOS) (tadalafil) November 2003 labeling	*Precautions:* Drug–drug interactions	Ketoconazole (400 mg daily), a selective and potent inhibitor of CYP3A4, increased tadalafil 20-mg single-dose exposure (AUC) by 312%. *Other CYP inhibitors*—Although specific interactions have not been studied, other CYP3A4 inhibitors, such as erythromycin, itraconazole, and "grapefruit" "juice," would likely increase tadalafil exposure.
CLARINEX® (Schering) (desloratadine) tablets, syrup, Reditabs® tablets August 2004 labeling	*Clinical Pharmacology:* Drug–drug interactions	Neither food nor "grapefruit" "juice" had an effect on the bioavailability (C_{max} and AUC) of desloratadine
COVERA-HS® (Searle) (verapamil hydrochloride) extended-release tablets July 2003 labeling	*Precautions:* Drug–drug interactions	"Grapefruit" "juice" may significantly increase concentrations of verapamil. "Grapefruit" "juice" given to nine healthy volunteers increased S- and R-verapamil AUC_{0-12} by 36% and 28%, respectively. Steady-state C_{max} and C_{min} of S-verapamil

(Continued)

Table 4 Labeling Examples of Drug–Grapefruit Juice Interactions (*Continued*)

Drug name	Labeling section	Labeling
		increased by 57% and 16.7%, respectively, with "grapefruit" "juice" compared to control. Similarly, C_{max} and C_{min} of R-verapamil increased by 40% and 13%, respectively. "Grapefruit" "juice" did not affect half-life, nor was there a significant change in AUC_{0-12} ratio R/S compared to control. "Grapefruit" "juice" did not cause a significant difference in the PK of norverapamil. This increase in verapamil plasma concentration is not expected to have any clinical consequence[b]
CRIXIVAN® (Merck) (indinavir sulfate) capsules May 2004 labeling	*Clinical Pharmacology*	AUC ratio (with/without coadministered drug) of Indinavir (90% CI): 0.73 (0.60, 0.87)
GENGRAF® (Abbott) (cyclosporine) capsules January 2003 labeling	*Dosage and Administration*	Grapefruit and "grapefruit" "juice" affect metabolism, increasing blood concentration of cyclosporine, and thus should be avoided
	Precautions	Patients should be advised to take Gengraf® on a consistent schedule with regard to time of day and relation to meals. Grapefruit and "grapefruit" "juice" affect metabolism, increasing blood concentration of cyclosporine, thus should be avoided[c]
INSPRA™ (Pfizer) (eplerenone) tablets October 2003 labeling	*Clinical Pharmacology*: Drug Interactions	"Grapefruit" "juice" caused only a small increase (about 25%) in exposure
Halcion (Pharmacia & Upjohn) (triazolam) May 1999 labeling	*Precautions*: Drug–drug interactions	Coadministration of "grapefruit" "juice" increased … the area under the curve by 48%

Drug	Label section	Description
KETEK™ (Aventis) (telithromycin) tablets March 2004 labeling	Drug–drug interactions	When telithromycin was given with 240 mL of "grapefruit" "juice" after an overnight fast to healthy subjects, the pharmacokinetics of telithromycin were not affected
NORVASC® (Pfizer) (amlodipine) tablets June 2003 labeling	*Precautions*: Drug–drug interactions	Coadministration of 240 mL of "grapefruit" "juice" with a single oral dose of amlodipine 10 mg in 20 healthy volunteers had no significant effect on the pharmacokinetics of amlodipine
ORAP® (Gate) (pimozide) tablets August 1999 labeling	*Precautions*: Information for patients	Because substances in "grapefruit" "juice" may inhibit the metabolism of pimozide by CYP 3A, patients should be advised to avoid "grapefruit" "juice"
PACERONE® (Upsher-Smith) (Amiodarone HCl) tablets August 2003 labeling	*Dosage and Administration*	Because "grapefruit" "juice" is known to inhibit CYP3A4-mediated metabolism of oral amiodarone in the intestinal mucosa, resulting in increased plasma levels of amiodarone, "grapefruit" "juice" should not be taken during treatment with oral amiodarone (see "*Precautions*: Drug interactions")
PLENDIL (AstraZeneca) (*felodipine*) September 2000 labeling	*Clinical Pharmacology*: Pharmacokinetics and metabolism *Precautions*: Drug–drug interactions	The bioavailability of felodipine was increased approximately twofold when taken with grapefruit juice. Orange juice does not appear to modify the kinetics of PLENDIL *Grapefruit juice*—Coadministration of felodipine with grapefruit juice resulted in more than twofold increase in the AUC and C_{max}, but no prolongation in the half-life of felodipine
PLETAL® (Otsuka America) (cilostazol) tablets May 2004 labeling	Pharmacokinetic and pharmacodynamic drug–drug interactions	"Grapefruit" "juice" increased the C_{max} of cilostazol by approximately 50%, but had no effect on AUC
PROGRAF® (Fujisawa) (tacrolimus) capsules July 2001 labeling	*Dosage and Administration*	Coadministered "grapefruit" "juice" has been reported to increase tacrolimus blood trough concentrations in liver transplant patients (see Drugs That May Alter Tacrolimus Concentrations)

(Continued)

Table 4 Labeling Examples of Drug–Grapefruit Juice Interactions (*Continued*)

Drug name	Labeling section	Labeling
RAPAMUNE® (Wyeth-Ayerst) (sirolimus) oral solution and tablets August 2004 labeling	*Dosage and Administration*	To minimize the variability of exposure to Rapamune, this drug should be taken consistently with or without food. "Grapefruit" "juice" reduces CYP3A4-mediated drug metabolism and potentially enhances P-gp–mediated drug countertransport from enterocytes of the small intestine. This juice must not be administered with Rapamune or used for dilution
SULAR® (First Horizon) (nisoldipine) extended release tablets March 2004 labeling	*Precautions*: Information for Patients	SULAR is an extended release tablet and should be swallowed whole. Tablets should not be chewed, divided, or crushed. SULAR should not be administered with a high-fat meal. "Grapefruit" "juice," which has been shown to increase significantly the bioavailability of nisoldipine and other dihydropyridine type calcium channel blockers, should not be taken with SULAR
TARGRETIN® (Ligand) (bexarotene) capsules April 2003 labeling	*Precautions*: Drug–drug interactions	On the basis of the metabolism of bexarotene by CYP3A4, ketoconazole, itraconazole, erythromycin, gemfibrozil, "grapefruit" "juice," and other inhibitors of CYP3A4 would be expected to lead to an increase in plasma bexarotene concentrations
TEGRETOL® (Novartis) (carbamazepine USP) tablet, suspension TEGRETOL®-XR (carbamazepine extended-release tablets) September 2003 labeling	*Precautions*: Drug–drug interactions	Drugs that have been shown, or would be expected, to increase plasma carbamazepine levels include cimetidine, danazol, diltiazem, macrolides, erythromycin, troleandomycin, clarithromycin, fluoxetine, fluvoxamine, nefazodone, loratadine, terfenadine, isoniazid, niacinamide, nicotinamide, propoxyphene, azoles (e.g., ketoconazole, itraconazole, and fluconazole), acetazolamide, verapamil, "grapefruit" "juice,"

TIKOSYN™ (Pfizer) (dofetilide) capsules December 1999 labeling	*Precautions*: Drug–drug interactions	protease inhibitors, and valproate Inhibitors of the CYP3A4 isoenzyme could increase systemic dofetilide exposure. Inhibitors of this isoenzyme (e.g., macrolide antibiotics, azole antifungal agents, protease inhibitors, serotonin reuptake inhibitors, amiodarone, cannabinoids, diltiazem, "grapefruit" "juice," nefazadone, norfloxacin, quinine, and zafirlukast) should be cautiously coadministered with TIKOSYN, because they can potentially increase dofetilide levels
VERSED (Roche) (midazolam) December 1998 labeling	Pharmacokinetics	Grapefruit juice (200 mL) increased AUC by 52%
VYTORIN™ 10/10 (Schering) (ezetimibe/simvastatin) July 2004 labeling	*Warnings*	Because VYTORIN contains simvastatin, the risk of myopathy/rhabdomyolysis is increased by concomitant use of VYTORIN with the following: Potent inhibitors of CYP3A4: Cyclosporine, itraconazole, ketoconazole, erythromycin, clarithromycin, HIV protease inhibitors, nefazodone, or large quantities of "grapefruit" "juice" (>1 quart daily), particularly with higher doses of VYTORIN (see "*Clinical Pharmacology*: Pharmacokinetics; *Precautions*: Drug Interactions, CYP3A4 Interactions")
XANAX® (Pharmacia & Upjohn) (alprazolam) tablets December 2001 labeling	*Precautions*: Drug–drug interactions	Drugs and other substances demonstrated to be CYP3A inhibitors on the basis of clinical studies involving benzodiazepines metabolized similarly to alprazolam or on the basis of in vitro studies with alprazolam or other benzodiazepines (caution is recommended during coadministration with alprazolam): Available data from clinical

(Continued)

Table 4 Labeling Examples of Drug–Grapefruit Juice Interactions (*Continued*)

Drug name	Labeling section	Labeling
		studies of benzodiazepines other than alprazolam suggest a possible drug interaction with alprazolam for the following: diltiazem, isoniazid, macrolide anti biotics such as erythromycin and cla rithromycin, and "grapefruit" "juice"
ZOCOR® Tablets (Merck) (simvastatin) February 2004 labeling	*Warnings*	The risk of myopathy/rhabdomyolysis is increased by concomitant use of simvastatin with the following: Potent inhibitors of CYP3A4—Cyclosporine, itraconazole, ketoconazole, erythromycin, clarithromycin, HIV protease inhibitors, nefazodone, or large quantities of "grapefruit" "juice" (greater than 1 quart daily), particularly with higher doses of simvastatin (see below: "*Clinical Pharmacology*: Pharmacokinetics; *Precautions*: Drug Interactions, CYP3A4 Interactions")
CIPRO® (Bayer) (ciprofloxacin) tablets suspension April 2004 labeling	*Dosage and Administration*	Ciprofloxacin should be administered at least 2 hours before or 6 hours after magnesium/aluminum antacids, or sucralfate, Videx® (didanosine) chewable/buffered tablets or pediatric powder for oral solution, or other prod- ucts containing calcium," iron, or zinc
	Precautions	That ciprofloxacin may be taken with or without meals and to drink fluids liberally. As with other quinolones, concurrent administration of ciprofloxacin with magnesium/aluminum antacids, or sucralfate, Videx® (didanosine) chewable/buffered tablets or pediatric powder, or with other products containing calcium," iron, or zinc should be avoided. Ciprofloxacin may be taken 2 hours before or 6 hours after taking these products.

Ciprofloxacin should not be taken with dairy products (like milk or yogurt) or calcium"-fortified juices alone, because absorption of ciprofloxacin may be significantly reduced; however, ciprofloxacin may be taken with a meal that contains these products

[a]Similar labeling language also in the labeling of FEMTRACE® (Warner Chilcott) (estradiol acetate tablets), August 2004; PREMARIN® (Wyeth-Ayerst) (conjugated estrogens tablets, USP), August 2004; and PREMPRO™ (Wyeth-Ayerst) (conjugated estrogens/medroxyprogesterone acetate tablets) PREMPHASE® (conjugated estrogens/medroxyprogesterone acetate tablets), April 2004.

[b]Similar labeling language also in the labeling of ISOPTIN® SR (Abbott) (verapamil HCl) sustained release oral tablets July 2003; and VERELAN® PM capsules (Schwarz) (verapamil hydrochloride) extended-release capsules controlled-onset, March 2003.

[c]Similar labeling language also in the labeling of NEORAL® SOFT GELATIN CAPSULES and SOLUTION (Novartis) (cyclosporine) MODIFIED; March 2004.

Abbreviations: AUC, area under the plasma concentration–time curve; CYP, cytochrome P450; HMG-CoA, 3-hydroxy-3-methylglutaryl coenzyme A.
Source: From Refs. 24, 26, 27.

interactions. Of these labels, half of them contain actual clinical data (e.g., ADALAT, ADVICOR, BILTRICIDE, CLARINEX, CONERA, CRIXI-VAN, INSPRA, KETEK, NORVASC, PACERONE, LETAL, PRO-GRAF, SULAR, and ZOCOR). All relevant literature data on grapefruit juice interactions with a particular drug product may be considered in the labeling of the drug product. For example, the latest package inserts for lovastatin (June 2002 version) and simvastatin (February 2004 version) include data from two clinical studies; one conducted by the sponsor and the other by an independent researcher. The results of the two studies differ widely, possibly because of the different study designs (timing and frequency of coadministration), and also because of variables that are difficult to control, such as the source, brand, lot-to-lot variation of the same brand, and the preparation procedure (including the extent of dilution by the consumers when using frozen concentrates) of the grapefruit juice. For both drug products, both sets of data have been included in the labeling (Table 4, "Clinical Pharmacology" section of the lovastatin labeling). Other labels include those based on theoretical interaction potential (e.g., CENESTIN®). Grapefruit juice has been considered as a "moderate CYP3A inhibitor" (5,20) that can be included with other moderate CYP3A inhibitors, such as erythromycin and diltiazem, as appropriate. Unlike most other CYP3A inhibitors, which affect both enteric and hepatic CYP3A, grapefruit juice appears to affect only enteric CYP3A; it would therefore be listed in the labeling only for drug products for oral administration and with low oral bioavailability.

Grapefruit Juice, Apple Juice, and Orange Juice Effects on Transporters

Grapefruit juice has been shown to inhibit P-gp transporter, resulting in increases in plasma levels of drugs that are substrates of P-gp transporter (see Chapter 7). Limited data have shown that grapefruit juice, as well as apple juice and orange juice, may inhibit organic anion transporting peptides (OATP), leading to decreased systemic exposure of drugs that are substrates of OATP. The overall effect of fruit juices on drugs that are substrates for both transporters may depend not only on the contribution of either transporter and other clearance pathways to the drugs' overall clearance, but also on other variables, including the amount, the type, and frequency of juices being consumed. Until more data are available, current labeling for known substrates of both transporters that are not substrates of CYP3A is to recommend taking these drug products with "water" (e.g., Table 4, ALLEGRA-D® 24 HOUR).

Calcium-Fortified Orange Juice Effect on Bioavailability

Chemical complexation of the fluoroquinolones with the calcium ion may play a major role in the reduced absorption and decreased plasma levels when calcium-fortified orange juice was coadministered with ciprofloxacin. The current labeling for Cipro (ciprofloxacin) tablets has warnings against the use of these products with calcium-fortified orange juice.

CONCLUSIONS

Drug–drug interactions have been a significant cause of adverse drug reactions (34). Various guidance documents for industry and for reviewers have stressed the importance of evaluating drug–drug interactions during drug development (4,17,18,20).

With increased understanding of how certain dietary supplements (e.g., St. John's wort) and juices (e.g., grapefruit juice) affect the systemic exposure of drug products, it is possible to anticipate an interaction with a drug based on the drug's clearance pathway and label the drug products accordingly. But while the potential for an interaction can be understood, it is much harder to describe the effect quantitatively or recommend dose modifications or usage. Dietary supplements or juices have multiple unknown components that are not well defined and vary from product to product and are used at very different doses and in a very variable time with relationship to drug use. Current labeling recommendations therefore urge avoidance of the coadministration of a drug and a dietary supplement or food that interacts with it in a clinically significant way (Tables 3A, 3B, 4), rather than adjustment of the drug dose or dosing interval, a recommendation that is common for dealing with drug–drug interactions (Tables 2A and 2B).

Despite the increased understanding and documentation of drug interactions in the labeling and in letters to "dear health care professionals," adverse reactions resulting from well-recognized drug–drug interactions continue to be reported (35–37). The increased use of dietary supplements with significant drug interaction potential increases the propensity for adverse drug reactions.

To better translate information into practice, Center for Drug Evaluation and Research (CDER) has published a final rule (38) on the physician's labeling format. When drug interactions that are significant, or their absence when they are expected to occur, would appear in labeling "Highlights," in addition to being included in the main body of the labeling (20). In addition, a proposed revision (20,22) of the 1999 drug interaction guidance (18) includes a proposal to use a classification system for CYP3A inhibitors (including grapefruit juice) in the labeling, in an effort to improve the consistency of labeling language and to highlight key drug interactions (20,22,23,25). Additional risk management tools have been proposed (39) for particularly serious situations, including use of medication guides and restricted distribution.

With continued improvement in our understanding of the mechanisms of interactions and contributions of additional patient factors (e.g., genetics and gender), the risks associated with these interactions can be better predicted, assessed, and managed to reduce the frequency of clinically significant adverse drug reactions.

REFERENCES

1. Huang S-M, Lesko LJ. Drug-drug, drug-dietary supplement and drug-citrus fruit and other food interactions–what have we learned? J Clin Pharmacol 2004; 44(6):559–69.
2. Huang S-M, Miller M, Toigo T, et al. Evaluation of drugs in women: regulatory perspective–in Section 11, Drug Metabolism/Clinical pharmacology (section editor: Schwartz J). In: Legato M, ed. Principles of Gender-Specific Medicine. Academic Press, 2004:848–859.
3. Huang S-M, Hall SD, Watkins P, et al. Drug interactions with herbal products & grapefruit juice: a conference report. Clin Pharmacol Ther 2004; 75(1):1–12.
4. Manual of Policy and Procedures (MAPP 400.4): Clinical Pharmacology and Biopharmaceutics Review Template, http://www.fda.gov/cder/mapp/4000.4.pdf, April 2004 (last accessed December 29, 2004).
5. Bjornsson TD, Callaghan JT, Einolf HJ, et al. The conduct of in vitro and in vivo drug-drug interaction studies: a Pharmaceutical Research and Manufacturers of America (PhRMA) perspective. Drug Metab Dispos 2003; 31(7): 815–832; J Clin Pharmacol 2003; 43(5):443–469.
6. Tucker T, Houston JB, Huang S-M. Optimizing drug development: strategies to assess drug metabolism/transporter interaction potential—toward a consensus. Clin Pharmacol Ther 2001; 70, 103; Br J Clin Pharmacol 2001; 52, 107; Eur J Pharm Sci 2001; 13, 417; Pharm Res 2001; 18, 1071.
7. Huang S-M, Lesko LJ, Williams RL. Assessment of the quality and quantity of drug-drug interaction studies in NDA submissions: study design and data analysis issues. J Clin Pharmacol 1999; 39:1006–1014.
8. Huang S-M, Honig P, Lesko LJ, Temple R, Williams R. An integrated approach to drug-drug interactions–a regulatory perspective. In: Rodrigues AD, ed. Drug-Drug Interactions: From Basic Pharmacokinetic Concepts to Marketing Issues. Marcel Dekker, 2001 (Chapter 18).
9. Yuan R, Madani S, Wei XX, Reynolds K, Huang SM. Evaluation of cytochrome P450 probe substrates commonly used by the pharmaceutical industry to study in vitro drug interactions. Drug Metab Dispos 2002; 30(12):1311–1319.
10. Huang S-M. Clinical drug-drug interactions. In: Krishna R, ed. Pharmacokinetic Applications in Drug Development : Kluwer Academic/Plenum Publishers, 2003.
11. Lu AYH, Huang S-M. In vitro drug metabolism studies during development of new drugs. In: Sahajwalla C, ed. New Drug Development, New York: Marcell Dekker, 2004:87–110.
12. Prueksaritanont T, Zhao JJ, Ma B, et al. Mechanistic studies on metabolic interactions between gemfibrozil and statins. Pharmacol Exp Ther 2002; 301(3): 1042–1051.
13. Mizuno N, Niwa T, Yotsumoto Y, Sugiyama Y. Impact of drug transporter studies on drug discovery and development. Pharmacol Rev 2003; 55:425–461.

14. Lin JH. Drug-drug interaction mediated by inhibition and induction of P-glycoprotein. Adv Drug Deliv Rev 2003; 55(1):53–81.
15. Dresser GK, Bailey DG, Leake BF, et al. Fruit juices inhibit organic anion transporting polypeptide-mediated uptake to decrease the oral availability of fexofenadine. Clin Pharmacol Ther 2002; 71:11–20.
16. Zhang L, Strong J, Qiu W, Lesko LJ, Huang S-M. Scientific perspectives on drug transporters and their role in drug interactions, Mol. Pharm, epublication: http://pubs.acs.org/cgi-bin/sample.cgi/mp0hbp/asap/pdf/mpo50095h.pdf (accessed January 27, 2006).
17. Guidance for industry: drug metabolism/drug interactions in the drug development process: studies in vitro. Internet: http://www.fda.gov/cder, April, 1997 (last accessed December 29, 2004).
18. Guidance for industry: in vivo metabolism/drug interactions: study design, data analysis and recommendation for dosing and labeling, Internet: http://www.fda.gov/cder, December, 1999 (last accessed December 29, 2004).
19. Guidance for industry: exposure-response relationship, study design, data analysis, and regulatory applications, April 2003. Internet: http://www.fda.gov/cder, posted May 2003 (last accessed December 29, 2004).
20. Drug Interaction Concept paper: http://www.fda.gov/ohrms/dockets/ac/04/briefing/2004-4079B1_04_Topic2-TabA.pdf; presented at the Food and Drug Administration Advisory Committee for Pharmaceutical Sciences and Clinical Pharmacology Subcommittee Meeting, November 3, 2004, http://www.fda.gov/ohrms/dockets/ac/04/briefing/2004-4079b1.htm; slides are available: http://www.fda.gov/ohrms/dockets/ac/04/slides/2004-4079s1.htm and http://www.fda.gov/ohrms/dockets/ac/04/slides/2004-4079S1_06_Huang. ppt (last accessed December 29, 2004).
21. Draft guidance for Industry: labeling for human prescription drug and biological products-implementing the new content and format requirements: http://www.fda.gov/cder/guidance/6005 dft.pdf (accessed January 27, 2006).
22. Draft guidance for industry: drug interaction studies-study design, data analysis, and implications for dosing and labeling: http://www.fda.gov/cder/guidance/index.htm (to be published in 2006).
23. Drug interactions at FDA website: http://www.fda.gov/cder/drug/druginteractions/default.htm (to be active in 2006).
24. Physicians' Desk Reference at http://pdrel.thomsonhc.com/pdrel/librarian (last accessed December 29, 2004).
25. Food and Drug Administration Advisory Committee for pharmaceutical sciences and Clinical Pharmacology Subcommittee meeting. Issues and challenges in the evaluation and labeling of drug interaction potentials of NME. Rockville, MD, April 23, 2003; http://www.fda.gov/ohrms/dockets/ac/03/slides/3947s2.htm; http://www.fda.gov/ohrms/dockets/ac/03/transcripts/3947T2.htm (last accessed December 29, 2004).
26. A catalog of FDA approved drug products, http://www.accessdata.fda.gov/scripts/cder/drugsatfda/ (last accessed December 29, 2004).
27. CDER New and Generic Drug Approvals: 1998–2004, http://www.fda.gov/cder/approval/index.htm (last accessed December 29, 2004).

28. Chen MC, Huang S-M, Mozersky R, Beitz J, Honig P. Drug interactions involving St. John's Wort–data from FDA's adverse reaction reporting system. Presented at the American Association of Pharmaceutical Scientists Annual Meeting, Denver CO, October 2001.
29. Guidance for industry: labeling for combined oral contraceptives, March 2004. Internet: http://www.fda.gov/cder/guidance/5197dft.pdf (last accessed December 29, 2004).
30. FTC Warning, http://www.ftc.gov/opa/2001/06/cureall.htm (last accessed December 29, 2004).
31. Piazza T, Huang S-M, Hepp P. FDA evaluation of drug grapefruit interaction labeling. Presented at the American College of Clinical Pharmacology Annual Meeting, San Francisco, CA, September 2002, and FDA science forum, Washington, D.C., April 2003.
32. Wei X, Park M, Ahn H. American Association of Pharmaceutical Scientists Fourth Annual Meeting and Exposition, New Orleans, November 14, 1999.
33. Park M, Wei X, Green M, Chang N. FDA Science Forum presentation, Washington, D.C., MD, February 2000.
34. Leape LL, Bates DW, Cullen DJ, et al. Systems analysis of adverse drug events. ADE Prevention Study Group. JAMA 1995; 274(1):35–43.
35. Burkhart GA, Sevka MJ, Temple R, Honig PK. Temporal decline in filling prescriptions for terfenadine closely in time with those for either ketoconazole or erythromycin. Clin Pharmacol Ther 1997; 61(1):93–96.
36. Smalley W, Shatin D, Wysowski DK, et al. Contraindicated use of cisapride: impact of food and drug administration regulatory action. JAMA 2000; 284(23):3036–3039, comment in JAMA 2000; 284(23):3047–3049.
37. Juurlink DN, Mamdani M, Kopp A, Laupacis A, Redelmeier DA. Drug-drug interactions among elderly patients hospitalized for drug toxicity. JAMA 2003; 289(13):1652–1658.
38. Final rule: Requirements on the content and format of labeling for human prescription drug and biological product, effective June 30, 2006, http://www.fda.gov/OHRMS/DOCKETS/98fr/00n-1269-nfr0001-01.pdf; http://www.fda.gov/OHRMS/DOCKETS/98fr/00n-1269-nfr0001-02.pdf; http://www.fda.gov/OHRMS/DOCKETS/98fr/00n-1269-nfr0001-03.pdf (accessed January 27, 2006)
39. Food and Drug Administration Concept Paper: Premarketing Risk Assessment. March 3, 2003, http://www.fda.gov/cder/meeting/riskManageI.htm; http://www.fda.gov/cder/meeting/riskManageII.htm; http://www.fda.gov/cder/meeting/riskManageIII.htm (last accessed December 29, 2004).

11

FDA Perspectives on the Use of Postmarketing Reporting Systems to Evaluate Drug Interactions with CAHP*

Lori A. Love

Office of Regulatory Affairs, Food and Drug Administration, Rockville, Maryland, U.S.A.

INTRODUCTION

In the United States, the use of products, including botanicals, thought to fall within the realm of complementary and alternative medicine is very common. It is difficult to obtain reliable estimates of use or to compare many of the current publications in this area because of diverse definitions for categorizing these products (e.g., dietary supplement, food supplement, herbal medicine, natural remedy, traditional medicine, etc.) in both the United States and elsewhere. A recent report on the use of complementary and alternative medicine by U.S. adults in 2002 indicated that approximately 19% of the population used "nonvitamin, nonmineral, and natural products," 19% used folk medicine, and 3% used megavitamin therapy in the past 12 months (1).

In this chapter, all of these types of products are collectively referred to as "complementary and alternative health products" (CAHP). The regulatory classification of individual products, even those containing the same or similar botanical ingredients, may be different and can influence the

---

*The views presented in this chapter are the author's and do not necessarily reflect those of the Food and Drug Administration.

safety of the product as is briefly discussed below. More in-depth information concerning the regulatory classification of botanical products is discussed in Chapters 14 and 15 of this book (2,3).

REGULATORY CLASSIFICATION OF BOTANICAL PRODUCTS

Botanical products, including those containing herbs, may be marketed as foods, dietary supplements, or drugs in the United States. Claims made by the manufacturer, particularly on the product label and labeling (information accompanying the product), determine how a product is regulated in the United States, and not necessarily what ingredients the product contains, how the doctor prescribes it, or how the consumer uses it. A product's regulatory classification is important because it determines what safety and effectiveness standards apply, the types of data needed to make this determination, and who makes the determination.

Products that make claims on their labels or labeling that state or suggest that it can treat, cure, prevent, mitigate symptoms, or diagnose a disease are drugs [prescription and over-the-counter (OTC) drugs] in the United States. Drugs must be shown to be safe and effective prior to marketing, and the Food and Drug Administration (FDA) makes these determinations. There are very specific requirements for drug manufacture and marketing. These include factors such as the purity, potency, and formulation of the ingredients in the finished drug, and the kinds of information that can or must appear on the product label (e.g., product claims, safety information, or warnings).

Conventionally, foods are items ingested for flavor, taste, aroma, or nutrition. The standards for foods primarily involve the safety and suitability of the food to meet nutritional needs, rather than safety and effectiveness as a form of treatment. Furthermore, the current standards for manufacturing or holding foods are mainly sanitation standards. In the United States, dietary supplements are a special category of foods as defined under the Dietary Supplement Health and Education Act of 1994. Unlike prescription and OTC medicines, dietary supplements are not reviewed by the FDA before marketing. Manufacturers also do not need to register before producing or selling their products. Manufacturers of dietary supplements are legally responsible for assuring the safety of their marketed products, and the FDA has the responsibility to take action against unsafe dietary supplement products after they reach the market. Except in the case of a new dietary ingredient, where the law requires premarket review for safety data and other information, a firm does not have to provide the FDA with the evidence that shows that its product is safe and effective. The FDA intends to publish minimum standards for manufacturing dietary supplements, which will focus on practices that ensure the identity, purity, quality, strength, and composition of dietary supplements. Dietary supplements can make claims about the effect of a product on the structure or function of the body, but may not make "disease" claims.

Worldwide, the majority of commercially available finished medical botanical products are regulated as drugs, although the raw botanicals themselves may be commercially available and fall outside regulatory schemes (4). In contrast, in the United States, the majority of marketed botanical products with any type of health information are sold as dietary supplements. Despite being labeled as a dietary supplement, botanical products with disease claims are unapproved drugs, because their safety and efficacy for a particular indication have not been proven prior to marketing. Currently there are a few botanicals in OTC drug products, but no prescription drug products in the United States. This situation may ultimately change, because a number of new drug applications on botanical products have been submitted to the FDA (3).

SAFETY CONCERNS RELATED TO BOTANICALS

As noted by numerous recent publications, the use of CAHP has increased dramatically in recent years, with echinacea, ginseng, ginkgo biloba, garlic, glucosamine, St. John's wort, peppermint, fish oils/omega fatty acids, ginger, and soy being the most commonly used products for health reasons (1). Safety concerns related to botanicals fall into two general areas—those related to populations using them and those related to the actual product or its ingredients.

There are a number of reasons to be concerned about the potential safety of such widespread use of CAHP. These products are frequently used by vulnerable populations, including older adults, those with chronic disorders, children, and women during pregnancy and lactation (5–10). These products are also used by patients to treat a variety of chronic disorders that are difficult to medically manage (e.g., anxiety, depression, dementia and memory impairment, headache, weight loss, back disorders, chronic pain, prostatic hypertrophy, and cancer) (1,11,12). Choice of a particular product for a particular condition is usually based on the claims made for the product and anecdotes of "historical" use, rather than conclusive scientific evidence that establishes the safety and efficacy of a particular product for a particular condition.

Concurrent use of CAHP with prescription medicines is common, with reported frequencies ranging from about 20% (13,14) to 43% (15). Less is known about potential interactions with OTC medications, but this too is of concern, particularly with the increasing switch of prescription drugs to OTC status. In addition, as with other types of CAHP, there are issues related to the recognition and monitoring of adverse events related to OTC drug products (16,17). Concurrent use of CAHP with OTC and prescription drug products can result in therapeutic failures or adverse events, as is increasingly noted from recent publications (summarized in Chapters 2, 5, and 6) (18–26).

Although many supplements are commonly advertised as being "natural," this does not make them automatically safer or better than drugs or synthetic ingredients. In many cases, there is much less credible information about the effects of particular natural products or their ingredients, and there is more product variability. Product quality and variability are known safety concerns (27,28). Natural products can contain anything found in our environment—including pesticides, bacteria, molds, heavy metals, and other poisons—as has been documented in the literature.

IDENTIFICATION AND EVALUATION OF POTENTIAL PRODUCT INTERACTIONS

Consumers frequently do not tell their health providers about their use of CAHP, health providers often fail to ask about the use of such products (13), and most of the purchases of these products occur outside a pharmacy—all of these factors enhance the likelihood of adverse product interactions and make detection of such interactions much more difficult.

Identification and evaluation of potential interactions is also difficult because there is a paucity of reliable scientific information about the effects of ingredients in CAHP, and this difficulty is compounded by product-related factors: many of the products are multi-ingredient, and as noted above there can be wide variability in the quality and consistency of ingredients and products. A number of recent reviews have tried to evaluate the credibility of data as it relates to drug–CAHP interactions (29), but these are limited to the published literature and do not consider information available in various adverse event reporting systems (e.g., FDA systems, Poison Control Centers). Because adverse events are underreported, and even fewer will ever be published in the scientific literature, it is not possible to estimate the true magnitude or significance of the drug–CAPH interactions, which is likely far greater than any current published estimates. Consequently, the results from these studies should be used with caution because the lack of documented cases in the scientific literature does not mean that a particular CAHP is safe or that interactions with drugs have not occurred or will not occur. It is critical, therefore, that health professional be cognizant of the use of CAHP by their patients and be on the alert for potential interactions. Health professionals would also increase the knowledge in this area if they diligently reported suspected adverse events.

ADVERSE EVENT REPORTING AT FDA: THE MEDWATCH PROGRAM

MedWatch is an umbrella program developed by the FDA to enhance the reporting of serious adverse events by health professionals, which are suspected to be related to the use of FDA-regulated products (www.fda.gov/

medwatch/report/hcp.htm). Within the FDA, there are many different systems at various levels in the agency, which deal with adverse event reports (AERs), including mandatory (active) and voluntary (passive) surveillance, which may have different infrastructure and system requirements. The particular system utilized depends upon the regulatory authority for the particular product. There is no central system based on the type of ingredients (i.e., botanical); the AER goes ultimately to the center with regulatory responsibility for the particular product. Consequently, more than one center in the FDA may have information about particular product interactions; for instance, an adverse event associated with a dietary supplement might be voluntarily reported by a consumer (sent to the FDA's Center for Food Safety and Applied Nutrition) or the adverse event might be a mandatory report from a drug manufacturer where a CAHP is listed as a concurrent exposure (sent to the FDA's Center for Drug Evaluation and Research).

The FDA considers postmarketing surveillance, which includes adverse event reporting, as one of the most useful indicators or signals of potential safety problems associated with a product. Although premarketing clinical studies can reveal certain safety problems, a major portion of the information concerning product safety becomes known only after marketing, with widespread use in "real life" situations. Postmarketing surveillance can either be active, such as in mandatory reporting by manufacturers of adverse events, or can utilize more passive systems, including voluntary reporting of adverse events, evaluation of consumer use data, etc. For certain drugs (those subject to the new drug approval process), it is mandatory that the manufacturers report adverse events to the FDA. Additionally, health professionals may voluntarily report adverse events associated with medical products. For other drugs, including many OTC drugs, reporting is currently voluntary.

In general, most systems used to evaluate adverse events associated with foods are passive or voluntary and are in their infancy when compared to the more formal and elaborate pharmacoepidemiologic systems that exist for certain types of drugs. The FDA learns about problems with foods, including dietary supplements, through a wide variety of sources, including the FDA MedWatch program for health professionals' reporting of adverse events. Other reporters of adverse events include consumers, state and local health departments, professional societies, other federal agencies or groups, and industry representatives that contact the FDA via multiple mechanisms (written and electronic correspondence, telephone, etc.). There have been increasing calls from health professionals and certain members of Congress to require dietary supplements manufacturers to report serious adverse events to the FDA. The recent Institute of Medicine Report on dietary supplement safety also recommended that Congress amend the Dietary Supplement Health and Education Act (DSHEA) to require manufacturers and distributors to report to the FDA in a timely manner any serious adverse events associated with the use of its marketed products.

ADVERSE EVENTS AND RISK MANAGEMENT

The FDA plays an important public health role in the identification and management of health risks associated with the use of products that it regulates. An important function of postmarketing surveillance systems is signal generation (i.e., the identification of new or emerging health risks) (30). Signals from adverse event information become apparent in a variety of ways. These include the emergence of a specific pattern of signs and symptoms, which is occurring with the use of a particular product or ingredient, an increasing number of adverse events or a change in the pattern, seriousness, or severity of adverse events observed with the use of a particular product or ingredient, or the occurrence of an adverse event that is unexpected with the use of a particular product. These systems are important because they can provide data not found or available prior to marketing on adverse effects seen in special groups, adverse effects that occur with relative infrequency, and adverse effects that develop with chronic use or exhibit latency.

For all the recognized advantages of using adverse event reporting as a component of pharmacovigilance of drug interactions, including those occurring with botanical products, there are also well-recognized limitations to current reporting systems, which are generally "passive" in nature. These include substantial and unquantified underreporting, frequent incomplete or inaccurate information in submitted reports, lack of exposure data, inability to detect adverse events with a long latency period, and the absence of a control group for the specific exposure.

A number of variables influence the likelihood of an adverse event being reported. These include the length of time that a product has been marketed, the market share, experience and sophistication of the population using the product, and publicity about adverse events. Currently there is little incentive for health professional reporting of adverse events, which partially underlies the problem with underreporting. Lack of exposure data and the issue of underreporting preclude estimation of incidence rates. Causality assessment is difficult or impossible because of the quality of the data received and the lack of a comparator (control) group. Finally, comparisons of product safety cannot be directly obtained from adverse event data.

When signals become apparent from the routine review of data in an adverse event reporting, additional elements of risk assessment are implemented, generally on a case-by-case basis, to provide the agency with adequate information to appropriately manage any public health risks. These additional elements may include clinical or scientific evaluation of all adverse events reported as associated with a particular product or ingredient; market surveys to gather information on product use (directions for use, warnings, populations using product, etc.); sample analyses, where appropriate, to identify particular substances in a product, the amount of a substance, etc.; independent scientific and clinical reviews from scientists in other Centers, or outside the agency; and expert scientific advisory committees.

This information serves as the basis of any FDA actions to mitigate risk. These actions, depending on the nature and severity of the identified risks, may include changes in the product's warnings or directions for use, education of the public (consumer, health professional, industry), or withdrawal of the product from the market. Because of the very limited amount of information that is available to the FDA at premarketing or first marketing, the majority of the FDA's efforts related to dietary supplement safety are focused in the postmarketing period. Any efforts to improve the safe use of CAHP, therefore, will include mechanisms to improve the type, quality, and availability of data that are available on these products. Such efforts could include more centralized electronic databases for scientific data, including that obtained from postmarketing surveillance of adverse events. Because we are in an era of limited resources, such efforts will require the coordinated efforts of federal agencies, academia, other public health groups, and industry to be successful.

REFERENCES

1. Barnes PM, Powell-Griner E, McFann K, Nahin RL. Complementary and alternative medicine use among adults: United States, 2002. Adv Data 2004; 343:1–19.
2. Hoffman FA. Botanicals as drugs: a US perspective. In: Lam YW, Huang S-M, Hall SD, eds. Herbal Supplements – Drug Interactions. Taylor & Francis, 2006.
3. Chen S. Development of herbal products as pharmaceutical agents—new regulatory approaches and review process at U.S. FDA. In: Lam YW, Huang S-M, Hall SD, eds. Herbal Supplements—Drug Interactions. Taylor & Francis, 2006.
4. WHO issues guidelines for herbal medicines. Bull World Health Organ 2004; 82(3):238.
5. Foster DF, Phillips RS, Hamel MB, Eisenberg DM. Alternative medicine use in older Americans. J Am Geriatr Soc 2000; 48(12):1560–1565.
6. Schilter B, Andersson C, Anton R, et al. Guidance for the safety assessment of botanicals and botanical preparations for use in food and food supplements. Food Chem Toxicol 2003; 41(12):1625–1649.
7. Al Windi A, Elmfeldt D, Svardsudd K. The relationship between age, gender, well-being and symptoms, and the use of pharmaceuticals, herbal medicines and self-care products in a Swedish municipality. Eur J Clin Pharmacol 2000; 56(4):311–317.
8. Pitetti R, Singh S, Hornyak D, Garcia SE, Herr S. Complementary and alternative medicine use in children. Pediatr Emerg Care 2001; 17(3):165–169.
9. Nordeng H, Havnen GC. Use of herbal drugs in pregnancy: a survey among 400 Norwegian women. Pharmacoepidemiol Drug Saf 2004; 13(6):371–380.

10. Kristoffersen SS, Atkin PA, Shenfield GM. Uptake of alternative medicine. Lancet 1996; 347(9006):972.

11. Astin JA. Why patients use alternative medicine: results of a national study. JAMA 1998; 279(19):1548–1553.

12. Barqawi A, Gamito E, O'Donnell C, Crawford ED. Herbal and vitamin supplement use in a prostate cancer screening population. Urology 2004; 63(2): 288–292.

13. Eisenberg DM, Davis RB, Ettner SL, et al. Trends in alternative medicine use in the United States, 1990–1997: results of a follow-up national survey. JAMA 1998; 280(18):1569–1575.

14. Kaufman DW, Kelly JP, Rosenberg L, Anderson TE, Mitchell AA. Recent patterns of medication use in the ambulatory adult population of the United States: the Slone survey. JAMA 2002; 287(3):337–344.

15. Peng CC, Glassman PA, Trilli LE, Hayes-Hunter J, Good CB. Incidence and severity of potential drug-dietary supplement interactions in primary care patients: an exploratory study of 2 outpatient practices. Arch Intern Med 2004; 164(6):630–636.

16. Bond C, Hannaford P. Issues related to monitoring the safety of over-the-counter (OTC) medicines. Drug Safety 2003; 26(15):1065–1074.

17. Barnes J, Mills SY, Abbot NC, Willoughby M, Ernst E. Different standards for reporting ADRs to herbal remedies and conventional OTC medicines: face-to-face interviews with 515 users of herbal remedies. Br J Clin Pharmacol 1998; 45(5):496–500.

18. Lam VWF, Huang S-M. Drug Interactions with Herbal Products; Francis Lam and Shiew-Mei Huang. In: Lam YW, Huang S-M, Hall SD, eds. Herbal Supplements – Drug Interactions. Taylor & Francis, 2006.

19. Lam VWF, Ernst E. Garlic, ginkgo and ginseng: herb-drug interactions. In: Lam YW, Huang S-M, Hall SD, eds. Herbal Supplements—Drug Interactions. Taylor & Francis, 2006.

20. Lam VWF, Qu M. A review of Chinese herb-drug interactions. In: Lam YW, Huang S-M, Hall SD, eds. Herbal Supplements—Drug Interactions. Taylor & Francis, 2006.

21. Izzo AA. Drug interactions with St. John's Wort (Hypericum perforatum): a review of the clinical evidence. Int J Clin Pharmacol Ther 2004; 42(3):139–148.

22. Jiang X, Williams KM, Liauw WS, et al. Effect of St John's wort and ginseng on the pharmacokinetics and pharmacodynamics of warfarin in healthy subjects. Br J Clin Pharmacol 2004; 57(5):592–599.

23. Tannergren C, Engman H, Knutson L, Hedeland M, Bondesson U, Lennernas H. St John's wort decreases the bioavailability of R- and S-verapamil through induction of the first-pass metabolism. Clin Pharmacol Ther 2004; 75(4):298–309.

24. Alscher DM, Klotz U. Drug interaction of herbal tea containing St. John's wort with cyclosporine. Transpl Int 2003; 16(7):543–544.

25. Hall SD, Wang Z, Huang SM, et al. The interaction between St John's wort and an oral contraceptive. Clin Pharmacol Ther 2003; 74(6):525–535.

26. Mai I, Stormer E, Bauer S, Kruger H, Budde K, Roots I. Impact of St John's wort treatment on the pharmacokinetics of tacrolimus and mycophenolic acid in renal transplant patients. Nephrol Dial Transplant 2003; 18(4):819–822.

27. Fong HH. Integration of herbal medicine into modern medical practices: issues and prospects. Integr Cancer Ther 2002; 1(3):287–293.
28. Chadwick LR, Fong HHS. Herb quality assurance and standardization in herb-drug interaction evaluation and documentation. In: Lam YW, Huang S-M, Hall SD, eds. Herbal Supplements—Drug Interactions. Taylor & Francis, 2006.
29. Williamson EM. Drug interactions between herbal and prescription medicines. Drug Safety 2003; 26(15):1075–1092.
30. Ahmad SR. Adverse drug event monitoring at the Food and Drug Administration. J Gen Intern Med 2003; 18(1):57–60.

12

St. John's Wort Drug Interaction Reports from FDA's Postmarketing AERS

Min-Chu Chen

Office of Drug Safety, Center for Drug Evaluation and Research (CDER), Food and Drug Administration, Silver Spring, Maryland, U.S.A.

INTRODUCTION

St. John's wort is a member of the genus *Hypericum*, which has 400 species worldwide in Europe, West Asia, North Africa, North America, and Australia (2). In the Western United States, the use of St. John's wort is especially prevalent in Northern California and Southern Oregon. The commercially available product contains hypericum dry extracts or their by-products prepared from flowers gathered during the time of blooming or from dried parts above ground. These extracts differ in varying degrees, based on their composition, from the following major natural product groups listed with suggested biological activities:

Major natural product groups	Suggested biological activities
Dianthrone derivatives: Hypericin, pseudohypericin, anthranol, photohypericin, hypericodehydrodianthrone	Photodynamic, antidepressant [monoamine oxidase inhibitor (MAOI)], antiviral
Flavanols: Catechin polymers (condensed tannins), leucocyanidin, epicatechin	Astringent, anti-inflammatory, styptic, antiviral

(Continued)

285

Major natural product groups	Suggested biological activities
Falvinoids: Hyperoside (hyperin), quercetin, rutin	Capillary-strengthening, anti-inflammatory, diuretic, cholagogic, dilates coronary arteries, sedative, tumor inhibition, antitumor, antidiarrheal
Xanthones	Generally antidepressant, antitubercular, choleretic, diuretic, antimicrobial, antiviral, and cardiotonic activity
Phloroglucinol derivatives: hyperforin	Antibacterial (*Staphylococcus aureus*)
Essential oil components	Antifungal

In modern European medicine, St. John's wort extracts are included in many over-the-counter and prescription drugs for management of mild depression, and have clinical implications for bed-wetting and nightmares in children. The extracts are included in diuretic preparations and the oil is taken orally using a teaspoon to help heal gastritis, gastric ulcers, and inflammatory conditions of the colon. The oil is also used extensively externally in burn and wound remedies.

Recent reports in animal studies by Rolli et al. (7) and Muller et al. (8) show that clinically used hypericum extract inhibited the synaptic reuptake of 5-hydroxytryptamine (5-HT), noradrenaline, and dopamine with an inhibition concentration at 50% (IC_{50}) around 2 µg/mL. The bioactive substance responsible for the inhibition is identified as hyperforin, from a study by Muller et al. (9). The effect of hypericin as an inhibitor of MAO-A has not been confirmed (10); however, other ingredients such as flavonoid aglycone, quercetin, and quercitrin have been shown to inhibit MAO-A (11). Overall significant benefits of St. John's wort for mild depression compared to a placebo (12), or equivalent efficacy compared to tricyclic antidepressants (maprotiline, imipramine, and amitriptyline) (13), in mild-to-moderate depression have been reported. However, cautious interpretation of these studies is warranted due to methodological weaknesses. Most tested preparations varied in several major ingredients. An advantage hypericum has over other antidepressants is its favorable side-effect profile. Hypericum has been shown to be well tolerated in patients with the incidence of adverse reactions similar to that of a placebo (13). The most common adverse effects reported after short-term therapy are gastrointestinal symptoms, dizziness/confusion, and tiredness/sedation.

DRUG INTERACTIONS WITH ST. JOHN'S WORT

There were multiple official regulatory warnings regarding the risk of increased drug levels of CYP3A4 substrates as a result of interactions with

St. John's wort (1,3–6). For example, the U.S. Food and Drug Administration (FDA) published a Public Health Advisory in 2000, alerting about the risk of drug interaction with indinavir, antiretroviral agents, and other drugs used to treat heart disease, depression, seizure, certain cancers, transplant rejection, and oral contraceptives. The European Agency for the Evaluation of Medicinal Products (EMEA) issued a Public Statement in 2000, on the risk of drug interactions between *H. perforatum* (St. John's wort) and cyclosporine, digoxin, oral contraceptives, theophylline, warfarin, and antiretroviral medicinal products such as protease inhibitors (PIs) and non-nucleoside reverse transcriptase inhibitors such as zidovudine, didanosine, and zalcitabine. The Australia Therapeutic Goods Administration published a Media Release in 2000 on interactions with indinavir, cyclosporine, warfarin, digoxin, theophylline, PIs, HIV non-nucleoside reverse transcriptase inhibitors, anticonvulsants, oral contraceptives, nefazodone, selective serotonin-reuptake inhibitors (SSRIs) such as citalopram, fluoxetine, fluvoxamine, paroxetine, sertraline, and antimigraine drugs. The Canadians marketed St. John's wort products as food, without health claims. The Irish Medicines Board subjected St. John's wort to prescription control. New Zealand's Medsafe issued a media release statement for St. John's wort interactions with antiepileptic drugs, PIs, immunosuppressive agents, antidepressants, antimigraine drugs, and oral contraceptives.

The FDA's Adverse Event Reporting System (AERS) at the Center for Drug Evaluation and Research (CDER) is an electronic database that currently contains over three million reports of suspected drug-related adverse events, both serious and nonserious outcomes, from all marketed drugs since 1969, which have been submitted to the agency. The reports are initiated on a voluntary basis from both United States and foreign sources that include both health care professionals and consumers and submitted to manufacturers or directly to the FDA. It is important to note that AERS reports are usually of variable quality and completeness and do not necessarily imply a direct causal relationship between drug exposure and the adverse event(s). In some cases, an analysis of such reports may suggest that they are the consequence of the treated underlying disease, other concurrent medical conditions, and/or concomitant medical product treatment. In addition, due to the voluntary nature of reporting, it is not possible to determine the actual incidence of drug-related events or determine the actual degree of risk associated with drug usage. Moreover, due to differences in reporting of adverse events for different type of drugs and other factors affecting reporting, a quantitative comparison of risk between products is highly problematic.

Up to 2001, AERS indicated up to 39 case reports of possible drug interactions between St. John's wort and a prescription drug. In these case reports, the potential drug interactions occurred mostly with oral contraceptives, antidepressants, cyclosporine, and sildenafil. All cases were reported between 1997 and 2000. Most of the reported cases were in females (24), with an age range between 17 and 73 (mean 42.5) years of age. Four reported hospitalization as a serious outcome. Examples of reported drug interactions with St. John's wort are summarized below.

Cyclosporine

Coadministration of St. John's wort with cyclosporine has resulted in a significant reduction in cyclosporine concentrations, which has led to graft rejection. Decreased cyclosporine drug levels were reported in five cases. Two cases from the United States, one from Australia, and two from Switzerland reported decreased cyclosporine levels or decreased therapeutic response while on St. John's wort concomitantly. The age ranges and doses of cyclosporine used in these five patients, where the data was reported, were 26 to 62 and 200 to 250 mg, respectively. Dose of St. John's wort was 300 mg in one case and 600 mg in another, but unspecified in three cases. Time to onset ranged from two to seven weeks after St. John's wort administration, and was unspecified in one case. The Australian case reported that cyclosporine levels returned to within normal range two weeks after stopping St. John's wort. The two Swiss cases documented endomyocardial rejection with concurrent St. John's wort therapy.

Oral Contraceptive Hormones

The metabolism of the components of oral contraceptives, ethinyl estradiol and norethindrone, is thought to be mediated at least in part by intestinal and hepatic CYP3A. St. John's wort significantly increased the oral clearance of norethindrone and decreased the peak serum concentration of norethindrone (refer to Chapters 2 and 4 for more information). Likewise, the elimination half-life of ethinyl estradiol was significantly reduced, therefore potentially reducing oral contraceptive efficacy or even failure. The most frequently reported hormones possibly interacting with St. John's wort were levonorgestrel in combination with estradiol through increased 3A4 metabolism. There were ten case reports of breakthrough bleeding while Alesse-28 and St. John's wort product were used concomitantly. The bleeding occurred from nine days to four months after Alesse-28 was started. The bleeding continued up to seven days while taking Alesse. Age ranged from 33 to 53 ($n = 7$, mean 41). Two patients were instructed to double the doses of Alesse-28 for an unspecified number of days and the bleeding stopped. One discontinued the use of Alesse-28. One patient became pregnant and had a miscarriage. This subject resumed taking St. John's wort and Alesse-28 and conceived again.

There were three reports of breakthrough bleeding while patients were on norgestimate and ethinyl estradiol (Ortho-Cyclen). A 29-year-old female took Ortho-Cyclen 28 tablets for a few months and experienced moderate breakthrough bleeding and some abdominal pain. She began taking two capsules of St. John's wort 10 days prior to her breakthrough bleeding. A 25-year-old female had been taking Ortho-Cyclen for years. She started taking St. John's wort for 30 days and experienced a lot of breakthrough bleeding. She is led to believe that St. John's wort decreased the efficacy of the oral contraceptive. A female of unknown age taking Ortho-Cyclen experienced breakthrough bleeding 17 days after starting St. John's wort.

There was one report in a 22-year-old female of irregular menses and unintended pregnancy while on levonorgestrel and St. John's wort with unspecified dose or indication. A 32-year-old female developed PMS symptoms, breakthrough bleeding, and unintended pregnancy while taking St. John's wort about the same time that she was taking levonorgestrel and ethinyl estradiol.

Antidepressants

For venlafaxine, fluvoxamine, and fluoxetine, the most frequently reported adverse events while on St. John's wort were hypertension and potential serotonin syndrome. There were no reports of lack of effect for these SSRIs, although St. John's wort may decrease the drug levels by inducing 3A4. Because St. John's wort inhibits reuptake of serotonin, noradrenaline, dopamine, and MAO, these events were likely associated with increased serotonin and/or adrenaline levels. Possibly under a similar mechanism, addition of St. John's wort to the MAOI phenelzine was associated with hypertensive crisis in one case, and with mild serotonin syndrome in another patient taking the tricyclic, doxepine. It is unclear whether sertraline had any drug interaction with St. John's wort, although four cases reported depression or intermittent ineffectiveness. According to the labeling, sertraline goes through extensive first-pass *N*-demethylation and the extent of 3A4 inhibition by sertraline is not likely to be of clinical significance.

One case from the United States and one from the United Kingdom reported hypertension and manic reaction, respectively, while on venlaflaxine and St. John's wort concomitantly. The case of hypertension from the United Kingdom was a 56-year-old male who had taken venlafaxine 300 mg daily for management of depression. Prior to consuming St. John's wort, the patient's blood pressure readings were 120/82 mmHg and five weeks after St. John's wort blood pressures were elevated at 180/115 mmHg and 165/112 mmHg. A 29-year-old male received Effexor 150 mg for the treatment of dysrhythmia. He decreased the dose and started taking St. John's wort, three tablets daily or every other day, without his prescribing physician's knowledge. He experienced a hypomanic episode that was described as sleeping poorly and feeling "wired" for two days with a lot of "energy" and inability to relax or calm down. A literature report from France described "serotonin syndrome" experienced by a 32-year-old male patient as malaise with anxiety, excessive sweating, chills, and tachycardia four days after St. John's wort therapy while on venlafaxine. St. John's wort dose was interrupted on day 4, and the symptoms regressed in three days without modifying the dosage of the antidepressant.

There were two cases of hypertension from the United States, or possible serotonin syndrome reported with fluvoxamine while on St. John's wort concomitantly. A 44-year-old male with obsessive-compulsive disorder received fluvoxamine and experienced severe hypertensive crisis (160–170/120 mmHg) after two tablets of St. John's wort. The physician stated that the reaction was probably due to the combination of fluvoxamine and St. John's wort, which has MAOI activity. A 38-year-old male was on fluvoxamine for approximately two months and hypericum 600 mg daily for approximately two weeks before reporting possible serotonin syndrome with severe bitemporal headache. He was hospitalized to rule out myocardial infarction. There were no electrocardiogram (EKG) changes or apparent causative pathology. Symptoms resolved on discontinuation of both drugs.

A 73-year-old female was treated with fluoxetine for depression for a long period of time and had a history of hypertension managed with multiple concomitant drugs: digoxin, enalapril, aspirin, isosorbide, amlodipine, carvedilol, metformin, and furosemide. The patient was treated with hypericum extract 425 mg for one time. Half an hour to one hour after the first dose, the patient experienced a hypertensive crisis (270/130 mmHg) during her stay in a rehabilitation center. The event was treated with nifedipine and abated (with blood pressures decreasing to 160/96 mmHg).

Five cases (ages 36, 48, 48 and 60 and one unknown; three males and two females) reported intermittent ineffectiveness with sertraline, including complaints of "does not seem to be working," anxiety attack, or worsening depression. In four cases, symptoms occurred after sertraline was added to the continuing St. John's wort therapy. In contrast to reports with other antidepressants, these cases did not report hypertension or possible serotonin syndrome. It is uncertain if the occasional events were possibly associated with the patients' unstable psychiatric status following sertraline therapy, or due to potential sertraline-related adverse events.

Potential drug interaction between sertraline and St. John's wort cannot be ruled out in one case that experienced manic depressive disorder symptoms one to two weeks after St. John's wort was started into sertraline therapy. The patient was treated with an antipsychotic and has had no problems after discontinuing St. John's wort and decreasing the sertraline dose.

Sildenafil

Four cases of lack of effect or impotence were reported in patients using sildenafil while on St. John's wort and other concomitant drugs (what are they? Are any of them significant from the standpoint of drug interaction?). The age range of the four male patients was between 55 to 73 years. Viagra doses were all 50 mg p.r.n. The St. John's wort dose was 600 mg daily in one case but unspecified in the other three cases. One case reported that Viagra did not work, but provided no additional details. Another two cases experienced facial flushing, headache, and ineffective Viagra treatment. One case indicated that Viagra 50 mg was used several times with only partial erection. The dose was increased to 100 mg with similar results. The fourth case summarized below had no other concomitant drug listed and indicated that the Viagra worked without St. John's wort, but did not work when St. John's wort was taken.

A physician reported that a 60-year-old male started sildenafil 50 mg while he was also taking 600 mg of St. John's wort daily for depression. When the patient increased the dose of St. John's wort to 1200 to 1800 mg daily for unknown reasons, the sildenafil was reported to be partially effective. Patient increased the dose of sildenafil to 100 mg but it was completely ineffective. The physician suspected that a drug interaction caused the adverse events. No other significant medical history was noted.

Anticonvulsants—Carbamazepine

There were two reported cases with carbamazepine. One case was that of a 17-year-old female who reported increased levels of carbamazepine following three months of St. John's wort and carbamazepine 200 mg b.i.d. with a baseline level of 4.7 µg/mL. She became nauseated with flu-like symptoms on 12/5/98. After experiencing a seizure, dizziness, and disorientation the next day, she was hospitalized with a carbamazepine level of 36 µg/mL.

Another case was a female who reported with complaints of increased incidence of "muscle twitching" episodes during daytime hours. These included "slapping leg and turning head to right." Patient was on valproic acid and carbamazepine and St. John's wort was started 50 days prior to the occurrence of adverse events. No carbamazepine levels were reported.

Because carbamazepine is also a CYP450 3A4 inducer, the role of St. John's wort is not clear from these two cases because only one case reported increased carbamazepine levels.

CONCLUSION

The available case reports in the FDA AERS support the published literature that there are pharmacokinetic interactions between St. John's wort and CYP3A4 and/or *p*-glycoprotein substrates, such as cyclosporine, levonorgestrel/estradiol and sildenafil, and pharmacodynamic interactions with the SSRIs or MAOI. Subsequent clinical studies including those conducted via a CDER clinical pharmacology research cooperative agreement (14–16) provided mechanistic basis of many of these interactions (refer to Chapter 4).

REFERENCES

1. Roby CA, Anderson GD, Kantor E, et al. St John's Wort: effect on CYP3A4 activity. Clin Pharmacol Ther 2000; 67(5):451–457.
2. St. John's Wort (*Hypericum perforatum* L.): A Review. Christopher Hobbs-Health World Online, 1996.
3. Breidenbach T, Hoffman MW, Becker T, et al. Drug interaction of St. John's Wort with cyclosporin. Lancet 2000; 355:1912.
4. Johne A, Brockmoller J, Bauer S, et al. Pharmacokinetic interaction of digoxin with an herbal extract from St John's wort (*Hypericum perforatum*). Clin Pharmacol Ther 1999; 66:338–345.
5. Linde K, Ramirez G, Mulrow CD, et al. St John's wort for depression — an overview and meta-analysis of randomized clinical trials. BMJ 1996; 313:258–261.
6. Jobst K, McIntyre M, St. George D, et al. Safety of ST John's wort (*Hypericum perforatum*). Lancet 2000; 355:575.
7. Rollie M, et al. Effects of hypericum extract LI 160 on neurotransmitter receptor binding and synapsomal uptake system. Pharmacopsychiatry 1995; 28:207–210.
8. Muller WE, Rollie M, Schafer C, et al. Effects of hypericum extract LI 160 in biochemical models of antidepressant activity. Pharmacopsychiatry 1997; 30(suppl 2):102–107.
9. Muller WE, Singer A, Wonnemann M, et al. Hyperforin represents the neuro-transmitter reuptake inhibiting constituent of hypericum extract. Pharmacopsychiatry 1998; 31(suppl 1):16–21.
10. Suzuki O, Katsumata Y, Oyo M, et al. Inhibition of monoamine oxidate by hypericin. Plant Medica 1984; 50:272–274.
11. Sommer H, Harrer G, et al. Placebo-controlled double blind study examining the effectiveness of a hypericum preparation in 105 mildly depressed patients. J Ger Psych Neurol 1994; 7:9–11.
12. Vorbach EU, Hubner WD, Amoldt KH, et al. Effectiveness and tolerance of the hypericum extract LI 160 in comparison with imipramine: randomized double blind study with 135 outpatients. J Ger Psychiat Neurol 1994; 7(suppl 1):S19–S23.
13. Ernst E, et al. Adverse effects profile of the herbal antidepressant St John's wort. Eur J Clin Pharmacol 1998; 54:589–594.
14. Wang Z, Gorski JC, Hamman MA, Huang SM, Lesko LJ, Hall SD. The effects of St John's wort (*Hypericum perforatum*) on human cytochrome P450 activity. Clin Pharmacol Ther 2001; 70(4):317–326.
15. Wang Z, Hamman MA, Huang SM, Lesko LJ, Hall SD. Effect of St John's wort on the pharmacokinetics of fexofenadine. Clin Pharmacol Ther 2002; 71(6):414–420.
16. Hall SD, Wang Z, Huang S-M, et al. The interaction between St John's wort and an oral contraceptive. Clin Pharmacol Ther 2003; 74(6):525–535.

13

Grapefruit Juice Interaction Reports from FDA's Postmarketing AERS

Toni Piazza-Hepp

Division of Surveillance, Research and Communication Support Office of Drug Safety, Center for Drug Evaluation and Research (CDER), Food and Drug Administration, Silver Spring, Maryland, U.S.A.

INTRODUCTION

Communication to the public of medical product risks, such as drug–grapefruit juice interaction, is an important aspect of public health agency work. Health Canada, for example, advised the public in 2002 (1) not to consume grapefruit products with medications used for certain medical conditions, such as anxiety, depression, and others. In the United States, the Food and Drug Administration (FDA) includes documented information on drug–grapefruit juice interaction in individual product labeling [also known as the package insert (PI)]. The process that the FDA uses to include such interactions in product labeling is reviewed in Chapter 10.

Information in the PI is typically based on the studies submitted by a drug's manufacturer. The FDA has also utilized spontaneous adverse event case reports as a tool in the evaluation of drug–grapefruit juice interaction labeling. Other sources of data that contribute to labeled information include studies or case reports from the medical literature.

SPONTANEOUS ADVERSE EVENT CASE REPORTS

To identify case reports containing information on drug and grapefruit juice interaction, the Adverse Event Reporting System (AERS) (2) database was searched in April 2004 for any mention of a grapefruit-containing product (e.g., grapefruit, grapefruit juice, grapefruit seed) as either a "suspect" (the product that is suspected by the reporter to have caused the event) or a "concomitant" (other medical products that the patient was receiving at the same time) product. It must be understood that the FDA does not receive all reports of adverse events and product interactions that occur in medical practice. This is particularly true for a product such as grapefruit juice. First, there is no regulatory requirement to submit food (such as grapefruit juice)–related adverse events to the FDA. Further, grapefruit juice is not generally considered a "medical product," so it is possible that a reporter describing a "drug" adverse event report concerning such an interaction may not list "grapefruit juice" in either of the "medical product" blocks on the MedWatch (3) form. Thus, all reports that mention grapefruit juice in the AERS database might not have been located.

The grapefruit juice search described above identified 186 cases in the AERS database. At that point, we had a group of cases that could describe drug–grapefruit juice interaction. However, as with all searches in AERS for spontaneous case reports, each patient case must be scrutinized further, using either a case definition or a set of criteria to better focus on the safety concern of interest. The following criteria were chosen to better identify reports that were more likely to describe an interaction between a drug product and grapefruit juice:

1. The patient was documented to be stable on the drug product prior to receiving grapefruit juice, and,
2. The adverse event occurred after the initiation of grapefruit juice, is a known effect of the drug, and is usually dose-related. Allergic reaction events, lack of drug effect, and events describing gastrointestinal upset after grapefruit juice consumption were not included.

or,

1. The patient was documented to be consuming grapefruit juice each day prior to starting drug therapy, or started grapefruit juice and the drug product at the same time, and,
2. The adverse event (as described in #2 above) occurred upon initiation of drug therapy, and,
3. The adverse event resolved upon retention of same dose of drug with discontinuation of grapefruit juice.

Among the original 186, forty case reports were identified that met the criteria. Thirty-three were from the United States, and seven were reported from foreign countries. Drug names and types of events described are listed in Table 1. Three case reports are presented below.

Table 1   Cases of Possible Drug–Grapefruit Interaction

Drug	Events
Amlodipine	Peripheral edema, asthenia, hypotension
Amlodipine	Dyspnea, anxiety, hypertension
Amlodipine	Dizziness
Amlodipine	Hypotension
Amlodipine	Head "fullness," strange sensations
Amlodipine	Hypotension, asthenia (feeling of tiredness)
Amlodipine	Dizziness, tachycardia, lightheadedness
Amlodipine	Near syncope
Amlodipine	Atrial fibrillation, ventricular tachycardia
Amlodipine	Increased LFTs and bilirubin
Amlodipine	Dizziness, asthenia
Amlodipine	Hypotension, syncope
Astemizole	Syncope, atrioventricular block
Atorvastatin	Anxiety
Atorvastatin	Epistaxis
Atorvastatin	Gingival bleeding
Atorvastatin	Myalgia, asthenia
Atorvastatin	Dizziness, nausea
Atorvastatin	Myalgia, myasthenia
Atorvastatin	Arm/shoulder pain
Atorvastatin	Paresthesia
Atorvastatin/azithromycin	Increased LFTs and bilirubin
Bupropion	Hypertensive crisis
Doxazosin	Near syncope
Estrogens, conjugated	Fluid retention
Gabapentin	Dizziness, syncope, slurred speech
Lisinopril	Headache, nausea, dizziness
Lisinopril	Dizziness, syncope, seizure
Lovastatin	Rhabdomyolysis
Nifedipine	Pedal edema
Nifedipine	Hypotension, gait abnormal
Nifedipine	Eye swelling, foggy feeling, headache
Nifedipine	Tiredness, asthenia
Nifedipine	Tachycardia
Nifedipine	Dizziness, asthenia, gingivitis
Nifedipine	Asthenia, dizziness, vertigo, disorientation
Risperidone/fluoxetine	Somnolence, fatigue
Sertraline	Sweating
Sibutramine	Insomnia
Verapamil	Palpitations, flushing, malaise, facial redness

Abbreviation: LFTs, liver function tests.

Case 1

A 60-year-old male patient with hypertension, chronic lower extremity venous stasis/edema, renal insufficiency, non–insulin dependent diabetes mellitus, and a familial history of hyperlipidemia had been receiving lovastatin, 40 mg tablet, twice a day for 5 to 10 years. Other therapy included gemfibrozil (600 mg b.i.d.), amlodipine, and an oral hypoglycemic agent. Early in the year, the patient's creatinine was 3.5 mg/dL. In October, the patient began drinking grapefruit juice in the morning for the first time in his life. During this time, the patient denied any strenuous exercise. Two weeks later, the patient was in so much pain that he went to an emergency room where his creatine phosphokinase was greater than 40,000 U/L. He was admitted to the hospital with a diagnosis of rhabdomyolysis. Therapy with lovastatin and gemfibrozil was discontinued. During that time, his creatinine increased to about 5.0 mg/dL. The patient was discharged from the hospital after approximately one week and was considered to be recovering. The physician felt that the patient's rhabdomyolysis was caused by the interaction of the grapefruit juice with lovastatin and gemfibrozil.

Case 2

A 92-year-old female with hypertension had been taking nifedipine 30 mg daily for four years. While traveling in Florida, she took her nifedipine with grapefruit juice and experienced extreme fatigue, dizziness, vertigo, decreased appetite, and disorientation. She was hospitalized for three to four days, the grapefruit juice was stopped, and she recovered. After returning home from Florida, she took her nifedipine with grapefruit juice again and experienced a similar but milder reaction. Her pharmacist suspected an interaction between nifedipine and grapefruit juice.

Case 3

A 62-year-old female with a history of systemic lupus erythematosis, osteoporisis, angina pectoris, and renal failure began taking amlodipine. She had also been taking lisinopril and spironolactone for an unknown duration. A year later, she started eating grapefruit every day. She fell down after developing disturbance of consciousness for a few minutes. Four days later, she developed generalized fatigue and was admitted the next day to the hospital for shock symptoms consisting of decreased blood pressure, clouded consciousness, and vomiting. Her medications were discontinued, and she was treated for the shock symptoms. The patient recovered. Her physician suspected an interaction between amlodipine and grapefruit.

CASE REPORTS COMPARED TO LABELING

The next step in the assessment was to check the current status of product labeling for drug–grapefruit juice interaction. The Physicians' Desk Reference (PDR Electronic Library^{TM}) (4) was utilized as a tool for this purpose. An online query in April 2004 for "grapefruit" was performed, which identified relevant labeling. An important limitation of this strategy is that not all products are included in the PDR, so this search was not expected to identify 100% of drug product labeling containing information on grapefruit. Further information on grapefruit labeling for drugs is presented in Table 4 of Chapter 10.

There were 24 ingredients identified in the PDR online search, which described documented or theoretical effects of grapefruit consumption; these are listed in Table 2. The information was contained in a variety of labeling sections: "Clinical Pharmacology," "Warnings," "Precautions," and "Dosage and Administration." For most drugs, placement of the information was in the Precautions/Drug Interactions section. The following

Table 2 Drugs with Labeling for Grapefruit Interaction

Alprazolam
Amiodarone
Amlodipine
Aripiprazole
Bexarotene
Budesonide
Cilostazol
Cyclosporine
Desloratadine
Dofetilide
Enalapril
Estradiol
Estrogens, conjugated
Felodipine
Indinavir
Lovastatin
Nifedipine
Nisoldipine
Pimozide
Simvastatin
Sirolimus
Tacrolimus
Tadalafil
Verapamil

Source: PDR Electronic Library, 2004.

three labeling examples were chosen to illustrate the range of information on drug–grapefruit interaction available.

Lovastatin (Mevacor)

Clinical Pharmacology

Lovastatin is a substrate for cytochrome P450 isoform 3A4 (CYP3A4) (see Precautions, *Drug Interactions*). Grapefruit juice contains one or more components that inhibit CYP3A4 and can increase the plasma concentrations of drugs metabolized by CYP3A4. In one study, 10 subjects consumed 200 mL of double-strength grapefruit juice (one can of frozen concentrate diluted with one rather than three cans of water) three times daily for two days and an additional 200 mL double-strength grapefruit juice together with and 30 and 90 minutes following a single dose of 80 mg lovastatin on the third day. This regimen of grapefruit juice resulted in a mean increase in the serum concentration of lovastatin and its (beta)-hydroxyacid metabolite (as measured by the area under the concentration–time curve) of 15-fold and 5-fold, respectively (as measured using a chemical assay—high performance liquid chromatography). In a second study, 15 subjects consumed one 8 oz glass of single-strength grapefruit juice (one can of frozen concentrate diluted with three cans of water) with breakfast for three consecutive days and a single dose of 40 mg lovastatin in the evening of the third day. This regimen of grapefruit juice resulted in a mean increase in the plasma concentration (as measured by the area under the concentration–time curve) of active and total hydroxymethylglutaryl coenzyme A (HMG-CoA) reductase inhibitory activity [using an enzyme inhibition assay both before (for active inhibitors) and after (for total inhibitors) base hydrolysis] of 1.34-fold and 1.36-fold, respectively, and of lovastatin and its (beta)-hydroxyacid metabolite (measured using a chemical assay—liquid chromatography/tandem mass spectrometry—different from that used in the first study) of 1.94-fold and 1.57-fold, respectively. The effect of the difference in amounts of grapefruit juice in these two studies of lovastatin pharmacokinetics has not been studied.

Warnings

Myopathy caused by drug interactions: The incidence and severity of myopathy are increased by concomitant administration of HMG-CoA reductase inhibitors with drugs that can cause myopathy when given alone, such as gemfibrozil and other fibrates, and lipid-lowering doses (greater than or equal to 1 g/day) of niacin (nicotonic acid).

In addition, the risk of myopathy may be increased by high levels of HMG-CoA reductase inhibitory activity in plasma. Lovastatin is metabolized by the CYP3A4. Potent inhibitors of this metabolic pathway can raise the plasma levels of HMG-CoA reductase inhibitory activity and may increase the risk of myopathy. These include cyclosporine; the azole antifungals itraconazole and ketoconazole; the macrolide antibiotics erythromycin and clarithromycin; HIV protease inhibitors; the antidepressant nefazodone; and large quantities of grapefruit juice (greater than 1 quart daily) (see below; Clinical Pharmacology, *Pharmacokinetics*; Precautions, *Drug Interactions*; and Dosage and Administration).

Precautions/Drug Interactions

CYP3A4 interactions: Lovastatin has no CYP3A4 inhibitory activity; therefore, it is not expected to affect the plasma concentrations of other drugs metabolized by CYP3A4. However, lovastatin itself is a substrate for CYP3A4. Potent inhibitors of CYP3A4 may increase the risk of myopathy by increasing the plasma concentration of HMG-CoA reductase inhibitory activity during lovastatin therapy. These inhibitors include cyclosporine, itraconazole, ketoconazole, erythromycin, clarithromycin, HIV protease inhibitors, nefazodone, and large quantities of grapefruit juice (greater than 1 quart daily) (see Clinical Pharmacology, *Pharmacokinetics* and Warnings, *Skeletal Muscle*).

Grapefruit juice contains one or more components that inhibit CYP3A4 and can increase the plasma concentrations of drugs metabolized by CYP3A4. Large quantities of grapefruit juice (greater than 1 quart daily) significantly increase the serum concentrations of lovastatin and its (beta)-hydroxyacid metabolite during lovastatin therapy and should be avoided (see Clinical Pharmacology, *Pharmacokinetics* and Warnings, *Skeletal Muscle*).

Nifedipine (Procardia)

Clinical Pharmacology

Coadministration of nifedipine and grapefruit juice resulted in an approximately twofold increase in nifedipine area under the curve (AUC) and C_{max} with no change in half-life. The increased plasma concentrations are most likely due to the inhibition of CYP3A4-related first-pass metabolism.

Precautions/Other Interactions

Grapefruit juice: Coadministration of nifedipine and grapefruit juice resulted in an approximately twofold increase in nifedipine AUC and C_{max} with no change in half-life. The increased plasma concentrations are most likely due to the inhibition of CYP3A4-related first-pass metabolism. Coadministration of nifedipine and grapefruit juice is to be avoided.

Dosage and Administration

Coadministration of nifedipine and grapefruit juice is to be avoided (see Clinical Pharmacology and Precautions: Other Interactions).

Aripiprazole (Abilify)

Precautions/Drug Interactions

Other strong inhibitors of CYP3A4 (itraconazole) would be expected to have similar effects and need similar dose reductions; weaker inhibitors (erythromycin and grapefruit juice) have not been studied.

PLAUSIBILITY OF DRUG–GRAPEFRUIT JUICE INTERACTION

When assessing cases identified in AERS, the plausibility of the drug–grapefruit juice interaction is also considered, based on the current knowledge of the mechanism of this interaction (discussed in Chapter 7). Drugs that are likely to interact with grapefruit juice would have to be given orally, be a substrate for metabolism by CYP3A4, and have a relatively low bioavailability due to extensive presystemic extraction (first-pass metabolism) by CYP3A4 (5,6).

The next step would be to compare the drugs identified in the AERS search with current labeling to check for potential drug–grapefruit juice interactions meriting further investigation and the possible need for labeling updates. One of the drugs is no longer marketed (astemizole). The following list categorizes the remaining drugs identified in the AERS cases in relation to product labeling.

1. Appropriate information on grapefruit juice interaction appears in product labeling: estrogens, lovastatin, nifedipine, and verapamil.
2. No information in product labeling, but low plausibility of grapefruit juice interaction: bupropion, doxazosin, gabapentin, lisinopril, risperidone, sertraline, and sibutramine.
3. Product labeling indicates lack of grapefruit juice interaction, but plausibility of interaction: amlodipine.
4. No information in product labeling, but plausibility of grapefruit interaction: atorvastatin.

This screening process indicated that the majority of drugs identified in the AERS cases contain appropriate information in their product labeling with the exception of the two drugs in categories 3 and 4. As described in Chapter 10, other available resources, such as the literature (see Chapter 7) and drug interaction studies submitted by manufacturers, will be sought to evaluate the need for labeling revisions for these two products. This process illustrates how the FDA continuously works with drug manufacturers to determine which drug products need revisions to their labeling to reflect accurate and clinically relevant information on drug–grapefruit juice interactions. This process has resulted in a number of changes to drug product labeling addressing grapefruit juice interaction in recent years (Chapter 10).

Drugs that are already labeled for grapefruit juice interaction can also be reviewed to evaluate labeling for similar products, such as those that have a similar pharmacokinetic profile and are in the same drug class. For example, current labeling for tadalafil (4) states that it is likely that grapefruit juice would increase tadalafil exposure. Two other drugs in this class, vardenafil and sildenafil, also appear to be sensitive substrates of CYP3A. This is suggested by high (10–49-fold) increases in AUC for these two drugs compared to a 2.2-fold increase with tadalafil after coadministration of strong CYP3A inhibitors such as ketoconazole and ritonavir. In addition, both have low oral bioavailability. There was one case of sildenafil–grapefruit juice interaction among the original 186 AERS cases that did not meet the specific criteria described above; however, the report (presented below) was suggestive of an interaction. The FDA is evaluating the labeling for these two products to ensure that proper grapefruit interaction information is included.

A 52-year-old male with impotence experienced hypotension several hours after taking sildenafil 100 mg. The patient took sildenafil with grapefruit juice. He was also taking a mixture of dietary flavinoids (Privex CV®) and triamterene/hydrochlorothiazide. The reporting pharmacist did not state if the patient took sildenafil alone without problems before this episode.

CONCLUSION

Spontaneous case reports have been an important addition to literature reports and manufacturer-submitted clinical studies to help the FDA continuously evaluate product labeling for drug–grapefruit interaction.

REFERENCES

1. Health Canada is advising Canadians not to take certain drugs with grapefruit juice: http://www.hc-sc.gc.ca/english/protection/warnings/2002/2002_49e.htm.
2. The Adverse Event Reporting System (AERS): http://www.fda.gov/cder/aers/default.htm.
3. www.fda.gov\medwatch.
4. Physicians' Desk Reference: http://pdrel.thomsonhc.com/pdrel/librarian (accessed April, 2004).
5. Kane GC, Lipsky JJ. Drug-grapefruit interactions. Mayo Clin Proc 2000; 75(9):933–942.
6. Greenblatt DJ, Patki KC, von Moltke LL, Shader RJ. Drug interactions with grapefruit juice: an update. J Clin Psychopharmacol 2001; 21(4):357–359.

14

Botanicals as Drugs: A U.S. Perspective

Freddie Ann Hoffman

HeteroGeneity, LLC, Washington, D.C., U.S.A.

INTRODUCTION

Nature, as a biochemist, is unparalleled. Mankind has harvested the benefits of her combinatorial talents for thousands of years as a source of novel medicinals. For more than half a century, however, natural products have been relegated to source materials for "chemical libraries" from which new "leads" are mined (1). In a grants announcement, the National Institutes of Health (NIH) stated: "Chemical libraries are a mainstay of drug discovery. Well-crafted libraries, consisting of collections of anywhere from a few compounds to millions of them, can help scientists sort quickly through a haystack of possibilities to find the shining needle that may be developed into a lifesaving drug" (2). Once an "active" or "new chemical entity" (NCE), is found, it is isolated, "optimized," and then screened in receptor assays for further clinical development. To enhance the odds of finding clinically useful NCEs, the pharmaceutical industry has developed modern techniques, which include proteomics, bioinformatics, "high-throughput" screening techniques, combinatorial chemistry, and computer-aided design and prediction of drug toxicity and metabolism. These new approaches are based upon increasing knowledge of receptor sites in normal and disease states.

But "botanicals" do not fit easily into this development paradigm. As a drug class, botanicals have no rival for their structural complexity or diversity of effects. Defined by their heterogeneity, botanicals have multiple actives, which in some cases are unknown and in others are too numerous to evaluate. Screening these products against individual receptor targets cannot begin to describe their rich activity profiles. Similar to biologic products, such as vaccines, the potential activity of botanicals as pharmaceutical products may be best illuminated in bioassays and, more importantly, in living systems.

Mainstream U.S. pharmaceutical development has thrived on regulatory policies that evolved over decades of experience with single NCEs. Therefore, the heterogeneous nature of botanicals engenders discomfort and uncertainty in those who are used to single-chemical entity drugs and the NCE regulatory structure. But the interest in botanicals and other heterogeneous products as pharmaceuticals has inspired a change in the U.S. perspective, resulting in a new regulatory paradigm that draws upon historical precedent and novel interpretations of regulatory policies. Only recently has the U.S. Food and Drug Administration (FDA) developed a regulatory definition of a "botanical," as any product that "contains ingredients of vegetable matter or its constituents as a finished product" (3). For the purposes of US regulation, botanicals include drug products derived from one or more plants, algae, or macroscopic fungi, but does not include a highly purified or chemically modified substance derived from such a source. In the United States, botanicals can be regulated as foods, drugs, biologics, cosmetics, and medical devices. However, no botanical "pharmaceuticals," or more precisely, botanical "new" drugs are being marketed at this time. A "new" drug is defined by the Federal Food, Drug and Cosmetic (FD&C) Act as any drug marketed after 1938 that is " . . . not generally recognized as safe (GRAS) and effective under the conditions prescribed, recommended or suggested in the labeling" or one that has become GRAS, but "which has not . . . been used to a material extent or for a material time" (FD&C Act, Section 201 p.). A "new" drug must be proven to be safe and effective for its intended use prior to marketing in the United States. To study a "new" drug, the product sponsor must file an "Investigational New Drug" (IND) application with the FDA, exempting the product from the requirements of safety and efficacy while it is being tested in an investigational setting. After sufficient evidence is obtained, the sponsor can submit the data to the FDA as part of a "New Drug Application" (NDA). If the information is deemed adequate, the FDA can approve the product for marketing.

Therefore, to be marketed as a pharmaceutical, a botanical must traverse the modern regulatory process resulting in an approved NDA. The fact that no botanical is currently "NDA-approved" has caused many to speculate whether a botanical could ever make it through the rigorous U.S. drug development process, and still others to ask "why" one would choose to pursue this avenue, given the panoply of regulatory options already available to botanicals in the United States.

REGULATORY OPTIONS

When asked to describe a "botanical" product, food products come quickly to the mind. Fruits, vegetables, grains, herbs and spices, condiments, and teas are easily recognized as products from plant sources. Dietary supplements, defined by the Dietary Supplement Health and Education Act (DSHEA) of 1994, belong to the regulatory category of food products permitted to contain ingredients that are " . . . herbs or other botanicals, . . . dietary substances or concentrates, metabolites, constituents, extracts, or combination of these ingredients . . . ." Products such as ginkgo, St. John's wort (SJW), and ginseng are examples of botanicals currently marketed in the United States as dietary supplements. Less commonly recognized as botanicals are the allergenic vaccines derived from grasses and pollens, which are regulated as biologics, and the dental alginates, poultices, and adhesives that are medical devices. Finally, botanicals are often ingredients of cosmetics, such as aloe-containing hand lotions and herbal shampoos.

HISTORICAL PERSPECTIVE

To understand the current regulatory milieu of botanicals as drugs in the United States, one must revisit their historical use. Botanical medicine is an integral part of U.S. history. The democratic processes that governed this new nation extended to the practice of the healing arts. At the beginning of the 19th century, no single medical profession existed. Samuel Thomson, who had no formal education, received a patent for his system of "botanic medicine," which he described in the "New Guide to Health," published in 1822. His followers, known as "Thomsonians," practiced a form of naturopathy using plant-based medicines such as *Lobelia inflata* or "Indian tobacco"—a violent emetic to purge the system of obstructions—and red pepper, to induce perspiration. After Thomson's death in 1843, his disciples formed another botanic sect, known as the "Eclectics," deriving their name from their assimilation of the "best" from the various schools of medicine that were developing at the time (4).

By 1900, most drugs in the United States were derived from natural sources. Ingredients were pulverized and extracted with hot water and alcohol, and administered in the form of teas, suspensions, emulsions, and syrups. Fine powders were prepared for pills or ointments. Ingredients were combined in proprietary mixtures called "patent" medicines. Hawked by their inventors as "cure-all" medicinals, these secret formulas were not only concocted by uneducated consumers, but were also sold directly to the unsuspecting public. Preparations often contained dangerous and addictive substances, such as morphine, cocaine, and opium, which resulted in severe and sometimes fatal reactions (5). In 1906, the first comprehensive federal legislation in the United States was passed to address the quality and safety of food and drug products.

This new law, known as the Pure Foods and Drugs Act, prevented the importation of "adulterated and spurious drugs and medicines," and required that all ingredients be identified on the drug label, thus ending the era of "secret" nostrums (6,7).

Passage of the 1906 act heralded the beginning of a new regulatory environment that would transform the U.S. drug industry. Many so-called drug "manufacturers" disappeared overnight, while others succeeded in complying with the new regulations (Fig. 1). Those who did change would grow into a new industry, gaining further momentum with the passage of the comprehensive 1938 FD&C Act. Fueled by the 1937 tragedy in which a hundred or so individuals died following ingestion of a tainted formulation of an "Elixir of Sulfanilamide," the new act now required that drugs be demonstrated as safe in animals and humans prior to being marketed. This new Act also considerably expanded the federal government's jurisdiction over the food and drug industries and has become the cornerstone of modern food and drug regulation in the United States (7).

By this time, however, botanicals as a product class had the reputation of being mostly palliative. Many had a slow onset of action and were used to treat signs and symptoms, without improving the underlying disease process. A notable exception was quinine, an extract of the bark of the South American cinchona tree, traditionally used to ward off the symptoms of malaria (8). One natural product, however, would irrevocably change the U.S. drug industry. From its discovery as a product of fermentation, to its isolation, purification, and synthesis, penicillin set the stage for an entirely new industry based on single chemical entities. Penicillin belonged

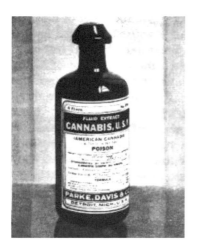

"Fluid Extract Cannabis, in common with other of our products that cannot be accurately assayed by chemical means, is tested physiologically and made to conform to a standard that has been found to be, in practice, reliable. Every package is stamped with the date of manufacture. Physiologic standardization was introduced **by Parke, Davis & Co.**

This fluid extract is prepared from *Cannabis sativa* grown in America. Extensive pharmacological and clinical tests have shown that its medicinal action cannot be distinguished from that of the fluid made from imported East Indian cannabis. Introduced to the medical profession by us.

Average dose, 1 1.2 mins. (0.1 cc). Narcotic, analgesic, sedative."

From the Parke, Davis & Company 1929-1930 physicians' catalog

Figure 1 Standardized botanical extracts. *Source*: Reprinted with permission of the Schaeffer Library of Drug Policy.

to a class of antibiotics that became known as the "miracle" drugs. Unlike the traditional botanicals, these drugs displayed a rapid onset of action and demonstrated remarkable therapeutic efficacy that would elevate the public's expectations for all future pharmaceuticals (9).

Following the passage of the FD&C Act, FDA was authorized to permit NDAs for "new" drugs, but the agency could not approve them affirmatively (see Section 505 of the FD&C Act). One such NDA was for the botanical rauwolfia (*Rauwolfia serpentina*), first marketed in the United States in 1953. Used in India for centuries, root of rauwolfia was sold in the United States as a treatment for hypertension. More than a dozen NDAs were subsequently recorded for the drug, all of which were discontinued by 1982, as better antihypertensives came to market (Table 1).

Table 1 NDAs for *Rauwolfia serpentina* (discontinued before January 1, 1982)

NDA number	Active ingredient	Dosage form; route	Strength	Proprietary name	Applicant
008842	*R. serpentina*	Tablet; oral	100 mg, 50 mg	Raudixin	Apothecon
009276	*R. serpentina*	Tablet; oral	100 mg, 50 mg	Hiwolfia	Bowman Pharms
009477	*R. serpentina*	Tablet; oral	100 mg, 50 mg	*R. serpentina*	Bundy
009926	*R. serpentina*	Tablet; oral	100 mg, 50 mg	Rauserpin	Ferndale Labs
009255	*R. serpentina*	Tablet; oral	100 mg, 50 mg	Wolfina	Forest Pharms
080498	*R. serpentina*	Tablet; oral	100 mg, 50 mg	*R. serpentina*	Halsey
009273	*R. serpentina*	Tablet; oral	100 mg, 50 mg	*R. serpentina*	Impax Labs
011521	*R. serpentina*	Tablet; oral	100 mg, 50 mg	*R. serpentina*	Ivax Pharms
009108	*R. serpentina*	Tablet; oral	100 mg, 50 mg	Rauval	Pal Pak
009278	*R. serpentina*	Tablet; oral	100 mg, 50 mg	Koglucoid	Panray
010581	*R. serpentina*	Tablet; oral	50 mg	Hyserpin	Phys Prods VA
080842	*R. serpentina*	Tablet; oral	100 mg, 50 mg	*R. serpentina*	Purepac Pharm
080583	*R. serpentina*	Tablet; oral	100 mg, 50 mg	*R. serpentina*	Pvt Form
080500	*R. serpentina*	Tablet; oral	100 mg, 50 mg	*R. serpentina*	Solvay
083444	*R. serpentina*	Tablet; oral	100 mg	*R. serpentina*	Tablicaps
083867	*R. serpentina*	Tablet; oral	50 mg	*R. serpentina*	Tablicaps
009668	*R. serpentina*	Tablet; oral	100 mg, 50 mg	*R. serpentina*	Valeant Pharm Intl
080914	*R. serpentina*	Tablet; oral	100 mg	*R. serpentina*	Watson Labs
080907	*R. serpentina*	Tablet; oral	50 mg	*R. serpentina*	Watson Labs

Abbreviation: NDA, new drug application.
Source: DHHS, FDA, Center for Drug Evaluation and Research: The Electronic Orange Book–Dec. 2003; Approved Drug Products with Therapeutic Equivalence Evaluations.

Passage of the Drug ("Kefauver–Harris") amendments in 1962 further tightened the federal government's control over the regulation of pharmaceuticals, increasing FDA's role in the testing of investigational drugs and providing the agency greater powers of enforcement. The legislation was precipitated by the thalidomide disaster that left hundreds of European infants malformed after their mothers took the drug as a sleeping aid during pregnancy. Drugs were now required to demonstrate proof of safety *and* efficacy for their labeled indications, prior to being marketed. Data collected from investigational studies would now be reviewed by FDA to determine whether the legal test of "substantial evidence" was met for approval. FDA was also required to review retrospectively all drugs that had entered the domestic market between 1938 and 1962. Those marketed under an NDA were reviewed by the Drug Efficacy Study Implementation or "DESI" program. Under DESI, more than 3400 drug products and 16,000 claims were reviewed. Thirty percent of the drugs lacked sufficient supporting evidence and were considered ineffective and removed from the U.S. market (10).

DESI also included 420 nonprescription ("over the counter" or "OTC") drugs, which had entered the US market through the "new" drug procedures during 1938 and 1962. OTC drugs not reviewed by the DESI program numbered in the hundreds of thousands and were considered to be "GRAS". The agency began its efficacy review of the OTC drugs in 1972. To conserve resources, FDA focused on active ingredients, which it grouped by therapeutic category. For each category, FDA promulgated regulations in the form of monographs, establishing conditions by which the ingredients were determined to be "generally recognized as effective" or "GRAE." Faced with the enormity of its task, FDA chose to limit its review to those ingredients that had U.S. marketing experience to support "material time" and "material extent" (11). As a result of the agency's narrow interpretation of the statute, many botanical ingredients were ineligible for inclusion in the OTC review, because at that time they were only being marketed outside of the United States (12). However, products that had entered the U.S. market prior to 1938 were exempt from review, and included botanicals such as senna, cascara, and witch hazel, which continue to be marketed as OTC drugs today.

COMPLEMENTARY AND ALTERNATIVE MEDICINE

During the 1980s, U.S. interest in botanicals resurfaced under the guise of "complementary and alternative medicine" (CAM). By this time, botanicals had lost considerable credibility. Proponents of "Laetrile"—a concoction of cyanogenic glycosides extracted from peach pits—drew media attention when the FDA began seizing the product as an "unapproved" drug and as "ineffective cancer treatment" (13). However, by 1991, in response to growing consumer interest, the U.S. Congress appropriated funds to the National

Institutes of Health for the establishment of a federal research program for the scientific evaluation of CAM. Now identified as one of the "biologically-based therapies," botanical medicine became a research priority for the new NIH Office of Alternative Medicine (OAM) (14).

This dramatic turnabout in the U.S. consumer attitude toward botanical medicine was not lost on foreign manufacturers. Many companies in Europe and Asia that had never stopped marketing botanicals were now eager to satisfy the growing U.S. demand. A rate-limiting step, however, was FDA's exclusion of foreign marketing experience as a threshhold criteria for inclusion in the OTC drug monograph process. Most botanicals had been discontinued from the US market in the earlier part of the century. Due to the 1962 amendments these same products would now have to undergo FDA approval as "new" drugs through the IND/NDA process—a process established based on single chemical entities. In July 1992, the European American Phytomedicine Coalition (EAPC), an alliance between the U.S. and European phytomedicine companies, submitted a petition to FDA requesting that foreign marketing histories be eligible for inclusion in the OTC review process. The agency took several years to respond to the petition, and when it did, its response was to request more information from the petitioners (11,15). This inaction led many in the industry to conclude that FDA either did not consider botanicals on equal footing with the single chemical entities, or would not seriously entertain their review under the IND/NDA process (16). According to Loren Israelsen, an attorney involved with the herb industry and EAPC cocounsel, "The issues raised by the EAPC are important policy considerations which deserve a thoughtful and affirmative response from FDA. We have tried to frame the problem and the solution squarely and FDA's silence is not only disappointing but gives support to the industry's belief that the Agency remains inflexible and unresponsive" (15).

FDA's inaction may have been responsible in part for efforts leading to the passage of DSHEA in October 1994. The new law addressed "herbs and other botanicals" in the context of nutritional supplement ingredients. Over the next six years, botanical supplement sales doubled, peaking at over US $4 billion in 2000 (17). Even so, the intent of Congress was clear from the language of DSHEA: unlike drugs, dietary supplements were not intended to diagnose, mitigate, treat, cure, or prevent disease, although similar to drugs they could make claims to "affect the structure or function of the body" [FD&C Act, Section 201(g)] (18).

A NEW REGULATORY PARADIGM

The legal limitations placed on dietary supplements with respect to disease claims did nothing to stem the increase in the consumer use of botanicals as an alternative means to prevent or treat disease conditions. A survey conducted in 1990 and repeated in 1997 found "herbal medicine" to be one of the leading alternative therapies responsible for a significant increase in CAM usage in the United States (19). In response to growing concerns over the safety and efficacy of botanicals, the OAM funded several grants that proposed to study botanicals for therapeutic indications. Although products could be purchased in local grocery and health-food stores, their evaluation as "new" drugs required that the trials be conducted under IND applications (20,21).

What criteria would the FDA use to determine whether the clinical trials could be allowed to proceed under an IND application? The test products were complex mixtures of botanical extracts with multiple or unknown actives. In the absence of a single known active, routine chemistry, pharmacology, and toxicology testing could not be easily conducted. The closest products resembling botanicals were biologics: vaccines and blood-derived products. Both product categories were defined by strict controls over the manufacturing process, rather than by chemical determination of the product in the final vial. Botanicals raised unique issues: not only were plant nomenclature and taxonomy not internationally harmonized, but also the common names for plants varied by country (22,23).

FDA needed a new regulatory paradigm—one that would be consistent with current drug law, but could also address the unique characteristics and status of botanicals as a heterogeneous class of pharmaceuticals (24). Over the next six years, the FDA developed a "Draft Guidance for Industry on Botanical Drug Products," published on August 10, 2000, and finalized in June 2004 (3) (see Chapter 15). The FDA would also amend its regulations to allow foreign marketing experience as a basis for including foreign-marketed botanicals in the OTC drug monograph process (25).

SELECTING A ROUTE TO MARKET

Although the new FDA guidance provides a broad outline for botanical drug development, it does not assume all botanicals to be drugs. Instead, manufacturers are presented with a "decision-tree" that describes the possible regulatory categories (3). How a product is regulated depends on several factors, which include product formulation and route of administration. Topically administered products can be sold as drugs, devices, or cosmetics, but not as foods or dietary supplements. Parenteral administration is reserved for drugs. Tablet or capsule formulations can be marketed as dietary supplements or drugs, but not as "conventional" foods.

Intrinsic safety can further define the regulatory possibilities. Foods, including dietary supplements, must be safe for the general public. Conventional foods are limited to ingredients that are "dietary," "GRAS," or approved food additives. In contrast, dietary supplements can contain both "dietary" ingredients and "new" dietary ingredients. "Dietary" ingredients must have been "present in the food supply in a form used for food, not chemically altered." Ingredients marketed in the United States after October 15, 1994, are considered to be "new dietary ingredients." "New" dietary ingredients must have "a 'history of use' or other evidence of safety ... that the new dietary ingredient would be reasonably expected to be safe under conditions of labeling." For products containing "new dietary ingredients," FDA must receive written notification at least 75 days prior to marketing, providing information to support the safety of the ingredients (18).

Unlike foods, including dietary supplements, the safety of a drug is based on a "benefit to risk ratio." "Benefit" is an assessment of the drug's efficacy, balanced against any negatives with respect to a particular indication in a target population (24). Thus, a drug that is deemed "safe" to treat leukemia may not be "safe" to treat osteoarthritis.

INTENDED USE

A defining principle of U.S. regulation is a product's "intended use." "Intended use" is determined by labeling claims. "Labeling" encompasses not only the required elements that make up the printed label on the bottle, but also any direct or implied claims made by the manufacturer or distributor in the product packaging, advertising, and promotional materials. "Intended use" defines the product category. For example, the FD&C Act defines drugs as "articles intended for use in the diagnosis, mitigation, treatment, cure or prevention of disease or to affect the structure or function of the body." Drug products may bear "disease," "sign," or "symptom-related" claims ("prevents migraine"; "lowers blood pressure"; and "relieves cough and fever").

Similar to drugs, dietary supplements can make claims to "affect the structure or function of the body." However, supplements are specifically prohibited from making "disease" claims. A dietary supplement bearing "structure or function" claims is also required to carry the following disclaimer on the product label: "The FDA has not evaluated this claim. This product is not intended to diagnose, mitigate, treat, cure or prevent disease" (19).

ADVANTAGES OF THE DRUG ROUTE

If a botanical is shown to reverse an abnormal test result, modify another drug's adverse event, or act synergistically with another modality, it will usually be best developed as a "drug." This is especially true if the botanical provides a distinct benefit for a patient population, but would pose safety concerns if used by the general public. In contrast to prevention, risk-reduction, or health-maintenance trials, therapeutic studies are often able to demonstrate clinical benefit with smaller numbers of subjects and with more tangible measures of outcome.

But sponsors, enticed by the low cost of market entry for dietary supplements, often dismiss the potential advantages of pharmaceutical development. Because the regulatory schema for a drug is significantly more complicated than that for foods, US law provides many protections for those who choose the pathway of drug development, not the least of which is the confidentiality of the process. From the filing of the IND through the NDA approval, exchanges between sponsors and FDA are kept confidential by the agency. This is in stark contrast to the very public process of food applications, petitions, and notifications.

Patents, trademarks, and copyrights provide additional proprietary protection, which may have a more profound impact on pharmaceuticals than on products sold in most other categories. Although food and cosmetic ingredients may be afforded some protection through composition and process patents, an underlying premise behind marketing of food products is their similarity to prior foods and ingredients with known histories of safe use. The further a "new dietary ingredient" strays from a traditional food ingredient, the more documentation will be necessary to ensure "safety," thus undermining the ease and minimal cost at which most food products are allowed to come to the market. In contrast, pharmaceuticals exploit differences, capitalizing on the nuances between molecular analogs and minor alterations in formulation, dosing, and usage. "New" drugs do not have "GRAS/E" status. Generic equivalents of "new" drugs usually enter the marketplace only after an innovator's patent protections have expired. Under the "Price Competition and Patent Term Restoration" Act (also known as the "Hatch-Waxman" Act), not only can the term of a drug's patent be extended or "restored" to account for market-time lost while the product is under regulatory review, but also it is in the FDA's purview to grant periods of marketing exclusivity during which the agency will not accept a competitive filing (26). For new clinical entities, the first product approved under an NDA can receive a five-year period of marketing exclusivity, and an additional five years is added to the expiration date of any patents. New indications, formulations, or routes of administration requiring additional clinical trials (beyond bioequivalency studies) are granted a three-year period of marketing exclusivity and patent term extension. Under the Orphan Drug Act of 1983, drugs for rare disorders for which the target indication occurs in less than 200,000 individuals annually in the United States, are granted the maximum term of seven years exclusivity and patent extension. Pediatric indications can provide an extra six months of protection. No similar provisions are available for dietary supplements or conventional foods.

Finally, "new" drug approval following the demonstration of safety and efficacy through the IND/NDA process brings with it an added benefit of medical and scientific acceptance that can significantly boost the marketing message. For a drug, clinical results may be conveyed in more direct language for advertising and promotion, rather than the restrictive wording delineated for supplement "structure or function" or "health" claims.

COST

The ongoing debate on U.S. drug development costs is another reason sponsors look to alternative development strategies for their products. At issue are recent estimates arrived at through a survey of 10 large pharmaceutical companies. Average development costs for an NCE were estimated at US $403 million (in 2000), and when the time between investment and marketing is added, costs totaled a mind-boggling US $802 million (27,28). The figures were based on new synthetic chemicals not previously tested in humans, reflecting costs from all NCE candidates tested, including those that had failed. From the tens of thousands of chemicals generated in the discovery process, only a few hundred made it through the screening process, leaving only a dozen or so to undergo animal safety testing. In one review, attrition rates were reportedly due to "safety issues" (20.2%), "toxicology concerns" (19.4%), and "disappointing clinical efficacy" (22.5%). Another 39% of candidates were terminated for business reasons and "other factors" (29). Cost increases often begin in the laboratory: "What big pharmaceutical companies have done is tested a lot of existing materials. But now they've run out of those materials. Today, you have to create new compounds and then test them" (30).

But botanical products do not have to be "created," and many have already been shown to produce potentially useful biological effects in humans. More importantly, documentation of safe use in the target species—humans—is a monumental step that can shorten the development time considerably (24,31).

Whether a particular botanical should be developed as a pharmaceutical depends on the product and the business objectives of the sponsor. Sponsors should be cognizant of the costs incurred in "Good Manufacturing Practices upgrades"—modifying the product's manufacturing standards either to meet U.S. drug standards or to move from a food to a pharmaceutical-grade product. Regardless of the extent of prior human use, a botanical drug will likely be required to undergo additional safety and efficacy testing (24,31). Undoubtedly, the majority of costs of drug development is incurred in the conduct of clinical trials (28,30). However, unlike NCEs, FDA may permit an initial study to be conducted with a product purchased "off-the-shelf" as a dietary supplement. A randomized, controlled "pilot" study may be the initial trial for a botanical drug under an IND, with an agreement between the agency and the product sponsor that at least one other large multicenter trial with a pharmaceutical-grade product will be conducted for the NDA, if initial results are promising (31). Animal toxicology testing may also be required to address safety questions that cannot be easily assessed in humans (24). Although not a requirement for foods, interactions of the botanical drug with other drugs and with foods must also be evaluated, depending on the indication and the potential for interactions.

Under the Prescription Drug User Fee Act, the FDA can levy fees for the review of applications containing clinical trial data, although waivers can be sought for nonprofit sponsors and small businesses.

WHOLE IS GREATER THAN THE PARTS

Whether a botanical should be pursued as a drug or whether it should be "mined" for its actives, depends on the botanical and its constituents. Isolation, purification, and synthesis of single active chemical moieties from natural products have produced a substantial number of the pharmaceuticals in use today. By some accounts, 62% of the current NCE anticancer drugs are nonsynthetic, and more than half of the antihypertensive drugs can be traced to natural product structures or mimics (32). Determining what is "active," however, is not always straightforward. Most botanical extracts yield legions of constituents with diverse biochemical profiles and pharmacologic effects. A constituent identified as "active" for one particular effect may be "inactive" for others. So-called "inactive" ingredients also may contribute to the biological effects of a product indirectly, through modulation of the actives.

To ensure lot-to-lot consistency, standardization of extracts often relies on constituents as "biomarkers" for plant identity and potency. SJW (*Hypericum perforatum*), a perennial shrub traditionally used as a mood enhancer and mild antidepressant, has been tested in dozens of clinical trials, with mixed results for efficacy. Some of its purported bioactive constituents include naphthodianthrones, including hypericin; flavonoids; phloroglucinols, including hyperforin; and essential oils. For many years, hypericin was presumed to be the active component. As a result most extracts were standardized based on hypericin concentration. Recent data, however, support other components such as hyperforin and the flavanoids, that may also contribute to the therapeutic efficacy of the SJW extracts (33–35). Because these secondary components were previously unaccounted for in the standardization of the former clinical test articles, and because these constituents are chemically unrelated to and their content within the plant varies independently of hypericin, it has been argued that the potency of these constituents in any particular batch was unlikely to be similar to that of other batches. This variability between batches could explain the observed differences in the clinical trial results (36).

For many botanicals, the "whole is greater than the parts." Indeed, individual constituents of an extract may actually produce contradictory effects. Oriental ginseng (*Panax ginseng*) root, widely used in traditional Chinese and Korean medicine, contains over 28 different ginsenosides. Although chemically similar in structure, various ginsenosides have been shown experimentally to produce opposite effects: hypothermia or hyperthermia, hypotension or hypertension, and hemolysis or inhibition of hemolysis—depending on the type of ginsenoside. One must, therefore, use caution in determining what is "active" and be aware that the properties—both positive and negative—of any particular constituent may not represent the biological activity of the extract as a whole (37,38).

In summary, botanicals are as diverse as nature itself. They bring a wealth of possibilities for innovative new drugs. As a result of the options available to botanical producers, a number of development approaches exist in the United States, but no single paradigm. While many botanicals are best sold as "foods," others will find a more promising future as pharmaceuticals. Those that are systematically studied in scientifically designed trials and are able to demonstrate consistent, clinically relevant biological activity may traverse the drug development process to achieve the status of "new" drugs—the "botanical pharmaceuticals."

REFERENCES

1. Mann J. Murder, Magic, and Medicine. Oxford University, 1994.
2. National Institutes of Health News. National Institute of General Medical Sciences Chemistry Center Grants to Expand Drug Discovery Toolkit. October 1, 2003.
3. Department of Health and Human Services, Food and Drug Administration. Center for Drug Evaluation and Research: Draft Guidance for Industry-Botanical Drug Products (http://www.fda.gov/cder/guidance/4592dft.htm. June, 2004).
4. Starr P. The Social Transformation of American Medicine. NY: Basic Books, Inc., 1982:50–52; 96.
5. Janssen W. Food and Drug Administration: The story of the laws behind the labels. FDA Consumer, June 1981.
6. Young J. The Toadstool Millionaires: A Social History of Patent Medicines in America Before Federal Regulation. Princeton Press, 1961.
7. Hutt R, Merrill R. Food and Drug Law–University Casebook Series. 2d ed. NY: The Foundation Press, Inc., 1991.
8. Honigsbaum M. The Fever Trail: In Search of the Cure for Malaria. Farrar, Straus & Giroux, 2001.
9. Lax E. The Mold in Dr. Florey's Coat: The Story of Penicillin and the Modern Age of Medical Miracles. Henry Holt & Company, 2004.
10. Food and Drug Administration; www.fda.gov.
11. Pinco R. Implications of FDA's proposal to include foreign marketing experience in the over-the-counter drug review process. Food Drug Law J 1998; 53:105–122.
12. Pape S, Kracov D, Rubin P. FDA Issues proposed regulations on foreign marketing data for OTC drug approvals. HerbalGram 2000; 48:40.
13. Young JH. Laetrile in historical perspective. In: Merkle GE, Petersen JC, eds. Politics, Science, and Cancer: The Laetrile Phenomenon. Boulder, CO: Westview Press, 1980.
14. National Institutes of Health, National Center for Complementary and Alternative Medicine (http://nccam.nih.gov/).

15. Blumenthal M. EAPC files petitions for OTC drug use for valerian and ginger. HerbalGram 1995; 35:19.
16. Bayne H. FDA publishes new draft guidance for botanical drug products. HerbalGram 2000; 50:68.
17. Nutr Bus J. www.nutritionbusiness.com.
18. Dietary Supplement Health and Education Act (DSHEA) Public Law 103–417 103rd Congress, October 1994.
19. Eisenberg D, Davis R, Ettner S, et al. Trends in alternative medicine use in the United States, 1990–1997. J Am Med Assoc 1998; 280:1569–1575.
20. Eskinazi D, Hoffman F. Progress in complementary and alternative medicine: contribution of the National Institutes of Health and the Food and Drug Administration. J Altern Complement Med 1999; 4(4):459–467.
21. Marwick C. Growing use of medicinal botanicals forces assessment by drug regulators. JAMA 1995; 273(8):607–609.
22. Reveal J. Proposals to Modify the International Code of Botanical Nomenclature: Suprageneric Names. Norton-Brown Herbarium, University of Maryland College Park, Maryland, USA (http://www.inform.umd.edu/PBIO/fam/articles.html).
23. Yuan M, Hong Y. Heterogeneity of Chinese medical herbs in Singapore assessed by fluorescence AFLP analysis. Am J Chin Med 2003; 31(5):773–779.
24. Wu K-M, Farrelly J, Birnkrant D, et al. Regulatory toxicology perspectives on the development of botanical drug products in the United States. Am J Ther 2004; 11(3):213–217.
25. Department of Health, Human Services, Food, Drug Administration. 21 CFR 330. Additional criteria and procedures for classifying over-the-counter drugs as generally recognized as safe and effective and not misbranded. Final Rule Fed Reg 2002; 67(15):3060–3076.
26. Drug Price Competition and Patent Term Restoration Act (Public Law 98-417) ["Hatch-Waxman"].
27. DiMasi J, Hansen R, Grabowski H. The price of innovation: new estimates of drug development costs. J Health Econ 2003; 22(2):151–185.
28. Pharmaceutical Research and Manufacturers Association–Quick Facts (http://www.phrma.org/publications/quickfacts/14.08.2001.278.cfm).
29. Frank R. Editorial-New estimates of drug development costs. J Health Econ 2003; 22:325–330.
30. Rogoski R. Technology, clinical trials drive up drug development costs. In Depth: Biotech J From the January 16, 2004 print edition.
31. Bindra J, Sciavolino F, MacLean D, et al. Back to nature: the alternative paradigm for drug development. In: Lin Y, ed. Drug Discovery and Traditional Chinese Medicine. Boston: Kluwer Academic Publishers, 2001, Chapter 16.
32. Newman DJ, Cragg GM, Snader KM. Natural products as sources of new drugs over the period 1981–2002. J Nat Prod 2003; 66(7):1022–1037.
33. Chatterjee S, Bhattacharya S, Wonnemann M, et al. Hyperforin as a possible antidepressant component of hypericum extracts. Life Sci 1998; 63:499–510.
34. Greeson J, Sanford B, Monti DA. St. John's wort (Hypericum perforatum): a review of the current pharmacological, toxicological, and clinical literature. Psychopharmacology 2001; 153:402–414.

35. Butterweck V, Christoffel V, Nahrstedt A, et al. Step by step removal of hyperforin and hypericin: activity profile of different hypericum preparations in behavioral models. Life Sci 2003; 73(5):627–639.

36. Goldman P. Herbal medicines today and the roots of modern pharmacology. Ann Intern Med 2001; 135(8 pt1):594–600.

37. Zhao R, McDaniel W. Ginseng improves strategic learning in normal and brain-damaged rats. NeuroReports 1998; 9:1619–1624.

38. Liu Z, Luo X, Sun Y, et al. Can ginsenosides protect human erythrocytes against free-radical-induced hemolysis? Biochim Biophys Acta 2002; 1572(1): 58–66.

15

Development of Botanical Products as Pharmaceutical Agents

New Regulatory Approaches and Review Process at U.S. FDA

Shaw T. Chen

Center for Drug Evaluation and Research (CDER), Food and Drug Administration, Silver Spring, Maryland, U.S.A.

INTRODUCTION

Botanical or herbal products have been used extensively as drug treatments in the complementary and alternative medical (CAM) system in many regions of the world, but have not been subjected to the same rigorous evaluation by regulatory agencies as that for modern nonbotanical pharmaceutical agents. To facilitate further development of new drugs from botanical sources, the Center for Drug Evaluation and Research (CDER) of U.S. Food and Drug Administration (FDA) has published a draft Guidance for Industry: Botanical Drug Product in August, 2000. The Guidance has since been published in its final form in June of 2004 (see link to the document given in Ref. 1). The new regulatory approaches in the Guidance take into consideration the unique features of the botanical drugs and the substantial past human experiences. Its major provisions will be summarized below.

To implement the new Guidance, the CDER established a new Botanical Review Team (BRT) dedicated to the review of botanical specific issues in new drug applications (NDAs). A new Manual of Policies and Procedures

(MAPP) for processing the botanical submissions in CDER has also been published for the application sponsors and the Agency review staff to follow. Information on the new MAPP and the BRT will be presented in the following pages, which can also be found in the FDA website (1).

THE REGULATORY OBJECTIVES

To support approval as a nonbotanical drug, adequate and well-controlled clinical studies are required. Not only must the treatment be shown to be effective, with real patient benefits in morbidity and/or mortality to justify the safety risk of adverse reactions as observed, but the clinical data must also provide practical instructions for use, which can be reasonably followed by health care professionals. There is no reason why these requirements should be different for botanical drugs, because patient suffering and treatment benefits are independent of medical theory or practice. Regardless of medical systems and terminology used, courses of diseases/conditions should be established and treatment effects must be clinically meaningful. Incorporation of alternative medical practice into the clinical studies will be acceptable if the new set of instructions derived from such studies will be practical.

The objective of the new FDA regulatory approaches to new botanical drug development is not to create an additional category of products different from dietary supplements or nonbotanical drugs. Instead, the goal is to confer the botanical new drugs the same degree of confidence in quality and clinical usefulness, as that of nonbotanical drugs, and ultimately to bring the botanical drugs into the mainstream medical use.

THE DISTINCTIVE FEATURES OF BOTANICALS

From a regulatory perspective, botanical drugs have some unique features that demand special considerations. Clinically, there is a large quantity of anecdotal experience about the efficacy, which is not supported by modern scientific data, nor can it easily be dismissed. Likewise, extensive human usages also suggest that most of the botanical preparations are possibly safe, but confidence in such presumed safety can only be based on mostly poorly documented data. The pre-existing availability of most botanical products, although not marketed as drugs, also creates difficulties in their regulation.

Concern about the quality of botanical products poses another regulatory challenge. Most botanical products are complex and variable mixtures of constituents too numerous to characterize individually. For many preparations, active ingredients have not been identified and it is thus difficult to quantify strength or potency of the botanical product. Because of the biological nature of botanical products, the assessment of their impurity and stability is often more problematic than that of nonbotanical pure drugs.

Beyond the natural mixtures in one part of a single plant, many botanical drugs are combinations of multiple botanical products. While the rationale of combining many plants is not easy to understand and contributions from ingredients remain to be elucidated, it is also not clear whether the ratio and composition have been optimized in many widely used formulations.

THE BOTANICAL GUIDANCE

In the Guidance, the botanical drug products are defined as those that contain as ingredients vegetable materials, which may include plant materials, algae, macroscopic fungi, or combinations thereof, that are *used as drugs*. It may be available as (but not limited to) a solution (e.g., tea), powder, tablet, capsule, elixir, topical, or injectable. In the current version, fermentation products, highly purified (or chemically modified) botanical substances, allergenic extracts and vaccines that contain botanical ingredients are excluded.

In essence, the Botanical Guidance provides that

- further purification of the botanical preparations is not required,
- identification of active ingredient(s) is not essential,
- chemistry, manufacturing and control (CMC) is extended to raw materials, not just regulations of drug substance and product, and
- nonclinical testing may be reduced or delayed for products with extensive history of human use.

It should be emphasized that, in the above new approaches, only different types of information are used in part of the safety assessment. This does not imply that overall standards for quality consistency and clinical efficacy/safety are more or less stringent than that of nonbotanical drugs.

In general, requirements in CMC and nonclinical studies for initiating a clinical study of botanical drugs depend to a large extent on the marketing history, known safety concerns (if any), the degree of modification from past use, and the scale of proposed clinical trials. For a small early phase study, animal toxicity may not be needed if the preparation and usage are the same as in prior human experiences. On the other hand, for large scale, more definitive trials, greater assurance in product quality, consistency, and reproducibility is necessary, as well as the safe use in the clinical setting of the protocol.

As evidence of prior human use, documentation of marketing history (with volume of sales) and review of past and current references, compendia, and literatures should be provided. It is understandable that many of these publications are in variable format and quality, and often do not consist of modern scientific data. In this respect, the Agency will accept all types of documentation for consideration and determine the validity of support in individual cases.

As noted above, all botanical drugs contain many potentially active molecular entities and many preparations are combinations of multiple parts/plants. Because the current policy on fixed-dose combination products requires demonstration of contribution to overall efficacy and safety from each active ingredient, it could be impractical or impossible for botanicals to comply with this regulation in the development as a drug product. This issue was not addressed in the current version of Botanical Guidance. While the Agency is considering revision of the fixed-dose combination regulation to accommodate the difficulties encountered by the botanical drugs, the sponsor is encouraged to consult the CDER for assistance.

For details of the Guidance, the readers are referred to the official FDA website for botanical drug review (1).

BOTANICAL REVIEW TEAM IN CENTER FOR DRUG EVALUATION AND RESEARCH

To acquire and consolidate regulatory experiences on botanical drugs, a dedicated BRT has been established in CDER. The BRT will provide scientific expertise on botanical issues to other reviewing staff to ensure consistent interpretation and implementation of the Botanical Guidance and related policies. In addition, the BRT has the following functions:

- Participates in all phases of reviews, meetings, and decision-making processes for all botanical drug applications and submissions as a collaborative scientific discipline, and serves as an expert resource for CDER on all botanical issues.
- Collects information, maintains a database of botanical applications, and performs periodic analysis on the status of botanical new drug development.
- Responds to external constituents who have general botanical drug development questions.
- Responds as the expert resource for CDER to issues and meeting requests from the Office of the Commissioner and interfaces on common botanical issues and fosters communication with the FDA Center for Food Safety and Applied Nutrition and the National Center for Complementary and Alternative Medicine and the Office of Dietary Supplements at the National Institutes of Health (NIH).
- Interfaces with external professional regulatory and scientific groups, makes presentations, and participates in workshops to promote and enhance botanical drug product development and knowledge.

The botanical reviews performed by the BRT cover the following area:

1. Medicinal plant biology: methods and problems in species identification; potential misuse of related but incorrect species.

2. Pharmacology and toxicology of medicinal plants used in the proposed studies: activities based on old, alternative theories and/or modern testing.
3. History of prior human uses: therapeutic effects in the CAM system; potential toxicities from past experience.

The BRT experts serve as members of the review teams, and provide scientific opinion on the botanical drug product in a role similar to that of other disciplines such as chemistry.

Currently, the BRT is a team of experts consisting of a medical officer as team leader, a pharmacognosy reviewer, and a project manager. The contact information is provided at the end of this chapter.

REVIEW PROCESSES FOR BOTANICAL APPLICATIONS

To implement the Botanical Guidance, a new set of review processes for botanical applications have been delineated in a new CDER MAPP (MAPP 6007.1 for Review of Botanical Drug Products).

As described in the MAPP, the BRT will respond only to general inquiries on botanical-related issues and interpretation of the Botanical Guidance and related policies. For questions about individual botanical drug product with specific clinical indication, the sponsor should submit the application to the new drug review divisions in charge of the therapeutic area in the CDER's Office of New Drugs, and the applications will remain under the divisions' administration. For specific botanical drug applications, all regulatory decisions will be the responsibilities of the new drug division and all regulatory actions will be issued by the division directors. Communication between sponsors and all review team members, including BRT staff, will be conducted through the project manager of the new drug division. As a member of the review team, the BRT experts provide scientific opinion on the botanical drug product in a role similar to that of experts in other disciplines.

In principle, all botanical submissions will be managed in the same manner as nonbotanical drug products by all review disciplines. That is, primary and secondary reviews in CMC, pharmacology/toxicology, biopharmaceutics, and clinical and statistical issues will be conducted by the respective primary reviewers and team leaders. To ensure consistency across different new drug review divisions, the supporting disciplines in CMC, pharmacology/toxicology, and biopharmaceutics have also designated one to three senior staff to serve as expert consultant(s) in botanical issues for the review divisions in each area.

These review processes for botanical applications have been tested in CDER with approximately 100 submissions. Collaborations between BRT and the new drug divisions have been smooth and productive.

BOTANICAL DRUG APPLICATIONS IN CENTER FOR DRUG EVALUATION AND RESEARCH

As of April 30, 2004, there are a total of 203 botanical drug applications in CDER, including 167 investigational new drug (IND) applications and 36 pre-IND consultations. At least 75% of the total botanical applications were submitted after 1999, and about two per month were received by the Agency recently.

Of these, 43% are commercial development programs and the remaining are academic research projects. These botanical submissions are distributed in all 14 therapeutic divisions, with most activities aggregated in the oncology, antiviral, and dermatology–dental drug areas (Fig. 1).

A great majority of botanical sponsors have taken advantage of the pre-IND consultation service provided by FDA. As a result, most IND applications were successful with initial submission and few (less than 20) were placed on clinical hold for safety concerns. However, despite the early success, many development programs and research projects have subsequently been suspended for various reasons. As of the above-mentioned cutoff date (April 30, 2004), nearly two-thirds (66%) of INDs still remain active (have not been placed on clinical hold, inactivated by FDA, or withdrawn by sponsor for lack of activities). To date, there have been no submissions of NDAs to FDA for marketing approval of botanical prescription drugs.

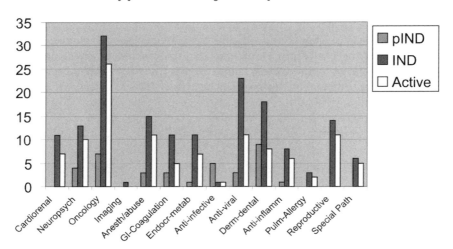

Figure 1   Numbers of IND applications (total and active) and pre-IND consultations in each of the New Drug Divisions in CDER. *Abbreviation*: IND, investigational new drug; CDER, Center for Drug Evaluation and Research.

CHALLENGES IN THE REVIEW OF BOTANICAL DRUG APPLICATIONS

Not surprisingly, quality of the botanical products is a frequent review issue in our regulatory experiences. Some sponsors had not presented accurate name/identification of the botanical plants and/or description of manufacturing processes. Because of the recent incidence of diethylstilbestrol containing PC-SPES, adulteration of botanicals with active chemical drugs has become a serious concern for both the study supporter (e.g., NIH) and the regulatory agency.

For many botanical preparations, there are often uncertainties in the identity of the plant species and/or consistency of botanical raw materials. Complicated manufacturing processes add further possible variation to the drug substance and final products. While most contamination problems unique to botanicals are resolvable, purity/potency and stability are more difficult technical issues, without knowing the identity of active ingredients.

Both the industry and the regulatory agency have realized that, as complex mixtures, it is usually difficult to define or characterize botanical preparations and differentiate among similar products. The tough task for the reviewing staff is thus finding out how to apply the set of regulations designed for highly pure, small molecular entities to a less well-defined botanical system. Apparently, some allowance of imprecision will be needed for CMC of botanical drugs without sacrificing the therapeutic consistency of different batches.

As provided in the Botanical Guidance, clinical studies have been permitted for many botanical preparations prior to a complete set of conventional animal toxicity testing. The decisions were not difficult for submissions with substantial and well-documented history of past human use. But some other applicants had not presented an adequate summary of the past human experiences and had failed even to document well-known toxicity of the herbal ingredients. Between these two extremes, how to adjust the requirements of animal toxicity data and substitute that with large quantity but poor quality of human experiences is another big challenge to the regulatory agency in the review of botanical applications.

As noted above, all available information on the historical use of botanical preparations will be accepted for safety consideration. But for FDA clinical reviewers, such experiences are often poorly documented and difficult to interpret or correlate with the paradigm of conventional (Western) medicine. In the alternative medical system, almost all the diagnoses to be treated with herbal medicine are defined in imprecise and foreign terms. Typically, one herbal medicine is indicated for numerous seemingly unrelated conditions, most of which are symptomatic relief without clear mechanisms. Furthermore, many botanicals are combinations of multiple herbs, but few references are available for the rationale of combining so many ingredients.

For these reasons, integrating all the background information into the over-all safety assessment for botanical applications has been difficult and required active participation of the BRT.

PROSPECTS OF FURTHER DEVELOPMENT

As noted above, there has been no botanical product approved as prescription new drug by the FDA. The slow pace of progress in botanical new drug development has been increasingly disappointing, possibly for the following reasons:

- The industry is still struggling with technical difficulties in bringing a complex and ill-defined system to comply with regulatory requirements set for precision of pure chemical drugs.
- Some of the diseases and conditions selected as indications for the botanical drugs are difficult to study. There are few exciting products to satisfy serious and unmet medical needs.
- Many sponsors were inexperienced in new drug development and unrealistic about the resources required for the complicated processes.
- There is no effective protection of intellectual property right and little incentive for further development of pre-existing preparations available on the market (albeit not yet as drugs).

Thus, while the Agency will in general use previous uncontrolled human experiences to expedite limited early stage testing to assess the therapeutic potential of herbal medicines, the overall progress has been slow. However, the technical difficulties in quality controls should be resolvable, and more clinical trials should be initiated. The sponsors of botanical applications should be prepared to go through a complicated scrutiny, the same as that for nonbotanical drugs, and plan ahead with an assessment of difficulties in clinical testing. Lastly, although market exclusivity may not be strictly enforceable for well-known botanical preparations, benefit of the first FDA-approved botanical drugs may still be significant but underestimated for the sponsor.

REFERENCE

1. The CDER Botanical Review Team website: http://www.fda.gov/cder/Offices/ODE_V_BRT/default.htm provides links to many useful FDA Guidances and related documents, including the Botanical Guidance and MAPP.

Index